BOTTOM LINE'S

REAL CAUSE

REAL CURE

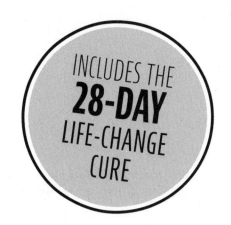

INCLUDES THE
28-DAY
LIFE-CHANGE
CURE

*Your Healing Toolkit to Find
and Fix the Root Causes of the
Most Common Health Problems
—and Feel Better Fast!*

REVISED AND UPDATED
JACOB TEITELBAUM, MD AND **BILL GOTTLIEB, CHC**

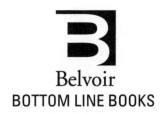

Belvoir
BOTTOM LINE BOOKS

Real Cause, Real Cure—Your Healing Toolkit to Find and Fix the Root Causes of the Most Common Health Problems

Bottom Line Books® is an imprint of Belvoir Media Group, LLC.

Belvoir

10   9   8   7   6   5   4   3   2   1

ISBN 978-0-88723-016-5

Bottom Line Books edition published by arrangement with Rodale Books, an imprint of the Crown Publishing Group, a division of Penguin Random House LLC. Original edition © 2011 Jacob Teitelbaum, MD, and Bill Gottlieb.

This book is intended as a reference volume only, not as a medical manual.

The information given here is designed to help you make informed decisions about your health. It is not intended as a substitute for any treatment that may have been prescribed by your doctor. If you suspect that you have a medical problem, we urge you to seek competent medical help.

Mention of specific companies, organizations, or authorities in this book does not imply endorsement by the author or publisher, nor does mention of specific companies, organizations, or authorities imply that they endorse this book, its author, or the publisher.

Internet addresses, products and telephone numbers given in this book were accurate at the time it went to press.

Bottom Line Books® is a registered trademark of Belvoir Media Group, LLC, 535 Connecticut Avenue, Norwalk, CT 06854-1713

Belvoir.com || BottomLineInc.com

Bottom Line Books® is an imprint of Belvoir Media Group, LLC, publisher of print and digital periodicals, books and online training programs. We are dedicated to bringing you the best information from the most knowledgeable sources in the world. Our goal is to help you gain greater wealth, better health, more wisdom, extra time and increased happiness.

Printed in the United States of America

To Laurie, my beautiful lady, my wife, my best friend,
and the love of my life;

My children, David, Amy, Shannon, Brittany, and Kelly,
and my grandchildren;

My mother, Sabina, and father, David,
whose unconditional love made this book possible;

The memories of Drs. Janet Travell, Hugh Riordan, and Billie Crook,
medical heroes and pioneers;

And to my patients, who have taught me
more than I can ever hope to teach them.

Jacob

To Julia, for her real love
Bill

Contents

Contents

PART 3—The 28-Day Life-Change Cure

Acknowledgments

From Jacob Teitelbaum:

would like to thank Bill Gottlieb. It has been a joy writing this book with him! So many have made this work possible that it is impossible to list them all. In truth, I have created nothing new; I have simply synthesized the wonderful work done by an army of hardworking and courageous physicians and healers. I would like to extend my sincerest thanks to: first and foremost, Cheryl Alberto and the rest of my staff. Their hard work, compassion, and dedication (and, I must admit, patience with me) are what made my work possible. The Anne Arundel Medical Center librarian, Joyce Miller. My wonderful and dedicated publicists, Dean Draznin and Terri Slater, and my webmaster, Richard Crouse, who are my teammates in making effective treatment and health available to everyone. Alan Weiss, MD, Bren Jacobson, and Jain Vaughn, best friends who keep me intellectually and spiritually honest while reminding me to keep my sense of humor. My many teachers, the real heroes and heroines in their fields, whose names could fill this book. They include William Crook, Max Boverman, Brugh Joy, Janet Travell, Hugh Riordan, Joseph Pizzorno, Melvyn Werbach, Sheri Lieberman, Neil Nathan, Robert Ivker, Tony Lebro, and Alan Gaby.

Special thanks to the Bottom Line team, especially our editor Marjory Abrams, who always uses the guiding star of what can best help people!

And finally and foremost, God and the universe, for the guidance and infinite blessings I have been given and for using me as an instrument for love and healing.

From Bill Gottlieb:

'd like to thank my coauthor, Jacob Teitelbaum, for his dedication to the health and happiness of his patients and everyone who desires a fuller life; for his creative and practical approach to comprehensive medicine; for his intelligence and insight; and for his warm and embracing heart. He was and is a pleasure to work with, and I feel grateful to know him as both a professional colleague and a dear friend. Thanks to Christine Tomasino, the literary agent for the original edition of the book and this update. And a warm thank you to Marjory Abrams and the team at Bottom Line Books, who decided to republish the book in an updated edition—my fifth title with Bottom Line. For over 20 years, I've worked closely with many editors at Bottom Line, writing articles for their newsletters and books—and regard them as part of my publishing family.

Introduction

I've been practicing medicine for more than 40 years and have treated more than 15,000 patients. But I'm not usually the first doctor my patients see. Typically, they've already been to doctor after doctor, seeking relief for their health problem—without success.

They've undergone medical tests that didn't detect the problem. (In fact, many were told that the results of their tests "proved" they *didn't* have a diagnosable disease, and that their very real pain and suffering was "all in your head." Sound familiar?) They were prescribed drugs that may have reduced symptoms to some extent (often creating a distressing new set of side effects).

But whatever the testing and treatment, the doctors they saw failed to detect the *real cause* of the health problem or implement the *real cure*. That's why these patients ended up in my office, often flying in from all over the world. And that's probably why you're reading this book.

If you're like the typical American, you have one or more ongoing health problems that doctors haven't been able to solve. Maybe it's an everyday problem such as fatigue, headaches, or insomnia—a problem so common and persistent that you figure you just have to "learn to live with it." Maybe it's a serious, chronic problem like diabetes, arthritis, or depression that is supposedly "under control" but never completely cured.

Well, if you have troubling health problems—your troubles may be over!

Real Cause, Real Cure pinpoints and explains the underlying and often-overlooked real causes of disease—and then offers dramatically effective natural treatments that will finally get to the root of not only your symptoms but also the condition itself.

Why Doesn't *My* Doctor Know About These Causes and Cures?

Now, since I'm a doctor, and I've written this book about real causes and real cures, you're probably asking yourself, "Why hasn't my doctor heard about them?"

The answer is relatively simple.

The real causes are based on a paradigm of *holistic medicine*, which sees the body and mind as a self-healing system that stays healthy when it's provided with the simple, natural factors of wellness, such as a wholesome, nutrient-packed diet and eight hours of nightly sleep. From the holistic perspective, the causes of disease are mostly the absence of these natural factors—absences common in modern life. On the other hand, the paradigm of *conventional medicine* treats the body and mind as a random collection of parts, and then zeroes in on the symptom with drugs or surgery—often ignoring the source of the problem. A real cause—a fundamental factor in the creation of disease—isn't a concept that fits the paradigm of modern medicine.

And the real cures found in this book—which are mostly natural treatments—aren't patentable; no one can claim exclusive ownership of vitamin C or garlic, for example. Therefore, these treatments are low cost—and drug companies won't pay for your physician to hear about them.

(The distorting, drug-dominating influence of the pharmaceutical industry has become so pervasive in medical research and practice that Marcia Angell, MD—the former editor-in-chief of the prestigious *New England Journal of Medicine* and currently on the faculty at Harvard Medical School—had this to say: "It is simply no longer possible to believe much of the clinical research that is published, or to rely on the judgment of trusted physicians or authoritative medical guidelines. I take no pleasure in this conclusion, which I reached slowly and reluctantly over my two decades as an editor of the *New England Journal of Medicine*.")

I'm not saying that drugs don't have a place in medicine; you'll find many prudent recommendations for drugs in this book. But they shouldn't have *first* place.

I'm a practitioner of what the late and wonderful Dr. Hugh Riordan liked to call "comprehensive medicine"—using the best of *all* natural and prescription therapies, based on what is safest and most effective rather than on what is most expensive and therefore most profitable. Comprehensive medicine is the type of medicine that you'll learn about in this book.

And that's great news—because there are hundreds, if not thousands, of highly effective natural treatments that most doctors don't know about. In fact, in my 40+ years as a physician I have come to find that there are very few problems that cannot be effectively treated by discovering their *real cause* and then applying a *real cure*. To achieve a real cure, you simply need to have real information. And I am happy to act as your advocate, sorting through the science to separate the real from the false.

How to Use This Book

There are many different ways to approach the wealth of information in this book.

You can start by reading about and understanding the real causes, as explained in Part I.

Or you can dive right into Part II—reading about the health conditions that concern you and your family. There, you'll find practical tips and remedies you can start using immediately—along with references to the information in Part I that can give you a deeper understanding of why those tips and remedies work.

Or you can start with Part III and the simple 28-Day Life-Change Cure, a plan that will leave you feeling great and having a life you love.

The most important point: Use *Real Cause, Real Cure* in the way that works best for you.

My goal is to have you start tuning in to your own feelings and body to see what feels best to you. An expert may be able to look at you and give you a fair guess as to what shoe size would fit you. But only by trying the shoes on and seeing what feels best to you can you really know. The same applies to health care advice, life in general—and the way you decide to use this book.

Ready to start? Let's do it!

Disclosure

Dear Reader,

I consider transparency about finances to be very important, especially for assessing health information from health professionals. (I would love to see fiscal transparency extend to politics and elsewhere as well!) In that spirit, *I am happy to supply the following information about my finances…*

Fiscal involvement with drug companies. As part of my dedication to promoting your health, I have a policy of not taking money from any pharmaceutical company.

Royalties from products and consulting. My royalties for products I've designed and consulting I currently offer for natural product companies go directly to a tax-exempt foundation. This foundation has many goals, including: making sure the public has access to optimal and accurate information on health and natural health; supporting research on natural therapies; and addressing international issues, such as childhood hunger. I donate my time to the foundation and other outreach work, so about two-thirds of my time is volunteer and unpaid.

My for-profit activities. I support myself and the work I do by treating patients and also from sales at my website (EndFatigue.com) of products from numerous companies that I find especially helpful. These products are also readily available from numerous retail stores and online. Purchasing from my website does help support me in the work I do—and I thank you!

My two products. I also personally produce two products: SHINE D-Ribose and Dr. Teitelbaum's Smart Energy. Profits from these products help support me, my work, and my outreach programs. At the time of this writing, I am also designing two studies on a new serum-based product that has shown dramatic promise for people with fibromyalgia. If the studies are successful, I may be financially involved in that company.

Love and Blessings,
Jacob Teitelbaum, MD

PART 1

The Real Causes

Nutritional Deficiencies

Optimize Nutrients, Optimize Health

With one-third of adults being obese and more than two-thirds overweight, Americans don't look like we have nutritional deficiencies—we look like we eat too much food. But extra calories don't necessarily translate into extra nutrients.

A study in the *American Journal of Clinical Nutrition* found that less than five percent of the study subjects got the government's Recommended Dietary Allowances (RDAs) for key minerals essential to health. In other words, fewer than one in 20 people were taking in the amount needed to avoid deficiencies, let alone the amount needed for optimal health and well-being. What's even more surprising, many of the study subjects worked at the U.S. Department of Agriculture in Beltsville, Maryland—one of the world's top nutritional research centers!

Other research, in the *Journal of the American College of Nutrition*, shows that nine out of 10 Americans fall short in the healthy intake of at least one vitamin, such as vitamins A, C, D and E.

Why are so many Americans deficient in vitamins and minerals? *There are several reasons...*

•**Too much sugar and white flour.** Added sugar, which is devoid of vitamins and minerals, accounts for 18 percent of the calories in the average American diet. Another 18 percent come from white flour, which has been stripped of bran, the grain's nutrient-rich outer covering. This all means that more than one-third of the total calories found in the typical American diet provide minuscule amounts of nutrients.

•**Too much processed food.** Not only does processed food deliver loads of energy-robbing refined carbs—it also often adds health-harming levels of artery-clogging trans fats and cell-poisoning artificial chemicals.

•**Not enough nutrient-rich whole foods.** In addition to eating too much of the wrong kinds of foods, we don't get enough of the right kinds. A report from the government's Centers

RDH (Requirement for Daily Healing)

If you feel overwhelmed by the avalanche of acronyms the government uses to describe the adequate intake of nutrients, you're not alone. You've got your RDA (Recommended Dietary Allowance), the government standard that's based on meeting the nutritional needs of 98 percent of the population. Then there's the AI (Adequate Intake), which applies to nutrients such as pantothenic acid that don't have enough scientific backup yet to set an RDA. And, oh yeah, there's the UL (Tolerable Upper Limit), which experts deem as the highest amount you can take without harm. And don't forget the DRI and the DV...

Actually, do forget about them. By definition, these intakes, allowances, requirements, and values are the lowest day-to-day intakes that will prevent deficiencies and a failure of the metabolic functions the nutrients support (such as the amount of iron needed to prevent anemia). These intakes are not aimed at achieving optimal health and well-being. They're so low that the RDA is sometimes called "Ridiculous Dietary Allowance."

So I recommend a different set of guidelines, which I call the RDH: Requirement for Daily Healing—the amount of each vitamin and mineral necessary to prevent and reverse disease and achieve glowing health. You'll find these optimal amounts accompanying each nutrient later in this chapter.

for Disease Control and Prevention (CDC) showed that nine out of 10 American adults don't eat the government's recommended daily servings of nutrient-rich fruits and vegetables. (And those requirements are already pretty scant: one-and-a-half to two cups of fruit, and two to three cups of vegetables.)

•**Too much modern life.** Unrelenting stress, air pollution, nutrient-depleted soil, chronic use of antacids, and diets overloaded with refined carbohydrates and saturated fat all drain the body of micronutrients or block their absorption.

What's the end result of widespread vitamin and mineral deficiencies? In a word: disease.

The Triage Theory

This state of disease due to nutritional deficiency is the basis of the "triage theory" of world-class scientist Bruce Ames, PhD, professor of biochemistry and molecular biology (emeritus) at the University of California, Berkeley, senior scientist at Children's Hospital Oakland Research Institute (CHORI) and director of their Nutrition & Metabolism Center, and the inventor of the Ames Test, the standard method used to determine whether a chemical can cause cancer. The triage theory says that the body copes with micronutrient deficiencies by using available vitamins and minerals to ensure day-to-day survival.

The result: The body's long-term needs are shortchanged, causing chronic diseases—specifically, the current plague of cancer, heart disease, type 2 diabetes, arthritis, osteoporosis, and Alzheimer's disease.

"Scientists have been evaluating the wrong factors in setting the RDAs," Dr. Ames told us. "They have been looking at adequate intake based on the acute but not the chronic effects of inadequate intake. So someone with an 'adequate' intake might seem perfectly healthy today—but he's setting himself up for chronic disease because of an ongoing deficiency of micronutrients. We need to be 'tuned up' with vitamins and minerals throughout life. Anytime we're not, we pay the price in long-term damage.

"Nutritionists say, 'If you eat a good diet, you'll get all the vitamins and minerals you need,'" Dr. Ames continued. "Well, I eat a good diet—but I also take a daily multivitamin/mineral supplement for insurance. I don't think any diet can be optimum in every micronutrient." (Dr. Ames is certainly living proof of his insurance policy—as of this update, he's in his nineties, and going strong!)

The daily micronutrient deficiencies that are likely causing long-term problems? Dr. Ames compiled the following list, and it reads a lot like the label of a typical multivitamin/mineral supplement!

- Acetyl-L-carnitine
- Alpha-lipoic acid
- Biotin
- Calcium
- Choline
- Cobalamin (vitamin B_{12})
- Copper
- Folate
- Iron
- Magnesium
- Niacin
- Omega-3 fatty acids
- Pantothenate
- Potassium
- Pyridoxine (vitamin B_6)
- Riboflavin (vitamin B_2)
- Selenium
- Thiamin (vitamin B_1)
- Vitamin D
- Zinc

In the following sections, you'll find a nutrient-by-nutrient guide to the level of vitamin and mineral supplementation that can prevent these deficiencies and—most important—optimize your health. For each nutrient, we also present the diseases that can be prevented, and sometimes cured, by treating a deficiency.

This is one of the longest chapters in the book. Why? Because I think that nutritional deficiency is the leading cause of so many modern illnesses and that simple nutritional support is one of the most powerful weapons in your self-care arsenal. (Later in the book, you'll find disease-by-disease reports on dozens of scientific studies that show—again and again—that suboptimal levels of nutrients can cause disease, and that supplementing the diet with one or more nutrients can help you recover from health problems, often dramatically.) By delving deeply into the link between nutrition and wellness, I hope to help you understand why nutritional supplementation is a must for your daily health regimen.

"All You Get from Taking Supplements Is Expensive Urine"

One reason I emphasize nutrition as an essential part of your self-care and self-healing is because there are so many "official" voices telling you that nutritional supplementation is a waste of your time and money.

A good example: the article *Should You Take Dietary Supplements*, from the National Institutes of Health, the government's main health agency. The articles states, "There's little evidence that any supplement can reverse the course of any chronic disease." False! There are tens of thousands of scientific studies showing supplements can reverse the course of disease—and you'll read the best of that evidence in this book.

Likewise, many so-called experts like to confuse people by making the "urine" statement above. (The statement is so often made that if you Google the phrase "expensive urine," you'll produce 30,000 hits!) Well, the oft-heard statement ignores the fact that the same thing happens to vitamins and other nutrients in food, so I guess you don't need to drink water either!

Let's start with a group of nutrients that are particularly crucial for good health: the antioxidants.

Antioxidant Vitamins

Oxygen is a double-edged sword: It's necessary for life and it's also incredibly toxic. That's because biochemical exposure to oxygen produces "free radicals" (also known as reactive oxygen species, or ROS)—rampaging molecules that set in motion an ongoing chain reaction of cellular damage. This oxidative stress is now understood to be a leading cause of chronic illness and premature aging. In fact, oxidative stress is one of the "evil twins" of chronic disease and aging, said the late James Joseph, PhD, who was an antioxidant researcher at Tufts University. (The other evil twin is chronic inflammation, which I discuss as a real cause in Chronic Inflammation on page 118.)

Excess oxidation causes disease. In fact, rust is a form of oxidation. But your body uses antioxidants to neutralize free radicals and limit oxidation. These nutrient superheroes can end the chain reaction, stop the cellular damage, and protect and improve your health.

Need an example of their power? Antioxidants help prevent age-related macular degeneration (ARMD), an eye disease caused by oxidation of the cells in the macula, the structure in the center of the retina that relays detailed images—such as those needed for reading this sentence—to the brain. About 11 million Americans have ARMD—13 percent of Americans over age 60, and 33 percent over age 80—and it's the leading cause of blindness in the United States. A scientific report in the journal *International Ophthalmology* reviewed all the studies on antioxidants and AMRD, and concluded that an antioxidant supplement can prevent ARMD, or slow its development. That's powerful medicine. Here's a list of the antioxidants you need in order to stay healthy.

The Problem with Antioxidant Research

A study in the *Journal of the American Medical Association* concluded that taking antioxidant supplements such as beta-carotene and vitamin E increased the risk of death by about five percent.

The study was a meta-analysis that analyzed the results of 68 other studies on antioxidants, involving more than 230,000 people. Critics quickly pointed out that many of the analyzed studies involved using antioxidants to treat heart disease and cancer—meaning the study participants were already pretty sick. Other critics said the studies in the analysis—involving many different age groups and levels of intake—were too dissimilar to combine.

Most important, from my perspective, the studies failed to acknowledge that these two much-studied antioxidants—vitamin E and beta-carotene—are part of larger families of nutrients (tocopherols and carotenoids, respectively). Giving super-high levels of any one type of vitamin E or carotenoid causes a relative deficiency of other types of vitamin E and carotenoids—which can likely cause health problems. To be effective and safe, nutrients need to be taken in balanced forms and amounts.

"This study does not advance our understanding," concluded Meir Stampfer, MD, DrPh, professor of epidemiology and nutrition and at the Harvard T.H. Chan School of Public Health. Dr. Stampfer also told the Associated Press that he planned to keep taking his vitamin supplement.

And Dr. Stampfer isn't alone. A survey in *Nutrition Journal* showed that 72 percent of doctors and 89 percent of nurses take nutritional supplements—and 80 percent recommend them to their patients. If your health care professional recommends a supplement, you're getting really good advice!

Vitamin C (RDH: 500 milligrams to 1,000 milligrams daily)

The C in vitamin C could stand for "classic." This nutrient has been and continues to be one of the most popular nutritional supplement in the United States, with most of us taking it to strengthen our immune systems and prevent colds. Vitamin C is also crucial in the creation of collagen, the protein responsible for firm, youthful skin and for maintaining the structure of other types of connective tissue, such as cartilage and tendons.

A classic study reported in the book *Vitamin C: Who Needs It?* by the late Emanuel Cheraskin, MD, DMD, found low vitamin C levels in 20 percent of healthy older people, 68 percent of older people with a disease, and 76 percent of people with cancer.

Good food sources include citrus fruits, broccoli, peppers, potatoes, leafy greens, and Brussels sprouts. (These foods will also help you absorb iron. In a study reported in the *American Journal of Clinical Nutrition*, researchers found that taking vitamin C with a meal boosted the absorption of iron by 2½ times.)

Recent research shows vitamin C may help prevent and/or treat…

- Allergies
- Anxiety
- Atrial fibrillation (irregular heart rhythms that increase the risk of a heart attack)
- Cataracts
- Circulation problems during prolonged sitting
- Cold sores
- Colds
- Colorectal cancer
- Depression
- Diabetes
- Fatigue
- Hearing loss
- Heart disease
- High blood pressure
- Infertility (male)
- Memory loss
- Muscle soreness after exercise
- Pollution toxicity
- Post-herpetic neuralgia (pain after a shingles infection)
- Post-surgical problems (slow healing and pain)
- Schizophrenia
- Stress-caused health problems
- Ulcers
- Urinary tract infections
- Wound healing

Vitamin E (RDH: 100 IU daily)

This powerful antioxidant protects the outer layer of the cell (called the membrane) from free radicals. And because it protects every cell in the body, it's a major key to overall health. It also boosts immunity by guarding the thymus gland, which manufactures the infection-fighting white blood cells named lymphocytes.

But a little vitamin E goes a long way. Research shows that intakes of more than 100 IU a day can be counterproductive, because too much of one antioxidant can stop the action of the others. If you take a higher level of vitamin E to treat a specific problem, do so for only a few months. Use a natural mixed tocopherol form rather than a synthetic if you're taking more than 100 IU a day. This delivers all the subtypes of vitamin E, including alpha- (the most abundant and active form), beta-, gamma-, and delta-tocopherols. Each subtype has a slightly different mode of action, and all are important.

When researchers at the Department of Nutrition and Health Sciences at the University of Nebraska tested people for blood levels of vitamin E, they found that nine out of 10 had low levels. "Most people do not meet current recommendations for intake" of vitamin E, said another team of researchers at the Jean Mayer U.S. Department of Agriculture Human Nutrition Research Center on Aging at Tufts University, in the *Journal of Nutrition*. Good food sources include vegetable oils, seeds, nuts, and whole grains.

Recent research shows vitamin E may help prevent and/or treat…

- ALS (amyotrophic lateral sclerosis)
- Alzheimer's disease
- Anemia
- Arthritis
- Asthma
- Breast cysts
- Cervical cancer
- Chemotherapy and radiation side effects
- COPD (chronic obstructive pulmonary disease)
- Dementia
- Diabetes
- Diabetic neuropathy (nerve pain)
- Gum disease (periodontitis)
- Heart disease
- Hepatitis C
- Memory loss
- Menstrual cramps and menstrual migraines
- Nonalcoholic fatty liver disease (also known as NASH, or nonalcoholic steatohepatitis)
- Parkinson's disease
- Peyronie's disease (bent penis from scar tissue)
- Polycystic ovary syndrome
- Prostate cancer
- Psoriasis (an inflammatory skin disease)
- Scleroderma (an autoimmune disease that hardens skin)
- Vitiligo (loss of skin coloration)

Vitamin A (RDH: 2,500 IU daily)

Vitamin A (retinol) plays a key role in vision, reproduction, immunity, and skin health. But, as with vitamin E, more isn't better. Birth defects can occur when pregnant women take more than 8,000 IU a day, and long-term doses of more than 50,000 IU a day can damage the liver. In fact, in my opinion, this is a rare case in which the RDA for men may be too high. (The RDA is 3,000 IU for men and 2,333 for women.) Studies show long-term intake of 5,000 IU (less than the supposedly safe "upper limit" of 10,000 IU) may lower bone density and increase the risk of fractures. Daily doses of more than 8,000 IU should be taken only with the approval and supervision of a qualified health practitioner.

High-dose vitamin A (often used with zinc, which can boost its therapeutic power) is used to treat acne, eczema, and other skin problems, as well as heavy menstrual periods during perimenopause, called dysfunctional uterine bleeding (DUB). The nutrient is also critical for preventing viral infections. Good food sources include colorful vegetables such as carrots, pumpkin, sweet potatoes, spinach, butternut squash, cantaloupe, mangoes, and leafy greens.

Beta-carotene (RDH: 2,500 IU daily)

The body turns carotenoids—the pigments that give plants their colors—into vitamin A. Beta-carotene is usually added to supplements, and like vitamin A, the right dose is helpful while too-high doses aren't. An intake of 25,000 IU or higher may increase the risk of cancer, and I recommend limiting intake to 5,000 IU daily. Good food sources include carrots, sweet potatoes, squash, spinach, apricots, green peppers, and leafy greens.

Recent research shows beta-carotene may help prevent and/or treat...

- Breast cancer
- Cystic fibrosis
- Heart disease
- High blood pressure
- HIV/AIDS

- Hostility
- Lung disease
- Memory loss
- Skin aging

Bioflavonoids (RDH: 500 milligrams daily)

This nutrient is a type of flavonoid, another compound that gives color to fruits and flowers. The richest source of bioflavonoids—quercetin, rutin, hesperidin, and naringin—is the inner lining (the white part) of citrus fruits. But the most researched of the bioflavonoids is quercetin, which can be found not only in citrus fruits, but also in all fruits and vegetables, particularly apples, onions, and parsley (as well as tea and red wine).

Recent research shows quercetin may help prevent and/or treat...

- Colds and flu
- Heart disease
- High blood pressure

- Prostatitis
- Sports fatigue
- Stroke

B Vitamins

The B vitamins are important for energy production, immunity, brain function, and much more—as you'll see in this B-by-B review. The RDAs for B vitamins are very suboptimal. The high doses of B vitamins in a good nutritional supplement are not only safe, they're downright crucial to health and well-being.

Vitamin B$_1$, or thiamin (RDH: 75 milligrams daily)

Thiamin is a must for energy production in the brain and the heart. Researchers in the Department of Nutrition at the University of North Carolina found low thiamin intake in many Americans between 60 and 80 years old, and concluded that most older U.S. citizens were likely to be deficient. "Many Americans do not consume the RDA of 1.5 mg," writes Michael Murray, ND, in *Encyclopedia of Nutritional Supplements*. Deficiencies are particularly common in people with heart failure or dementia, in alcoholics, in people living in long-term-care facilities, and after bariatric surgery for obesity.

Good food sources include soybeans, brown rice, sunflower seeds, peanuts, brewer's yeast, and wheat germ.

Recent research shows thiamin may help prevent and/or treat...

- •Anxiety
- •Back pain
- •Brain fog (lack of mental clarity)
- •Diabetic neuropathy (nerve damage from diabetes)

- •Fatigue
- •Kidney disease
- •Sudden infant death syndrome

Vitamin B$_2$, or riboflavin (RDH: 75 milligrams daily)

Riboflavin is crucial in the functioning of two enzymes that help produce energy for the body. "Suboptimal riboflavin status may be a problem in all age groups," concluded a team of researchers at the Northern Ireland Centre for Food and Health in a study published in the *American Journal of Clinical Nutrition*. (In this case, *status* is a technical word nutritional researchers use to indicate the blood level or dietary intake of a nutrient.)

Good food sources include whole grains, almonds, mushrooms, leafy green vegetables, soybeans, and organ meats.

Recent research shows riboflavin may help prevent and/or treat...

- •Cataracts
- •High blood pressure

- •Migraine headaches
- •Postpartum depression

Vitamin B$_3$, or niacin (RDH: 50 milligrams daily)

Because niacin is a key component of NADH—an enzyme that helps power mitochondria, the tiny energy factories in every cell—it plays a major role in the body's production of energy. It also helps metabolize fats, carbohydrates, and cholesterol, and it aids in the manufacture of several hormones.

For everyday use, I recommend the niacinamide form, as regular niacin can cause flushing—sudden, temporary widening of small blood vessels on the surface of the skin, leading to warm, tingling, itchy (and sometimes annoying) sensations in the face and trunk. Good food sources include eggs, fish, peanuts, legumes, whole grains, milk, avocados, and organ meats (such as liver).

Recent research shows niacin may help prevent or treat...

- •Alzheimer's disease
- •Diabetes

- •Kidney disease
- •Metabolic syndrome

Vitamin B$_5$, or pantothenic acid (RDH: 50 milligrams daily)

Pantothenic acid and its cousin pantethine play many key roles in the body, including ensuring the proper functioning of the adrenal glands, which generate stress and other hormones. The nutrient is also critical for the proper handling of fats—pantethine has a decades-long history as a treatment for lowering high blood fats and boosting good HDL cholesterol.

Good food sources of pantothenic acid include milk, fish, poultry, whole grains, legumes, sweet potatoes, broccoli, cauliflower, oranges, and strawberries.

Vitamin B$_6$, or pyridoxine (RDH: 40 milligrams to 85 milligrams daily)

Vitamin B$_6$ helps build proteins, neurotransmitters (chemicals that relay messages between brain cells), and hormones. In a study published in the *American Journal of Clinical Nutrition*, researchers at Tufts University reviewed data on blood levels of vitamin B$_6$ from the National Health and Nutrition Examination Survey. They concluded that even while consuming the RDA, "substantial proportions of some population subgroups" don't have "adequate vitamin B$_6$ status." They include women of reproductive age, especially current and former users of oral contraceptives, male smokers, African-American men, and people over 65.

They also found that nearly one in four people not using nutritional supplements had lower-than-acceptable blood levels of B$_6$. Among supplement users, only one in 10 had lower-than-acceptable levels. "The question our study raises," said the researchers, "is whether, due to aging, genetics, or exposures [to factors such as oral contraceptives], some population subgroups need supplements to achieve the current biochemical definition of adequate status." My answer: Yes!

Of particular interest to premenopausal women: The researchers found that 75 percent of women using oral contraceptives but not taking vitamin B$_6$ supplements were deficient in the nutrient. More than 25 years ago, holistic physicians recognized that birth control pills can cause B$_6$ deficiency (and accompanying depression). Maybe in another 25 years or so, conventional doctors will recommend that women on the Pill take vitamin B$_6$. If you're on the Pill, don't wait for them to do so!

Good food sources include whole grains, legumes, bananas, seeds and nuts, potatoes, Brussels sprouts, and cauliflower. Needless to say, I recommend that *everyone* supplement their diet with B$_6$ to guarantee not merely adequate but optimal blood levels of the nutrient.

Recent research shows vitamin B$_6$ may help prevent and/or treat...

- Carpal tunnel syndrome
- Fluid retention
- Macular degeneration
- Morning sickness
- Overweight
- Parkinson's disease
- Stressed-caused anxiety and depression
- Tardive dyskinesia (spasmodic facial movements as a side effect of long-term use of certain medications, such as for Parkinson's disease and schizophrenia)

Vitamin B$_{12}$, or cobalamin (RDH: 500 micrograms to 1,000 micrograms daily)

B$_{12}$ teams up with the B vitamin folate to help produce DNA, red blood cells, and the myelin sheath that insulates nerve cells. Because the nutrient is mostly found in animal foods such as meat, fish, eggs, and cheese, vegetarians are often advised to supplement with B_{12}—a recommendation I endorse. But just about everybody could do with extra B_{12}.

Technically, the B_{12} blood level is considered normal if it's over 208 picograms per deciliter. But a study in the *New England Journal of Medicine* shows that people can suffer severe (and even long-term) nerve and brain damage with levels as high as 300 picograms per deciliter. And a study in the *American Journal of Nutrition* showed that signs of B_{12} deficiency, such as tingling and numbness, can occur even with levels over 500 picograms per deciliter.

It's no surprise, then, that many people with "normal" blood levels of B_{12} see great improvement after B_{12} injections—a treatment considered by many "modern" doctors to be an archetype of old-fashioned, unscientific medicine. For example, my patients with chronic fatigue syndrome and fibromyalgia syndrome often respond dramatically to B_{12} injections, despite normal blood levels. (I suspect, however, that those in the medical establishment will be a little slow in admitting they were wrong about B_{12}. Instead, they will continue to believe that when people feel better on B_{12} shots, it's because they're deluded. They're not.)

Extra B_{12} from a supplement—at levels much higher than the RDA—is particularly important in those 65 and older, among whom suboptimal B_{12} is common. The body uses a molecule called intrinsic factor to absorb B_{12} in the small intestine, and intrinsic factor declines as you get older. In a study on older people in the *Archives of Internal Medicine*, researchers noted, "The lowest dose of oral B_{12} required to normalize mild vitamin B_{12} deficiency is more than 200 times greater than the recommended dietary allowance." They continued, "Clinical trials are currently assessing the effects of high doses of oral cobalamin on markers of cognitive function and depression. If such trials can demonstrate that the reported associations of vitamin B_{12} deficiency with cognitive impairment or depression are causal and reversible by treatment, the relevance of correction of vitamin B_{12} deficiency in older people could be substantial."

Instead of waiting 10 years for those studies to be completed…and replicated by other researchers…and their findings incorporated by the government into standard nutritional recommendations such as the RDA…I recommend getting 500 micrograms a day of B_{12} today.

Recent research shows vitamin B_{12} may help prevent and/or treat…

- Acne
- Autism
- Canker sores
- Celiac disease
- Dementia
- Depression
- Diabetes
- Eczema
- Hearing loss

- Heartburn and indigestion
- Hepatitis C
- Memory loss
- Neuropathy
- Parkinson's disease
- Pollution toxicity
- Schizophrenia
- Tinnitus

B_{12}: The Firefighter's Friend

Of 69 people treated for acute smoke inhalation (39 of whom were comatose), 50 survived after injection of a special form of vitamin B_{12} (*hydroxocobalamin*), reported researchers from the Division of Emergency Medicine at the University of Texas Health Science Center, in a report published in the journal *Annals of Emergency Medicine*. The vitamin works by countering cyanide poisoning from the smoke.

Folate, or folic acid (RDH: 400 micrograms daily)

Folate works with other B vitamins to manufacture DNA and guide the division of cells (crucial in the development of the fetus). The following factors drain your body of folate, putting you at risk for a deficiency: alcoholism; liver disease; taking anticonvulsant medications, such as *phenytoin* (Dilantin) for epilepsy; and kidney dialysis, a blood-purifying treatment for chronic kidney disease.

The word *folate* is derived from *folium*, which is Latin for "foliage." You can forage for that foliage in the produce section of your supermarket: green, leafy vegetables such as kale, spinach, and Swiss chard are rich in folate, as are cabbage, broccoli, and asparagus. Other good sources include beans, whole grains, nuts, and citrus fruits. Flour is fortified with folate, to help prevent birth defects caused by a low intake. However, an analysis of folate intake by experts at the National Institutes of Health showed that all "women of childbearing age" need to improve their folate intake.

A 1,000-microgram dose is the "daily upper limit" for supplements established by the U.S. government. That's because too much folate can mask a type of anemia that is a telltale sign of vitamin B_{12} deficiency—megaloblastic anemia, or overlarge red blood cells. And that untreated deficiency can permanently damage your nerves. However, this type of masking is not a risk if your supplement contains plenty of B_{12}.

Recent research shows folate may help prevent and/or treat...

- Alzheimer's disease
- Anemia
- Bipolar depression
- Cervical dysplasia
- Depression
- Heart disease
- High blood pressure
- Infertility (male)
- Memory loss
- Metabolic syndrome
- Migraine
- Neural tube defects
- Neuroblastoma (nerve cancer, the most common cancer in young children)
- Osteoporosis
- Polycystic ovary syndrome
- Schizophrenia
- Skin cancer
- Stroke

Biotin (RDH: 200 micrograms daily)

This B vitamin—produced in the gut by bacteria—is key in the production of enzymes that help digest and utilize sugar (glucose), fats, and amino acids (the building blocks of protein).

"A substantial proportion of pregnant women are marginally biotin deficient, and that deficiency may play a role in birth defects," said researchers from the University of Arkansas in the *Journal of Nutrition*.

I find biotin very effective for treating hair loss in women, though it takes about a year for full recovery. Biotin can also help build stronger nails and healthier skin. In one study, a daily biotin supplement of 2,500 micrograms increased nail thickness by 25 percent in nine out of 10 people with brittle nails.

Good food sources include brewer's yeast, soybeans, peanuts, walnuts, eggs, molasses, and milk.

Vitamin D (RDH: 2,000 IU daily)

Vitamin D deficiency is incredibly common: Seventy percent of whites, 90 percent of Latinos, and 97 percent of blacks in the United States have low blood levels of vitamin D, reported researchers at Harvard and the University of Colorado in the *Archives of Internal Medicine*. That's three out of four Americans with a vitamin D deficiency. Thirty years ago it was one out of 20!

This epidemic of vitamin D deficiency is finally getting the attention it deserves from the medical profession and the public. And that's an important development. Vitamin D deficiency—which is so easy to prevent—causes tens of thousands of unnecessary deaths every year in the United States, from heart disease, cancer, diabetes, dementia, falls, and the flu. Research now shows that these health problems are caused or complicated by vitamin D deficiency. (You can add arthritis, high blood pressure, osteoporosis, depression, insomnia, fibromyalgia, and multiple sclerosis to that list of D-deficiency conditions. And there are many more!)

Vitamin D is famous as the "sunshine vitamin" that helps the body absorb calcium, a mineral that's a must for bone health. But research now shows that vitamin D targets more than 2,000 genes—including genes that maintain the health of the heart, brain, immune system, and muscles.

Why has vitamin D deficiency increased so much in the past two decades? To answer that question, ask a dermatologist about the risks and benefits of sunshine. You'll no doubt be told to shield your skin from sunlight in order to prevent melanoma, a deadly skin cancer. But by blocking the sun, you block vitamin D. More than 90 percent of the vitamin D in your body is created by the sun striking your skin, which produces cholecalciferol…which turns into calcidiol (25-hydroxy vitamin D)…which your kidneys turn into calcitriol, the so-called active form of vitamin D. According to John Cannell, MD, CEO of the Vitamin D Council (an organization devoted to wiping out the worldwide epidemic of vitamin D deficiency), the skin produces approximately 10,000 IU of vitamin D in response to 20 to 30 minutes of summer sun exposure—16 times more than the U.S. government's RDA of 600 IU per day!

Along with Dr. Cannell—and many other experts, including Michael Holick, PhD, MD, a world-renowned vitamin D expert and author of *The Vitamin D Solution*—I don't believe the increase in melanoma rates (an increase that is itself debatable) is being caused by increased exposure to the sun. Most melanomas are not in sun-exposed areas—they are under our clothes. If there is an increase in rates of melanoma, I believe it is because of a fatty, salty, sugary diet, an environment saturated with toxic chemicals, and a population that is sleep deprived—all resulting in weakened immune systems.

"Repeated sunburns, especially in childhood and among redheads and very fair-skinned people, have been linked to melanoma, but there is no credible scientific evidence that moderate sun exposure causes it," Dr. Holick told us. "The problem has been that the American Academy of Dermatology has been unchallenged for 20 years. They have brainwashed the public at every level. I am advocating common sense—not prolonged sunbathing or tanning salons, but enough sunlight to make vitamin D."

The real cancer problem is *lack* of vitamin D, which study after study links to the development of cancer. Low vitamin D levels are also predictive of cancer severity and survival—those with the lowest levels do the worst. It is estimated that the advice to avoid sunshine doesn't prevent cancer—it causes an estimated 85,000 unnecessary cancer deaths every year! Sunshine is good for you. Avoid sunburn, not sunshine. Dr. Holick's general recommendation: during the summer months, five to 10 minutes a day of sun exposure to the arms and legs (not the face), to maintain healthy vitamin D levels throughout the year.

What level of nutritional supplementation is optimal? At least 1,000 IU a day is the recommendation of Heike A. Bischoff-Ferrari, MD, MPH, a researcher at the University of Zurich in Switzerland. However, Dr. Holick points out that in a study of healthy adults, supplements of 1,000 IU of vitamin D_3 a day given during the winter did not raise blood levels above the 30 nanograms per milliliter that experts say is the minimum for good health. Susan E. Brown, PhD, of the Center for Better Bones and author of *Better Bones, Better Body: Beyond Estrogen and Calcium*, recommends 2,000 IU a day as an ideal dosage. Dr. Cannell recommends 5,000 IU a day for people who don't get much exposure to sunlight. Although sunlight and supplements are the best ways to build blood levels of vitamin D, good food sources include salmon, sardines, eggs, and D-fortified foods such as milk and cereal.

A final point about this crucial nutrient: If you're taking 1,000 to 5,000 IU a day (and I think 1,000 IU a day in a multivitamin supplement is plenty), and your blood levels of vitamin D are *still* low…*don't* increase your dose of the vitamin. If intake is high but blood levels are low, it's likely because your body is converting the vitamin D in the supplement to *calcitriol*, a form of vitamin D that is not measured by standard tests. And too-high levels of calcitriol can cause immune dysfunction. (Some people might also have problems with vitamin D absorption, such as those with inflammatory bowel disease, celiac disease, or if you've had gastric bypass surgery.)

Bottom line: 5,000 IU daily is a safe upper limit—and plenty of D to get the job done.

Recent research shows vitamin D may help prevent and/or treat…

- Arthritis
- Asthma
- Breast cancer
- Colds and flu
- Colorectal cancer
- Diabetes
- Heart disease
- Lung cancer
- Multiple sclerosis
- Osteoporosis
- Prostate cancer
- Stroke

Vitamin K (RDH: 50 micrograms to 500 micrograms daily)

Like vitamins A and D, vitamin K is a fat-soluble nutrient (it's stored in body fat). And like vitamin E, it's not just one but actually many compounds. There's vitamin K_1 (*phylloquinone*) and vitamin K_2 (*menaquinone*)—and K_2 itself has more than a dozen forms, most of them created in the body from K_1. Vitamin K_1 helps the liver manufacture proteins that control blood clotting. Vitamin K_2 has many functions, including building collagen in bone and strengthening arteries.

Good food sources include leafy green vegetables, asparagus, green beans, and vegetable oils. But we're probably not getting enough of the nutrient, because many of us develop the chronic diseases that vitamin K can help prevent and treat. "Poor vitamin K nutrition has been linked to several chronic diseases," said researchers from Tufts University in the journal *Current Opinion in Clinical Nutrition & Metabolic Care*.

Recent research shows vitamin K may help prevent and treat…

- Alzheimer's disease
- Arthritis
- Cancer
- Diabetes
- Heart disease
- Osteoporosis

Minerals

Minerals rock your world. Without calcium, your bones would turn to dust. Without iron, you couldn't use oxygen. Without magnesium, your nerves would sputter and short out.

Generally speaking, minerals play two main roles in the body. Like vitamins, they pair up with enzymes, the biochemical sparkplugs that ignite the endless chemical reactions powering your body. Minerals are also building materials for essential structures such as bones and blood.

There are two types of minerals: major (of which you need more than 100 milligrams a day) and minor or trace (of which you need less than 100 milligrams a day). Needless to say, both types are very important for good health.

Potassium (RDH: 4,500+ milligrams daily)

Potassium (along with sodium and chloride) is an electrolyte—dissolved in water, it conducts electricity. That ability is a must for maintaining osmotic balance, the life-sustaining ratio of fluids on the inside and the outside of cells. Potassium also plays a key role in regulating pH, the all-important acid-alkaline balance of the body's chemistry. And potassium is crucial for the health of your muscles, nerves, heart, kidneys, and adrenal glands.

The Daily Value for adults for potassium is 4,700 milligrams, and the mineral is abundant in meat, vegetables, and fruit. But the average American's intake is about 1,755 milligrams. Along with too little potassium, most of us get too much sodium—four times more sodium than potassium. That potassium-to-sodium ratio is just the opposite of what our hunter-gatherer bodies were built for, said Nicolaos Madias, MD, of the Tufts University School of Medicine, in the *New England Journal of Medicine*.

The meat- and plant-rich diet of our Stone Age ancestors had 16 times more potassium than sodium, Dr. Madias explained. As a result, our kidneys evolved to *excrete* potassium and *retain* sodium. "This mechanism, however, is unfit for the sodium-rich and potassium-poor modern diet," he wrote. "The end result of the failure of the kidneys to adapt to the modern diet" is high blood pressure.

Research backs him up. Studies show that low intake of dietary potassium increases blood pressure levels by 7 points systolic (the upper number in a blood pressure reading) and 6 points diastolic (the lower number)—thereby increasing the risk of stroke by 28 percent. A diet that "approaches the high potassium-to-sodium ratio of the diet of human ancestors is a critical strategy for the prevention and treatment of hypertension," wrote Dr. Madias.

But don't count on supplements to supply the difference. The FDA restricts potassium in supplements to 99 milligrams (more requires a warning label) because the mineral can build up to toxic levels in people with chronic kidney disease (whose failed kidneys can't process the nutrient).

My advice: Daily, eat a potassium-rich banana…or drink a 12-ounce glass of potassium-rich coconut water, V8, or tomato juice…or eat half an avocado. Each of these supply about 500 mg of potassium.

Calcium (RDH: 1,000 milligrams from food)

Calcium is one of the few nutrients for which taking a supplement is actively promoted by "modern medicine," to prevent, slow, or stop osteoporosis. As you know by now, I'm a fervid supporter of the benefits of nutritional supplementation—but that doesn't include calcium! In fact, I think it has a very minor role in treating osteoporosis.

Dr. Susan Brown of the Better Bones Foundation points out that people in most areas of the world have lower calcium intakes than Americans *and* lower rates of osteoporosis. And, she says, studies show that calcium supplements reduce the risk of osteoporosis by only one percent to two percent. She thinks that other bone-building nutrients (such as vitamin D

The Calcium Conundrum

A "coronary artery calcium scan" is a test given to some people with heart disease to pinpoint their level of risk. This CT (computerized tomography) scan generates a "coronary calcium score"—the exact amount of calcium or "calcification" in your heart's arteries.

Calcium can harden and thicken blood vessels, making them less flexible and more prone to artery-clogging clots.

So why are calcium supplements—which add calcium to the system—a good idea? Maybe they're not, concluded a study from researchers at the University of Auckland in New Zealand. The researchers conducted a so-called meta-analysis of 15 studies involving more than 12,000 people with osteoporosis who took a calcium supplement to help prevent a bone fracture.

The result: Those who took the supplements increased their risk of a heart attack by 31 percent, compared with those who took a placebo. In another study, published in the *Journal of the American Heart Association*, taking 1,000 mg of supplemental calcium daily doubled the risk of stroke.)

Interestingly, the researchers in the New Zealand study found no increased risk from high dietary intake of calcium, only from a calcium supplement. And in the studies analyzed, participants took *just* a calcium supplement by itself. Calcium combined with vitamin D did not increase heart attacks.

"The likely adverse effects of calcium on cardiovascular events, taken together with its modest overall efficacy in reducing fracture (about 10 percent reduction in total fractures), suggest that a reassessment of the role of calcium supplementations in the prevention and treatment of osteoporosis is warranted," concluded the researchers.

Needless to say, a lot of other scientists criticized the study. (Scientists like to argue!) *They pointed out...*

- **There are more than 300 other studies** of calcium supplements that weren't included.

- **Seven of the 15 analyzed studies had either no or incomplete data** on whether or not the participants had heart attacks—and only five of the studies accounted for the estimated risk.

- **None of the analyzed studies were originally designed to measure cardiovascular (CV) risk,** and only eight of them had complete CV data.

"It's unfortunate that these researchers are making sweeping judgments about the value of calcium supplements by only assessing a handful of handpicked studies," opined one critic from the Council for Responsible Nutrition.

Still, the study reinforces what I've always thought about calcium supplements: High doses should not be taken for the prevention of osteoporosis unless they are combined and balanced with the heart-protective nutrients magnesium, vitamin D, and vitamin K. I also prefer that antacid tablets contain calcium, vitamin D, *and* magnesium.

Bottom line: I do continue to recommend calcium if you are diagnosed with osteopenia or osteoporosis, but only when used in balance with these other nutrients.

and vitamin K) are much more important than calcium. She also emphasizes the importance of reducing calcium-depleting lifestyle factors, such as eating excess protein, salt, fat, and sugar, and a lack of physical activity.

I agree with Dr. Brown: Low calcium is *not* the main cause of lower bone mineral density. I believe other nutrients, hormones, and lifestyle factors are much more important. However, if you've been diagnosed with low bone mineral density (BMD)—a BMD of -1 to -2.5 (osteopenia) or under -2.5 (osteoporosis)—I recommend a daily supplement of 400 to 1,000 milligrams of calcium, but only if taken with other key nutrients.

Many vitamins and minerals are helpful in building BMD, including well-known nutrients such as vitamin D and magnesium and little-known nutrients such as boron, silica, and strontium. (Strontium is nearly twice as effective as conventional osteoporosis medications in building bone and preventing fractures.)

I suggest my patients take three products: The Energy Revitalization System vitamin powder (Nature's Way, formerly Enzymatic Therapy) and Silica-20 (Terry Naturally) in the morning (follow manufacturer's suggested dose for both supplements), and 750 mg of strontium (Life Extension) at bedtime.

To maximize your calcium intake from food—the best way to get this mineral—eat one to two servings of dairy products, such as unsweetened yogurt, milk, and cheese, along with leafy green vegetables and canned salmon or sardines with bones. You can also get calcium from calcium-fortified foods, such as cereal, orange juice, and non-dairy milks.

Magnesium (RDH: supplement with 200 milligrams)

Magnesium is a must for more than 300 biochemical reactions. It relaxes muscles and steadies nerves. It stabilizes the heartbeat and strengthens bones. It regulates blood pressure and blood sugar. It lends a helping hand in energy production and immunity.

"Substantial numbers of U.S. adults fail to consume adequate magnesium in their diets," concluded a study in the *Journal of Nutrition*, which showed that the average American intake was nearly 20 percent below the Daily Value of 400 milligrams. And that low intake is linked to a parade of health problems. Fortunately, supplementing with magnesium can help reverse chronic disease and treat a number of conditions. In fact, in one 18-year study of 4,000 people, those with the highest dietary intake of magnesium had a 40 percent lower risk of dying from *any* cause, compared with those with the lowest intake.

Good food sources are legumes (beans and peas), seeds, nuts, whole grains, and leafy green vegetables. (Meat, fish, and dairy are low in magnesium, as are most processed foods.)

Recent research shows magnesium may help prevent and/or treat…

- Arrhythmia
- Asthma
- Attention-deficit/hyperactivity disorder (ADHD)
- Chronic obstructive pulmonary disease (COPD)
- Colon cancer
- Constipation
- Cystic fibrosis
- Depression
- Diabetes
- Diabetic foot ulcers
- Fibromyalgia
- Heart disease
- High blood pressure
- Low back pain
- Metabolic syndrome
- Migraine
- Muscle injury from exercise
- Osteoporosis
- Polycystic ovary syndrome (PCOS)
- Post-operative pain
- Stroke

Zinc (RDH: 15 milligrams to 25 milligrams daily)

Zinc lends a helping hand to more than 200 enzymes. It also helps produce several hormones from the thyroid gland, the sex glands, and the pancreas. Needless to say, it's crucial for the good health of a lot of body parts and systems, including your skin, immune system, senses, and (if you're a guy) prostate.

However, many people—including a lot of members of AARP!—don't get enough dietary zinc. An estimated 45 percent of adults over age 60 may have zinc intakes below recommended levels. Specific groups at risk include pregnant or breastfeeding women; people with immune dysfunction or chronic infections, such as those with fibromyalgia or AIDS; people with chronic inflammation, such as those with inflammatory bowel disease; people with chronic liver disease or chronic kidney disease; people with sickle-cell disease; vegetarians; and alcoholics.

Too little zinc can worsen those diseases—or cause new ones. "Mild zinc deficiencies" can lead to or worsen "immune deficiency, gastrointestinal problems, endocrine disorders, neurologic dysfunction, cancer, accelerated aging, degenerative disease, and more," declared a team of researchers in a scientific paper titled "The Ubiquitous Role of Zinc in Health and Disease."

A Mineral with Good Taste

Older people often lose their sense of taste—and their appetite along with it, leading to nutritional deficiencies. In a study by Irish researchers of 199 people ages 70 to 87, a daily supplement of 30 milligrams of zinc helped restore sensitivity to salty tastes.

The best food source is oysters (about eight times more than any other food). Other good sources include red meat, crab, lobster, and chicken. Plant foods with decent levels of zinc include whole grains, legumes, and nuts and seeds.

Recent research shows zinc may help prevent and/or treat…

- AIDS
- Alcoholism
- Anger
- Anxiety
- Attention-deficit/hyperactivity disorder (ADHD)
- Bad breath
- Burns
- Cancer
- Canker sores
- Colds
- Depression
- Diabetes and prediabetes
- Foot ulcers (diabetic)
- Gum disease
- Heart disease
- Macular degeneration
- Memory loss
- Mucosotis (ulceration of mucous membranes, caused by cancer treatment)
- Pneumonia
- Polycystic ovary syndrome (PCOS)
- Premenstrual syndrome (PMS)
- Rosacea
- Sickle-cell anemia
- Sleep problems
- Sore throat
- Stroke
- Taste problems
- Warts

Iron (RDH: 8 milligrams to 18 milligrams a day, from food)

Twenty percent of American women have iron-deficiency anemia—an iron level so low the body can't make enough hemoglobin, the protein that helps red blood cells carry oxygen to every tissue and cell. Suffocating from the inside out, you're weak, weary, and pale, and also likely to have an immune system in low gear, a broken thermostat (your hands and feet always feel cold), and a literally lame brain (with poor memory, concentration, and learning ability).

Another estimated 40 percent of women are iron deficient—lab tests don't show outright anemia, but their levels of iron are lower than is needed. (Studies now show that iron deficiency causes a mild version of symptoms once thought to be caused only by anemia.) Women are at particular risk for this problem because of iron-draining menstrual periods, iron-sapping pregnancies, and iron-poor diets. So why don't I recommend that women supplement their diets with iron?

Well, while too little iron is disease causing, so is too much! Extra iron generates inflammatory free radicals, increasing the risk of heart attack, stroke, arthritis, liver disease, and cancer. In fact, when many people have their iron levels tested (more about that test in a minute), they are found to have hemochromatosis, a genetic disease of excess iron. (If caught early, the disease is very easy to treat by removing blood regularly, like a blood donation; if caught late, it is disabling and even life threatening.)

The best way to know if you need extra iron (or if you have too much) is to have three common blood tests: iron level, total iron binding capacity (TIBC), and ferritin. But standard blood tests are often misinterpreted, with many people told they are "normal" when they're not. Interestingly, I've found that low iron levels that are technically considered "normal" can cause restless legs syndrome during sleep, a form of the condition called periodic limb movement disorder. Treating the iron deficiency can cure the disease and is as effective as—and much less expensive than—*ropinirole* (Requip), the drug typically used for the problem. Needless to say, most doctors know about only the expensive medication and not the inexpensive mineral.

For more insight and information about how to work with your doctor to determine if your iron levels are too low or too high, see "The Right Way to Test for an Iron Deficiency" below. In the meantime, good food sources include red meat, turkey, oysters, legumes, spinach, and iron-fortified cereals.

The Right Way to Test for an Iron Deficiency

If you have the symptoms of iron-deficiency anemia, your doctor will probably order an initial blood test (complete blood count, or CBC). If it shows low levels of hemoglobin—less than 11.1 grams per deciliter—your doctor will then test for ferritin, the protein that helps store iron in the body and the best indicator of long-term iron levels. Here's where the problem starts.

Most doctors will tell you that your ferritin is normal if it is over 9. However, accumulating scientific data and my clinical experience show that anyone with a ferritin level below 40 is a prime candidate for iron therapy. For example, research in the medical journal *Lancet* showed that infertile women whose ferritin levels were between 20 and 40 (so-called normal) were often able to become pregnant after they took an iron supplement. And hair loss in women—a widespread problem—is often reversed only when ferritin levels are above 100.

I also recommend your doctor perform two other tests to help detect iron deficiency: the iron level and the total iron binding capacity (TIBC). Individually, each of these tests is not useful…but together they are extremely telling. Dividing the iron level by the TIBC gives a percent saturation—and if your percent saturation is below 22 percent, you're a candidate for iron therapy. Some insurance companies balk at paying for all three tests, but I strongly suggest having them done. (Also, if both the ferritin and iron percent saturation tests are above normal, be sure your doctor tests for hemochromatosis, a disorder in which too much iron builds up in the blood.)

If your iron percent saturation is under 22 percent, or your ferritin is under 40, I recommend a daily iron supplement containing 25 milligrams to 35 milligrams. Take it on an empty stomach (bedtime is fine) with 500 milligrams of vitamin C, which aids iron absorption. In my experience, the best way to take this dosage is every other day, or three weeks on and one week off. Have your iron levels rechecked after three months of treatment.

Don't worry if your stools turn black. That's normal when you're taking iron. If they're black and very foul smelling, call your doctor immediately—that's a sign of internal bleeding.

Manganese (RDH: 2 milligrams to 4 milligrams daily)

Manganese plays a role in many enzymes, including those involved in blood sugar, energy production, and thyroid hormones. But it's particularly important for bone health—it helps form collagen (the protein substructure for minerals in bone) and also helps mineralize bones. Few Americans have an adequate intake of this nutrient.

There's not a lot of scientific research on manganese and health in people, but the little there is points to its importance. In one study published in the *European Journal of Cancer*, Chinese researchers discovered that a disruption in one of the manganese-containing enzymes (manganese superoxide dismutase, or MnSOD) nearly tripled the risk of breast cancer in women who had a low intake of antioxidants. The same disruption increased the risk of prostate cancer by 30 percent.

Finnish researchers found that the disruption in MnSOD also increased the risk of diabetic retinopathy, an eye disease in people with diabetes, according to a study in the *British Journal of Ophthalmology*. Good food sources include beets and beet greens, dark rye flour, raisin bran, peanuts, blackberries, loganberries, and fresh pineapple.

Boron (RDH: 2 milligrams to 3 milligrams daily)

Boron is an important bone-building cofactor—it helps vitamin D, calcium, and magnesium strengthen your skeleton and protect you against osteoporosis. "Low boron intakes result in impaired bone health, brain function, and immune response," said a team of researchers from the USDA's Grand Forks Human Nutrition Research Center in North Dakota, in the journal *Nutrition Reviews*. "Thus, low boron intake is a relevant nutritional concern, which diets rich in fruits, vegetables, nuts and pulses [beans and peas] can prevent."

However, most diets aren't rich in those foods, and a study shows that the average daily intake of boron in America is less than 2 milligrams, an amount I don't think is enough. Too little boron may make you particularly vulnerable to arthritis.

Writing in the journal *Environmental Health Perspectives*, a researcher in England claims that boron is a "safe and effective treatment for some forms of arthritis"—in fact, treatment with the mineral alleviated his own "arthritic pain and discomfort." He cites three studies on boron and arthritis. In one, researchers found lower levels of boron in the bones and synovial fluid (the lubricating fluid inside joints) of people with arthritis. In a population study, areas of the world where boron intake is 3 milligrams to 10 milligrams a day had an incidence of arthritis that was about one in 10 of the population, while areas where the intake was one milligram a day had an incidence of up to seven in 10. And in a clinical study on boron, researchers divided 20 people with arthritis into two groups, giving one group 6 milligrams a day of the mineral. The arthritis of 50 percent of those receiving boron improved, compared with only 10 percent of the placebo group. "Boron is an essential nutrient for healthy bones and joints," concluded the UK researcher.

Boron may be good for the brain, too. One researcher conducted an informal study, giving half his students boron and half of them a placebo. The boron group got better grades!

Copper (RDH: 500 micrograms daily)

Copper is good for you—and bad for you. It's a critical factor in the body's production of powerful antioxidants, such as superoxide dismutase. But it also triggers the production of free radicals and (like many minerals) is toxic in excess. For example, one study analyzed death rates in 4,000 men. Those with the highest blood levels of copper were 50 percent more likely to die from any cause, 40 percent more likely to die from cancer, and 30 percent more likely to die from cardiovascular disease. (If you find a penny and pick it up—don't chew on it!)

To strike an optimal balance of copper intake, I recommend 500 micrograms (0.5 milligram) a day.

Chromium (RDH: 200 micrograms to 500 micrograms daily)

Chromium buffs up your body's ability to use insulin, the hormone that moves glucose out of the bloodstream and into the cells. Chromium works in several ways. The mineral increases the number of insulin receptors, boosts an enzyme that helps those receptors work, and then blocks an enzyme that turns the receptors off.

"If chromium were a drug for diabetes, everybody would have touted it as a wonder drug," we were told by Richard Anderson, PhD, a researcher at the Beltsville Human Nutrition Research Center in Maryland who has authored more than 70 studies on chromium. But the scientific "consensus" is that (if chromium works at all) it works better to *control* diabetes than to *prevent* it. I advise using it for both. For example, a study shows that chromium supplements improve glucose metabolism in healthy young men.

The adequate intake for chromium is 20 to 35 micrograms for adults, and most adults get that—but many holistic health professionals (including myself) think 200 micrograms or more is optimal. Good food sources include meats and whole grains, along with broccoli, grape juice, orange juice, potatoes, and garlic.

Recent research shows chromium may help prevent and/or treat…

- Binge-eating disorder
- Depression (especially accompanied by anger)
- Diabetes
- Heart disease
- Menstrual problems
- Overweight
- Polycystic ovary syndrome

Molybdenum (RDH: 250 micrograms daily)

This mineral boosts the power of enzymes that aid in breaking down and eliminating toxic chemicals. It can be helpful in easing the symptoms of those with food allergies, especially sensitivity to the sulfites found in wine, beer, and dried fruits. Good food sources include whole grains and legumes. Molybdenum is a recent newcomer to the nutritional scene, so there aren't any human studies showing it can prevent and beat disease. But a recent review paper—from scientists at the USDA's Human Nutrition Research Center in Beltsville, Maryland, and the University of

Missouri—makes clear that the mineral might combat Wilson's Disease (an overaccumulation of copper), as well as cancer, arthritis, and cardiovascular disease.

Selenium (RDH: 55 micrograms daily)

Selenium combines with proteins to form selenoproteins, powerful antioxidant enzymes that help protect the membrane of every cell. Selenium is also critical for a healthy thyroid gland and a strong immune system.

In a study in the *American Journal of Clinical Nutrition*, researchers admitted how difficult it has been for nutritionists to determine "optimal selenium status" and found that adequate blood levels were achieved only by supplementing the diet with 50 micrograms of the mineral. (Supplements of 100 and 200 micrograms produced even better results.) And the researchers noted that achieving a truly optimal level is very important, because study after study has linked higher selenium levels to lower risk of dying from any cause, including cancer, heart disease, and stroke—the three leading killers of Americans. In fact, when French researchers studied nearly 1,400 older people for nine years, they found that those with the lowest blood selenium levels were 46 percent more likely to die of any cause. On the other hand, a study showed that higher selenium intakes were associated with a possible increased risk of diabetes. A good balance is to supplement with 55 micrograms a day.

The best food source of selenium is Brazil nuts, containing 10 times more selenium than a serving of almost any other food. In a study in the *American Journal of Clinical Nutrition*, people who ate two Brazil nuts a day for three months boosted blood selenium levels by 67 percent. Other good sources include beef, whole grains, fish (tuna and cod), turkey, chicken, eggs, and shellfish such as lobster, crab, clams, and oysters.

Recent research shows selenium may help prevent and/or treat...

- Benign prostatic hypertrophy
- Cancer
- Cervical dysplasia
- Hearing loss
- Heart disease
- HIV/AIDS
- Infertility
- Kidney disease
- Mild cognitive impairment
- Osteoporosis
- Polycystic ovary syndrome
- Schizophrenia
- Sepsis
- Stroke
- Thyroid disease

Iodine (RDH: 150 micrograms to 250 micrograms daily)

Maybe you think of iodine deficiency as a goiter-causing condition that no longer threatens Americans since table salt began to be fortified with the mineral. (A goiter is an enlarged thyroid gland.) But Americans should dine on more iodine. *Here's why...*

•**Flour is now fortified with bromine rather than iodine, decreasing iodine intake.** Meanwhile, iodine intakes have dropped by around 50 percent in the last 30 years. ("Iodine intakes in the USA have fallen in recent years," said a report in the journal *Proceedings of the Nutrition Society*.) In fact, bromine and other chemically related compounds added to food and water (the halides chlorine and fluorine) may actually *block* the activity of iodine.

•**Iodine's main role is to help manufacture thyroid hormones.** That's why a subclinical iodine deficiency—enough to prevent a goiter, but not enough for optimal health—can cause hypothyroidism, an underrecognized condition that I think is epidemic in America. (Its symptoms include fatigue, overweight, pain, and even infertility.) I discuss the cause of thyroid problems at length in Hormonal Imbalances on page 84, and in Hypothyroidism on page 254.

•**Iodine deficiency is a common trigger for breast tenderness and fibrocystic breast disease, and I routinely use iodine supplements in women with these problems.** Iodine levels are also low in women with breast cancer, and I routinely supplement the diets of my patients with breast cancer with 6,250 to 12,500 micrograms a day, using a form called tri-iodine.

•**A low intake of iodine during pregnancy is linked to lower IQs in children.** There is a "growing problem of iodine deficiency among women of gestational age in…industrial nations," said a team of Spanish researchers, who found 15 percent lower "development quotients" in 18-month-olds born to women with low iodine levels during pregnancy.

The best food source of the nutrient is seafood, particularly seaweed such as kelp. If you need more than the RDH for therapeutic reasons, I favor Tri-Iodine from Terry Naturally.

Amino Acids

Amino acids are the 22 links in the chainlike structure of proteins. And just as the 26 letters of the alphabet spell millions of different words, so the 22 amino acids make millions of different proteins. Your body manufactures 14 of those amino acids on its own. Eight others are "essential"—you get them only from food.

Without amino acids and proteins, your body wouldn't work. In fact, without amino acids, your body wouldn't exist. Amino acids are literally the stuff of life. And liveliness.

I've found amino acid supplements—particularly amino acids from a natural source, such as whey protein—can aid health in all kinds of ways. (Whey is the natural liquid by-product of cheese production.) As is the case with most nutrients, optimal levels of amino acids are good (and likely better than the RDA), but more is not always better. (For example, limit tyrosine supplementation to no more than 500 mg daily. More has been linked to an increased risk for diabetes.) Whey protein delivers a very balanced level of aminos. Another rich source of amino acids is eggs, with a balance of aminos resembling that found in the human body—plus, they're a perfect alternative to whey protein if you're allergic to milk. (You can read more about why I think eggs are a good-for-you food—rather than a risk factor for heart disease—in Heart Disease on page 239.) And if neither of those options appeal to you, rely on Clinical Essentials Multi-Vitamin & Minerals, from Terry Naturally, which supplies a complete range of aminos.

Recent studies on whey protein and its complement of amino acids show it can help…

- Increase the flexibility (youthfulness) of arterial walls
- Lower blood pressure
- Balance post-meal blood sugar levels in healthy people
- Control high blood sugar in diabetes
- Prevent bone loss and increase bone mineral density
- Preserve muscle mass (on average, people lose three percent to five percent of total muscle mass per decade, starting at age 30)
- Decrease fat mass
- Promote weight loss
- Stop the advance of fatty liver disease
- Prevent overeating (when used before a meal)
- Boost the level of the immune system's disease-fighting white blood cells
- Reduce allergic reactions in allergy-prone children
- Reduce crying time in colicky babies
- Decrease "airway reactivity" in children with asthma
- Help cut the incidence of colds by more than half
- Ease the symptoms of psoriasis, a disease of red, scaly, itchy skin
- Prevent side effects from antibiotics, such as diarrhea
- Maintain mental balance under stress
- Increase endurance and strength, and improve athletic performance
- Reduce muscle wear and tear from intense exercise
- Improve rehabilitation in frail, elderly people who have recently left the hospital, and after a hip fracture
- Improve the health of people with HIV/AIDS

Omega-3 Essential Fatty Acids

Amino acids are the building blocks of protein. Fatty acids are the building blocks of body fat, and they also provide the outer layering (membrane) of our cells. Fish oil is particularly rich in two vital omega-3 fatty acids: EPA (eicosapentaenoic acid) and DHA (docosahexaenoic acid). Decades of studies on fish oil and heart health, involving more than 40,000 people, show that fish oil can and does help prevent heart disease. Specifically, fish oil reduces triglycerides, blood fats that can hurt the heart; stabilizes plaque, which might otherwise break off and form an artery-clogging clot; thins the blood, helping to stop blood clots; generates more clot-dissolving, artery-relaxing nitric oxide; blocks the buildup of proteins that can harden arteries; lowers blood pressure; and reduces inflammation, the fuel of heart disease. (Whew!) "The good news about fish oil supplements isn't just hype," said Carl Lavie,

MD, medical director of cardiac rehabilitation and prevention at the John Ochsner Heart and Vascular Institute in New Orleans, who published a review paper on fish oil in the *Journal of the American College of Cardiology*. "We now have tremendous and compelling evidence from very large studies that demonstrate the protective benefits of omega-3 fish oil in multiple aspects of preventive cardiology."

Like Dr. Lavie, I strongly recommend you include oily fish in your diet or take fish oil supplements. Eating three to four servings a week of salmon gives you plenty of omega-3s. As for supplements, the good news is that a unique form of omega-3s from fish, called Vecto-mega, has a chemical structure identical to that found in salmon and dramatically increases absorption—so one to two tablets a day are plenty, instead of the typical eight to 16. Vecto-mega has all the good and none of the bad of fish oil.

Omega-3 fatty acids from fish not only protect the heart. They also strengthen the membrane of *every* cell in the body, particularly brain cells.

Recent research shows omega-3s can help prevent and/or treat…

- Age-related macular degeneration
- Alzheimer's disease
- Arrhythmia
- Arthritis
- Attention-deficit/ hyperactivity disorder
- Autism
- Autism spectrum disorder (ASD)
- Benign prostatic hyperplasia (BPH)
- Cancer
- Canker sores (aphthous ulcers)
- Crohn's disease
- Cystic fibrosis
- Hot flashes
- Infertility
- Memory loss
- Migraine
- Mild cognitive impairment
- Multiple sclerosis
- Muscle soreness after exercise
- Depression
- Diabetes
- Diabetic complications (foot ulcers, neuropathy, retinopathy)
- Dry eyes
- Eczema
- Epilepsy
- Fatty liver disease (NAFLD)
- Gum disease (periodontitis)
- Heart disease
- High blood pressure
- Hostility and aggressiveness
- Nicotine dependence
- Parkinson's disease
- Polycystic ovary syndrome (PCOS)
- Post-traumatic stress disorder (PTSD)
- Schizophrenia
- Skin aging

Your One-Stop Supplement

Perhaps you're thinking, *If I try to supplement my diet with all the nutrients Dr. Teitelbaum says are important, I'll have to take handfuls of supplements a couple of times a day.* And you could, if you wanted to.

But you can also obtain optimal levels of all the nutrients discussed in this chapter (except iron and fish oil) by mixing up just one drink each morning—using the Energy Revitalization System multivitamin powder made by Nature's Way. This single drink replaces more than 35 supplement pills.

I formulated this supplement, and like most of the products I am involved with, my royalties go to charity. This allows me to be unabashed in giving various treatments a thumbs-up or thumbs-down in my role as a patient advocate.

I lecture frequently to many of the world's leading nutritional and health experts, including the International and American Associations of Clinical Nutritionists' annual conference, and I routinely present them with this challenge: If any of you can find the nutrients in the Energy Revitalization System in less than 35 capsules, I'll give you $50. (Multiplied by the thousands of attendees I've lectured to, my risk is tens of thousands of dollars, so I don't make this challenge lightly.) To date, no one has successfully met the "capsule challenge"—and these are top nutritional experts. (But for those who don't like powders and prefer a pill, an excellent multivitamin is Clinical Essentials from Terry Naturally.)

The Right Amount

If you're well and looking to prevent disease, ½ to 1 scoop of the powder is plenty. If you're ill and looking for optimum nutritional support in treating and reversing disease, you can take the full scoop, which will get you to the full RDH of all the nutrients mentioned in this chapter.

Adjust the dose to whatever feels best to you. (I take ⅘ scoop each morning.) Because the supplement is a powder, you can take it many different ways. Some like to add it to yogurt. Others add the orange-flavored form (my wife's favorite) to 2 ounces of orange juice, 2 ounces of milk, and 4 ounces of water, producing an orange smoothie. I favor the berry flavor and simply add it to water. (I like to avoid the sugar in fruit juices.)

If you hand-mix rather than use a blender (which I do), put the powder in a dry glass and add 2 to 3 ounces of whatever liquid you're using, give it a few stirs until any lumps are gone, and then add the rest of the liquid. It's the most worthwhile 10 seconds you'll spend each day!

Don't Forget a Healthy Diet!

Although an excellent nutritional supplement is an important "insurance policy" to obtain optimal amounts of vitamins, minerals, and other micronutrients, eating a healthy diet is a key foundation of good health.

But when I say "healthy," I'm not talking about eliminating all the foods that might be bad for you. Such a diet is almost impossible to follow, as so many people find out when they try it. Dietary deprivation usually leads to so-called indulgence. Pleasurable moderation—including "indulging" in the foods you love to eat—is the key. As Mark Twain so aptly put it, "Moderation in all things—including moderation!" To stay healthy, all you have to do is eat a diet that is reasonably healthful. *My key recommendations…*

•**Eat lots of whole foods, including whole grains, fresh fruits (whole fruit, not fruit juice), and fresh vegetables, and minimize processed foods.** Following this one simple guideline will have amazing results—because the more unprocessed your diet, the healthier it is for you. Why? The closer the food is to its original form, the higher its nutritional value.

•**Increase water intake.** Water lubricates the body. You can tell you're adequately hydrated when your lips and mouth aren't dry. But you want your water to be pure, so you're not filling your body with toxins while slaking your thirst. The best way to ensure pure water is a good water filter in your home. I recommend the filter Multipure (with carbon block filtration systems) or a (more expensive) reverse-osmosis filter, which uses a different type of multistep system (the same type used to remove salt from seawater). You can also buy large jugs of water that have been purified by either carbon block filtration or reverse osmosis. What you want to wean off of is water from soft plastic bottles. Eventually, we'll realize that these were a mistake, adding unacceptable toxins to the water (not to mention its impact on the environment).

•**Minimize or eliminate sugar and other sweeteners from your diet.** As I explain at length in my book *The Complete Guide to Beating Sugar Addiction*, excess sugar can weaken your immune system; worsen pain; boost your blood pressure and cholesterol levels, increasing your risk of heart disease; lead to obesity; cause type 2 diabetes; and play a role in causing or complicating many other health problems and diseases, such as chronic fatigue syndrome, fibromyalgia, chronic sinusitis, irritable bowel syndrome, cancer, autoimmune diseases, candida and yeast infections, and attention-deficit/hyperactivity disorder.

For a healthy sugar substitute, you can use stevia (made from the leaves of the stevia plant, a sweet-tasting herb in the chrysanthemum family). The brands I like best are Now and Stevia Select. You can also use saccharin (Sweet'N Low), which has a long record of safety. I don't recommend aspartame, because some people experience severe reactions to it, including seizures, headaches, nausea, dizziness, depression, and more. (It's surprising to me that it ever received FDA approval for use.) I think the jury is still out on the safety of sucralose, which is sold as Splenda—animal studies show it can lower levels of friendly gut bacteria, and some people report digestive distress when they use it.

•**Remove excess caffeine from your diet.** Coffee drinkers are often caught in a vicious cycle. The energy boost from excess caffeine (along with skyrocketing adrenaline levels) is followed by an inevitable low, causing you to drink ever-increasing amounts of coffee to sustain your energy. If you're a coffee drinker and suffer from severe fatigue and anxiety, I recommend you stop drinking coffee completely for two to three months. (Substitute a morning glass of brewed tea—which has about half the caffeine—for your morning jump start.) If after that time you're feeling good, you can start drinking coffee again—but no more than two 12-ounce cups daily. As an alternative, try one to two cups a day of green or black tea, both of which are loaded with health-giving antioxidants.

Although I recommend stopping excess coffee completely, I don't recommend stopping it suddenly. To successfully reduce your coffee consumption, remove it from your diet gradually. Cut your intake in half every week, until you are down to one or two cups a day. For example, if you drink four cups a day, cut your intake to two cups a day the first week, and then to one

Preventing Supplement Side Effects

The most common side effects from nutritional supplements, occurring in a very small percentage of people, are gas, diarrhea, or an upset stomach. If this is a problem for you, try taking Nature's Way Energy Revitalization System powder with a meal or at bedtime.

Another strategy: Split the dose in two, taking ¼ to ½ scoop of the powder twice a day.

Some people don't have general digestive upset from a supplement but find the high levels of magnesium cause diarrhea. If you have that problem, there is a sustained-release magnesium supplement from Jigsaw Health that works well and doesn't cause the runs.

Nutritional supplements rich in the B vitamins turn the urine bright yellow; this is a normal (and good) sign that they are being absorbed. If you have kidney failure, take a nutritional supplement containing magnesium only with your doctor's approval and supervision; otherwise, magnesium levels may rise too high.

cup a day the second week. When you are down to one to two cups a day—enjoy it! (Or, as I mentioned earlier, switch to tea.)

I would note that chocolate, coffee, and tea, in moderation, are actually health foods. They come from plants that are chockful of healthy nutrients and have been shown to have numerous health benefits.

•**Limit alcohol consumption to one to two drinks daily.** Hundreds of studies show that the benefits of alcohol intake follow what scientists call a J curve. No alcohol intake (the left tip of the J) is less healthy than a moderate amount of intake (the bottom of the J). But as you increase alcohol intake beyond moderation, you begin to suffer negative effects (the line of the J on the right).

Bottom line: A moderate amount of alcohol intake (one drink a day) can be good for your heart (according to some studies), while a large amount is bad for your entire body.

I advise patients who drink more than three drinks daily to stop drinking alcohol completely for three months. If you decide to return alcohol to your diet at the end of that time, make two drinks a day your limit. One drink equals 5 ounces of wine, 12 ounces of beer, or 1½ ounces of whiskey or other "hard" liquor.

•**Follow your bliss.** Perhaps you're familiar with the famous advice given by Joseph Campbell, who wrote books about the lessons in ancient myths that could help guide our lives.

His main admonition: Follow your bliss. Well, I agree. Better than any expert, your body knows what's good for you and will tell you what's good for you—by making you feel good!

Poor Sleep

Good Night and Great Health

Let's board a time machine and travel back a century or so, to 1900. William McKinley is reelected president. The U.S. currency is placed on the gold standard. And the temperance crusader Carrie Nation is attacking saloons with her hatchet. But amid all the excitement, America's population of around 70 million people is sleeping quite soundly—snoozing an average of nine hours per night.

Yes, believe it or not, in the pre-TV, pre-Internet days of the early 20th century, Americans actually slept nine hours. Now let's re-board our time machine and return to the 24/7 reality of the 21st century. The American population has increased: There are more than 300 million of us. But American shut-eye has decreased—to an average of 6.8 hours a night, with 40 percent of us sleeping six hours or less—and only 28 percent of us sleeping eight hours or more. (Nine hours is considered abnormal.) And for tens of millions of us, that abbreviated trip to the Land of Nod isn't by choice.

An estimated 45 million Americans fit the official medical definition of chronic insomnia: having trouble falling asleep or staying asleep, or waking up too early, at least three times a month, for more than a month. Another 60 million have the same symptoms but less often. Meanwhile, many other types of sleep disorders, such as sleep apnea and restless legs syndrome, also wreck a good night's sleep. This all means there's a very good chance you're either troubled by sleeplessness or squeezing sleep to a minimum.

The Risk Factor We Forget

Well, it's time we Americans woke up to this little-known fact: Poor sleep is a real cause of disease (along with fatigue, lack of mental clarity, ongoing pain and achiness, and many other problems that don't qualify as "diseases" but are very troublesome). And good sleep is a real cure.

As you'll read in a minute, scientific study after study shows that lack of sleep is as much a disease risk factor as eating a sugary diet or never exercising. For most people, six to seven hours of sleep a night doesn't give the body enough time to repair and regenerate. And because every part of the body is worn out by the typical demands of the day and needs regular rest—your busy brain, your loyal heart muscle, your diligent digestive tract, and all the other organs and systems and tissues—every part of the body can start to break down when you're sleep deprived.

Your bank account can start to suffer, too. Researchers found that insomnia patients had more than three times the yearly health costs of non-insomniacs. In another study, researchers from the University of Minnesota, the University of Chicago, and other institutions surveyed the "health-related quality of life" of 397 people and found that those with "severe sleep disturbances" had six times the likelihood of having poor scores. And a 14-year study by researchers at the Pennsylvania State College of Medicine found that insomnia and sleep duration under six hours a night increased men's death rates up to *fivefold* compared to those with normal sleep.

Sleeping Pills Aren't the Answer

Only one-third of people with sleep problems discuss them with their doctor, and only seven percent of chronic insomniacs are treated for the problem. And most of those insomniacs are merely prescribed sleeping pills. (More than 20 million sleeping pill prescriptions are written in the United States every year, according to researchers from the University of North Carolina at Chapel Hill.) But sleeping pills are only a short-term solution, don't treat the causes of insomnia, often worsen sleep quality, and can have dangerous side effects, says Gregg Jacobs, PhD, a former professor at the Sleep Disorders Center at the University of Massachusetts Medical School and author of *Say Good Night to Insomnia*.

One survey showed that 38 percent of those who take sleeping pills do so for longer than the recommended two weeks (these drugs are intended as a short-term treatment, not a long-term solution). And 63 percent experience side effects, which can include fuzzy thinking and poorer driving performance the next day (sleep experts call this "next-day sedation"); worsened insomnia when the drug is stopped ("rebound"); the spooky side phenomena of "somnambulism," such as sleepwalking, sleep-related eating, and even sleep driving; psychosis (hallucinations and delusional thinking); severe allergic reactions; and even a higher risk of death.

In a seven-year study of more than 100,000 people, researchers from the University of Warwick Medical School in the UK compared death rates of those who had been prescribed sleeping pills to those who hadn't—and found those who took the pills had triple the risk of dying. This study is one of many that have linked sleeping pills to higher death rates, particularly from cancer, according to doctors from the University of California, San Diego and the Scripps Clinic Sleep Center, in a report in the *Journal of Sleep Research*. (Interestingly, the sleep medication Ambien was not associated with decreased longevity. But that doesn't make it harmless. When it's stopped, it can cause severe rebound insomnia—making it difficult to sleep for a week.)

As I discuss in Insomnia and Other Sleep Disorders on page 268, most people can cure their insomnia with natural sleep remedies instead of prescription drugs. Those remedies include proper "sleep hygiene" (such as not drinking coffee after 4:00 p.m. and not using your bed as a site for problem solving or work) and taking nutrients and herbs that calm the brain and induce sleep. However, I endorse the use of sleeping medication in treating chronic fatigue syndrome and fibromyalgia, which are nearly impossible to cure without first addressing the problem of severe, chronic insomnia.

For the rest of this chapter, I'll present the scientific evidence that proves insomnia can cause or complicate literally dozens of health conditions. I want you to be thoroughly convinced of this real cause, so you're inspired to implement the real cure!

Poor Sleep, Poor Health

What happens during the one-third or so of your life when you're asleep? Surprisingly, scientists don't really know. *But they theorize that sleep provides…*

•**Rest** for a body and mind worn out by the day's activity.

•**Repair,** as the sleeping body generates human growth hormone (HGH, also called the fountain-of-youth hormone), which fuels tissue growth in childhood and tissue repair in adults. In a study from researchers at the University of Chicago, reducing deep sleep by 90 minutes a night cut the production of HGH by 23 percent.

•**Mental and emotional maintenance,** as memories are filed and dreams process complicated emotions.

But even if scientists don't know exactly *how* sleep works to keep you healthy, they know *what* can happen when you don't get enough. You can get sick! *And in a lot of different ways…*

•**Anxiety and worry.** Researchers at the National Institutes of Health found that people who had trouble sleeping were nearly six times more likely to have an "anxiety disorder" such as generalized anxiety disorder (GAD)—near-constant worrying that's often out of proportion to the situation you're worried about. Researchers at the University of California, San Francisco found that insomnia was linked to "subclinical anxiety" (not bad enough to be diagnosed with GAD, but bad enough to bother you). Easing chronic insomnia may prevent anxiety, said Norwegian researchers, who conducted an 11-year study showing that insomniacs were three times as likely to have an anxiety disorder.

•**Brain shrinkage.** Dutch researchers measured brain volume in insomniacs who were otherwise psychologically healthy and found smaller amounts of gray matter in the left orbitofrontal cortex—the part of the brain linked to pleasure and rest. "This study suggests that there are additional risks of not treating insomnia, such as detrimental effects on the microstructure of the brain," said the editor of *Biological Psychiatry*, the journal in which the study appeared.

•**Burnout.** In this condition, you feel exhausted and disinterested because of long-term stress. (Nurses, psychologists, and people in other "helping professions" are particularly prone.) Israeli researchers reported in the *Journal of Psychosomatic Research* that insomniacs were

64 percent more likely to suffer from burnout. And in a study from France, researchers found that insomnia made it *14 times more likely* a person would suffer from burnout! In fact, concluded the researchers, "job strain represents a burnout risk factor only if associated with insomnia."

•**Depression.** Dutch researchers found that insomniacs were 42 percent more likely to be depressed. "Depressive disorder is strongly associated with sleep disturbances," concluded the researchers in the *Journal of Clinical Psychiatry*. And insomnia is not just a common symptom of depression, asserted researchers from Stanford University in a paper in *Current Psychiatry Reports*. Insomnia also can play a role in causing the illness, they wrote.

•**Diabetes.** In a study published in *Diabetes/Metabolism Research and Reviews*, scientists analyzed 10 years of health data, and found that people with chronic insomnia were 51 percent more likely to develop type 2 diabetes. One way that sleep loss may cause diabetes is by decreasing insulin sensitivity—the ability of cells to respond to insulin, the hormone that ushers glucose out of the bloodstream and into muscle and fat cells.

•**Emotional intelligence.** People with "emotional intelligence" are aware of their own emotions and the emotions of others, and that awareness positively influences their decisions and behaviors. Researchers at the Walter Reed Army Institute of Research found that sleep deprivation decreased emotional intelligence. In their study published in the journal *Sleep Medicine*, they also found that the sleep-deprived had lower scores on tests measuring several other positive psychological traits, such as assertiveness, independence, stress management skills, and positive thinking. Sleep loss, theorized the researchers, causes a "mild dysfunction" in the prefrontal lobe, the part of the brain that controls emotions and thinking.

•**Fibromyalgia syndrome (FMS).** This condition, caused by shortened, tightened muscles, is characterized by pain—sometimes chronic, sometimes intermittent, usually all over the body but sometimes only in specific areas. In a study in the journal *Pain*, researchers at the University of Connecticut School of Medicine evaluated 50 women with fibromyalgia and found that those who did not sleep well reported more pain; a night of poor sleep was followed by a more painful day; and a more painful day was followed by a night of poorer sleep (creating a vicious cycle all too familiar to the millions of people with fibromyalgia). Poor sleep also seemed to make pain more prominent, regardless of its intensity. And in a study in the *Clinical Journal of Pain*, people with fibromyalgia and insomnia were nearly four times more likely to take antidepressants, three times more likely to take muscle relaxants, and 59 percent more likely to take opioids.

•**Fitness.** People who are sleep deprived exercise less, and the smaller amount of exercise they do is less intense, reported German researchers in the *American Journal of Clinical Nutrition*. "The observed decrease in daytime physical activity may point to another potentially important behavioral mechanism for the health-impairing influence of sleep loss," they concluded. In other words: less sleep = less exercise = more illness.

•**Frailty syndrome.** This common problem among people 80 and older is characterized by loss of muscle mass and symptoms such as slower walking, weaker grip, exhaustion, and significant weight loss. It's often the first sign that a serious and perhaps life-ending illness is around the corner. Researchers at the Yale University School of Medicine studied 374 people with an average

age of 84 who were living at home and found that those with insomnia were 93 percent more likely to be frail. "Sleep-wake disturbances that present with daytime drowsiness" are linked to frailty, they concluded in the study published in the *Journal of the American Geriatrics Society*. And in a study from Mexican researchers, sleep problems tripled the rate of frailty among women aged 70 and older.

•**Heartburn (gastroesophageal reflux disease, or GERD).** In a study of nearly 25,000 people by Swedish researchers at the Karolinska Institute, those with sleep disturbances and insomnia were three times more likely to develop GERD. And those with GERD were 40 percent more likely to develop sleep problems. That makes the problem "bidirectional" the researchers wrote in the medical journal *Sleep*: insomnia causes heartburn; heartburn causes insomnia.

•**Heart disease and stroke.** Two researchers from Harvard Medical School analyzed all the most recent research on the link between insomnia and heart disease, publishing their results in the medical journal *Chest. They found that sleep problems increased the risk of…*
  •High blood pressure fourfold, or 400 percent
  •Heart attack by 45 percent
  •Heart failure by more than threefold, or 367 percent
  •Death from heart disease by 48 percent

The researchers found that sleep deprivation weakens the heart in several ways. It speeds heart rate (taxing the heart). It makes the rhythm of the heartbeat less variable (making the heart less responsive to challenges of all kinds, from stress to exercise). It generates stress hormones that damage the heart. It increases inflammation, a driving force in cardiovascular disease (and many other diseases, as you learned earlier). And it speeds the development of artery-clogging plaque.

•**Memory loss and other types of cognitive decline.** Researchers from the Sleep Research and Treatment Center at the Penn State College of Medicine gave nearly 2,000 people tests to measure mental abilities such as memory, speed of processing information, and the ability to switch attention from one task to another. People with the shortest sleep duration had the lowest scores. And in a study of nearly 5,200 people conducted by Finnish researchers, short sleep duration and daytime tiredness and fatigue were linked to "decreased cognitive function." (There are literally dozens of other studies showing the "cognitive consequences of sleep loss," as a team of researchers from the University of California, Berkeley, put it.)

Needless to say, the final step in memory and cognitive decline is dementia—and sleep problems increase the risk of dementia by 36 percent, according to a study in the journal *Alzheimer's & Dementia*.

•**Menopause problems.** In the journal *Menopause*, researchers compared menopausal women who had chronic insomnia with menopausal women who didn't and found that the poor sleepers had more emergency room visits, a 21 percent greater impairment in overall activity, lower scores on a "physical and mental summary" test, and 17 percent lower productivity at work. And researchers at the University of Maryland concluded that "bothersome menopausal symptoms" such as hot flashes may cause depression in menopausal women *because* those symptoms disturb sleep.

●**Overweight.** In a seven-year study of 1,300 women 40 to 60 years old, Finnish researchers linked sleep problems and weight problems. Those who had trouble falling asleep were 65 percent more likely to have "major weight gain" (11 pounds or more). Those who woke up several times during the night were 49 percent more likely to have put on lots of pounds. And those who had trouble staying asleep were 41 percent more likely to have gained extra weight. "To prevent major weight gain and obesity, sleep problems need to be taken into account," concluded the researchers in the *International Journal of Obesity*.

What does your bed have to do with your scale? Studies show that insomnia alters levels of ghrelin, a hormone that stimulates your appetite. It also lowers leptin, an appetite-suppressing hormone. People who sleep less also eat more calorie-laden fast food, reported researchers at the City University of New York. And researchers at Wake Forest University School of Medicine showed that women who sleep five hours or less a night have more visceral fat—the abdominal fat around the internal organs that is a risk factor for heart disease and diabetes.

Bottom line: Inadequate sleep can pack on the pounds. Overcoming insomnia can help you sleep your way to weight loss.

●**Pain (chronic).** Researchers from the University of North Texas studied 772 people and found that those with chronic insomnia had nearly three times the risk of chronic pain, according to a study in the journal *Sleep*. And in a study in the journal *Pain*, researchers at Johns Hopkins University School of Medicine found that burn victims who had insomnia when they were discharged from the hospital also had "significantly decreased improvement in pain and increased pain severity during long-term follow-up." The researchers concluded: "This study provides support for a long-term…reciprocal interaction between insomnia and pain."

Over 35 years, I've effectively treated thousands of chronic pain patients and found that eight hours of sleep is a must for making the pain go away.

●**Post-traumatic stress disorder (PTSD).** In PTSD, chronic anxiety is triggered by a traumatic event, such as war, a serious car accident, or an assault. And nine out of 10 people with PTSD also have sleep problems such as insomnia, sleep apnea, and nightmares, according to a scientific report from researchers at the University of California, San Diego, the University of California, San Francisco, and the National Center for PTSD. And, say those researchers, sleep disorders make some of the symptoms of PTSD—depression, substance abuse, impaired daily functioning, poor health, and suicide risk—a lot worse.

●**Productivity at work.** People with insomnia have "significantly worse productivity, performance, and safety outcomes" at work, reported a study in the *Journal of Occupational and Environmental Medicine*. Daytime fatigue from insomnia costs nearly $2,000 a year per employee in productivity losses. In a study from Canada, people with insomnia had 32 percent more absenteeism, 70 percent more reduced productivity, and 49 percent more accidents at work. In studies by Norwegian researchers, those with insomnia were twice as likely to take sick leave and four times as likely to receive a disability pension from the country's National Insurance

OSA and RLS: The Other Sleep Disorders

Insomnia isn't the only common sleep disorder that causes fatigue and other health problems. There's also obstructive sleep apnea (OSA) and restless legs syndrome (RLS), which now is called periodic limb movement disorder (PLMD) when it occurs only at night. Both are common causes of falling asleep during the day—particularly when watching TV or driving.

In OSA (a condition common among older, overweight men), the soft tissue at the back of the throat plugs the airway during sleep, repeatedly cutting off breathing—and repeatedly waking up the sleeper. OSA is linked to higher risk of heart disease, stroke, type 2 diabetes, depression, and erectile dysfunction—and a five-times-higher risk of dying from any cause.

Both RLS and PLMD cause unpleasant sensations in your legs, and your legs get "jumpy." RLS/PLMD has been linked to high blood pressure, heart disease, stroke, blood sugar problems, overweight, depression, anxiety, hot flashes during menopause, kidney disease, liver disease, migraine headaches, tinnitus (ringing in the ears), erectile dysfunction, attention-deficit/hyperactivity disorder (in children and adults), chronic neck pain, dizziness, and (no surprise) poorer "health-related quality of life." In one study, women with RLS and daytime sleepiness had an 85 percent higher risk of dying from any cause.

Could you have one of these problems and don't know it? Possibly. Ask your bed partner if your legs are jumpy or if you snore. Sleeping alone? Use your cell phone to record yourself sleeping. You can find real cures for both of these sleep disorders in Insomnia and Other Sleep Disorders on pages 268–77.

Administration. And in a study of 3,000 workers, published in the journal *Sleep Health*, insomnia was the "strongest predictor" of poor productivity at work.

•**Stroke.** In a scientific paper in the journal *Expert Review of Neurotherapeutics*, researchers link sleep problems other than sleep apnea to a 20 percent increased risk of stroke. As for sleep apnea itself, the researchers found it triples the risk of stroke.

•**Suicide.** In a 10-year study of more than 14,000 people ages 67 to 90, researchers at Florida State University linked sleep complaints to a higher rate of committing suicide. In another study, sleep problems were a more important factor in "suicidal ideation" (thinking about suicide) than either depression or hopelessness.

•**Urinary problems.** Researchers at the University of North Texas found that those with chronic insomnia had nearly double the risk of urinary problems.

After reading about all these health problems that lack of sleep can cause, go ahead and take a nap. And after you wake up, turn to Insomnia and Other Sleep Disorders on page 268, where you'll find a wide variety of easy-to-implement real cures for this real cause.

Inactivity

Tell Sickness to Take a Hike

W e're hardly the first to make the following point, but it's a point worth making again (and again): *If exercise were a pill, everyone would take it.*

That's because exercise can effectively help prevent or treat just about every health problem out there. Get ready for a long list.

•**Aging: Keeps you youthful all your life.** Needless to say, death is usually the result of aging. In a 20-year study involving more than 5,000 older men, the fittest had a 38 percent lower risk of dying from any cause during the study, reported researchers in the journal *Circulation*. And men who weren't fit but became fit lowered their risk by 35 percent. Exercise (along with sex and sleep) stimulates the production of human growth hormone (HGH), the so-called fountain-of-youth hormone that melts fat, builds muscle, and helps you feel and look younger.

•**Alzheimer's disease: Reduces risk by one-third.** Ten minutes of walking a day is linked to a 32 percent lower risk of developing Alzheimer's, reported researchers from the University of Washington. Research also shows that regular exercise sharpened the minds of seniors with mild cognitive impairment, the mental decline that precedes Alzheimer's. No drug can do that!

•**Arthritis: Builds muscle that makes a difference.** Women with the strongest thighs had a 30 percent lower risk of developing osteoarthritis of the knee (the most common kind), reported researchers from the University of Iowa.

•**Asthma: Soothes symptoms.** In a study published in the *Journal of Asthma*, an international team of researchers found that light exercise, three times a week, reduced asthma episodes by 56 percent. In another study in the journal *Chest*, three months of regular exercise decreased symptoms dramatically in 50 people with asthma and lessened anxiety and depression.

•**Cancer: Prevents and protects.** A large and growing body of scientific research shows that exercise can help prevent cancer and cancer recurrence and ease the side effects of cancer treatment. *For example, studies show regular exercise can lower the risk of...*

- •Prostate cancer by 35 percent
- •Endometrial cancer by 23 percent
- •Breast cancer by 16 percent
- •The recurrence of breast cancer by 56 percent
- •Dying from colon cancer (if you have it) by 53 percent
- •Dying from any cancer (if you have it) by 53 percent

•**Chronic fatigue syndrome (CFS): Gives more energy.** In a review of seven studies on CFS and exercise, European researchers found that regular exercise reduced fatigue, and improved sleep, daily physical functioning, and general health. (Energy production is limited when you have this condition, so exercising beyond what is comfortable is counterproductive.)

•**Depression: Works as an antidepressant.** In a review of dozens of studies, involving nearly 50,000 people, researchers found that exercise reduced levels of depression by more than 50 percent. In one study, walking worked just as well as an antidepressant drug in relieving depression, according to researchers in the Department of Psychiatry and Behavioral Sciences at Duke University.

•**Diabetes: Radically reduces risk.** Regular exercise lowers your risk of developing diabetes by up to 53 percent, studies show. And exercise can be as effective as any drug in regulating the high blood sugar levels of diabetes.

•**Falls: Helps achieve balance.** Every year, more than 30 percent of people age 65 and over fall—with one in 10 seriously injured and nearly 13,000 killed. Research shows that many different types of regular exercise—including walking, dancing, strength training, and tai chi—can help seniors stay on their feet.

•**Fibromyalgia: Relieves pain.** Regular water exercise decreased pain and improved health in a group of 30 women with fibromyalgia, reported an international team of researchers in the journal *Rheumatology*. And in a review of all the studies on fibromyalgia and water exercise, Canadian researchers found it not only decreased pain, but also reduced stiffness, built strength, and improved physical functioning. (Exercise is not a solution for this illness. But if you have fibromyalgia, it's important to do as much as you're able to maintain your conditioning. The key words here are "as you're able." Don't overdo!)

•**Gallstones: Cuts the risk of surgery.** Researchers from China analyzed data from 16 studies on exercise and gallstone disease and found that regular exercise decreased risk by over 20 percent. In a study of more than 60,000 women, those who regularly participated in "recreational physical activity" (such as walking or bicycling) were 31 percent less likely to have gallstone surgery compared with sedentary women, reported researchers from the Harvard T.H. Chan School of Public Health in the *New England Journal of Medicine*. And in a study of more than 45,000 men, those who watched television for more than 40 hours a week had a three-times-higher risk of painful gallbladder attacks compared with men watching TV less than six hours a week. "Thirty-four percent of symptomatic gallstone disease in men could be prevented by increasing exercise to 30 minutes, five times a week," concluded the researchers in the *Annals of Internal Medicine*.

•**Heart disease: Prevents the first attack…or the second.** Regular exercise reduces the risk of having a heart attack by 27 percent, reported Italian researchers in the *European Journal of Cardiovascular Prevention & Rehabilitation*. And regular exercise after a heart attack reduces the risk of dying by 31 percent, concluded a study in the medical journal *BMJ*.

•**High blood pressure: Provides the perfect prescription.** In people with high blood pressure, exercise (either walking on a treadmill or resistance training) reduced blood pressure for up to seven hours after the exercise session, reported Brazilian researchers in the *Journal of Strength and Conditioning Research*. These types of exercises would be a helpful "prescription" for anyone with high blood pressure, they concluded. (I recommend a walk in the sunshine, as you'll read about on page 53 of this chapter. Sunshine helps the body make vitamin D, which also helps lower blood pressure.)

•**Immune problems: Turns your natural killer cells loose.** In research on exercise and immunity, led by David Nieman, PhD, director of the Human Performance Lab at the North Carolina Research Campus and author of *Exercise Testing and Prescription*, scientists studied more than 1,000 people during the fall and winter. They found that those who exercised a total of 150 minutes a week (such as five 30-minute walks) had 43 percent fewer colds and bouts of the flu than inactive people. "This difference is greater in magnitude than could be achieved with any drug," Dr. Nieman told us. The reason it works: Exercise boosts circulating levels of virus-killing immune cells, such as natural killer cells. But, he said, the effect lasts only a few hours, which is why you have to exercise regularly to supercharge your immune system.

•**Insomnia: Helps you fall asleep faster.** Researchers from Boston University analyzed data from 66 studies on exercise and sleep—and found that exercise helped people fall asleep faster, improved total sleep time, and led to more restful sleep.

•**Menopausal symptoms: Cools hot flashes.** Women who had greater levels of physical activity had fewer menopausal symptoms, such as hot flashes, reported researchers from Pennsylvania State University in the journal *Maturitas*. In another study, from researchers at Harvard University and several other institutions and published in the journal *Menopause,* menopausal women who exercised regularly had fewer problems with sleep and were less depressed.

•**Multiple sclerosis: Improves quality of life.** In one study, Swiss researchers at the University of Basel looked at 46 people with multiple sclerosis (an autoimmune disease that gradually destroys the protective covering of nerves, causing a range of physical, mental, and emotional problems). Those who exercised regularly for three weeks had deeper sleep, less depression, less fatigue, and less numbness and tingling (paresthesia).

•**Osteoporosis: Strengthens bones.** "Exercise is effective in preserving bone mass, preventing fractures, and improving the quality of life in patients with osteoporosis," reported Japanese doctors who reviewed decades of research on exercise and osteoporosis.

•**Overweight: Keeps pounds off.** It's relatively easy to *lose* weight—most veteran dieters have done it many times. But only about five percent of people who shed pounds keep them off for good. Researchers at the University of Pittsburgh studied 201 overweight women who had lost 10 percent of their total body weight. They found that those who successfully kept it off after two years were those who exercised the most (4.5 hours per week). And in a scientific paper, titled *Is Regular Exercise an Effective Strategy for Weight Loss Maintenance?*, researchers from the University of Colorado point out that studies show "a program of regular exercise" is a "key characteristic of those who have been successful with weight loss maintenance."

•**Stress: Shields you from the damage.** "People with high exercise levels exhibit less health problems when they encounter stress," concluded a team of Swiss researchers who reviewed 30 years of research on stress and health. And in a study by an international team of researchers, exercise decreased anxiety in people with "stress-related disorders."

•**Stroke: Protects your brain.** Brisk walking for 30 minutes, 6 days a week, reduces the risk of stroke by 30 percent, reported researchers from Harvard Medical School in the *Journal of the American Medical Association*.

If everyone engaged in regular moderate physical activity, there would be 250,000 fewer deaths every year in America, wrote researchers from the Mayo Clinic and several other institutions in the *Mayo Clinic Proceedings*. They urged doctors to prescribe physical activity to inactive people.

Why Workouts Work

There's a simple explanation for why inactivity is a real cause and exercise is a real cure: Our bodies were made to move!

Our genes are an inheritance from the Late Paleolithic period of 10,000 years ago, when we were hunter-gatherers—and really, really active. We walked (or fled) everywhere, and our "sedentary" hours were confined to mealtime and bedtime. This is what scientists call our genotype: the instructions in our genetic code, the biological command that says, "Take a hike—a long hike!"

What happens when you don't shape up for General Gene? He assigns you to the hospital! In other words, you're likely to end up as one of the more than 130 million Americans with a chronic condition such as cardiovascular disease, type 2 diabetes, or cancer, conditions that account for more than 75 percent of all health costs in the United States. These chronic illnesses have many causes, but one of the big ones is chronic inactivity.

Well, desks and TVs (and cars and endless other "you-won't-have-to-lift-a-finger" conveniences) are permanent facts of modern life. But that doesn't mean you can't give your genes a big lift.

"Daily physical activity normalizes gene expression toward patterns established to maintain survival in the Late Paleolithic era," wrote Manu Chakravarthy, MD, PhD, of the University of Medicine and Dentistry of New Jersey, in the *Journal of Physiology*.

To paraphrase: Use it or lose it! But to do that, you probably have to *start* exercising regularly. Because if you're anything like the typical American, you're not exercising now.

Our National Vegetable: The Couch Potato

Only 15 percent of American adults meet the standard exercise recommendation of 30 minutes or more of moderate-intensity physical activity (such as a brisk walk) most days of the week, reported researchers from the U.S. Department of Health and Human Services. Forty percent of adults never exercise. Another study produced an equally sedentary statistic: The average American adult gets about two minutes a day of vigorous physical activity, the kind you get from jogging or playing singles tennis. And among folks who decide to join the fit-minded, most typically don't do so for long: Studies show that 50 percent of people who start a regular exercise program drop out within six months.

What's a body to do? Well, first you have to think of exercise as every bit as important as eating and sleeping (and you probably find at least a little time every day for those activities).

The good news: There are easy, effective ways to develop the exercise habit. Here are my recommendations, along with those of some of the top exercise experts in North America.

The Secret of Workout Willpower

For many people, the hardest thing about exercise is getting started—having the willpower to work out. To find out the best ways to motivate yourself to move, we talked to one of the world's top experts on the subject, Kathleen Martin Ginis, PhD, a professor in the School of Health and Exercise Sciences at the University of British Columbia in Canada. Dr. Ginis is a proponent of a school of thinking about willpower developed by psychologist Roy Baumeister, PhD, at Florida State University, called the "limited strength model of self-regulation." (*Self-regulation* is a technical term that psychologists use for *willpower.*)

The key idea is that using your willpower is a lot like using your muscles when you lift weights. Like your muscles, your willpower has limited strength. Like your muscles, when you use your willpower over and over, it weakens and then stops working entirely. And like your muscles, you have to rest your willpower—you have to give it time to recover—before you can use it again. What does that have to do with exercise?

Imagine you've been using your willpower all day. You stopped yourself from pressing the "Snooze" button on your alarm and actually got out of bed on the first ring. You resisted eating that doughnut midmorning. You plowed through mountains of paperwork you didn't really want to do. You forced yourself to listen to your spouse tell about his day, even though you were in the mood for relaxing in front of the TV. But when it came time to put on and lace up your walking shoes…and walk out the door…and haul your body around the block—forget about it! Your willpower had gone AWOL. But Dr. Ginis told us that you can work *with* your willpower to make sure there's enough around so that when you decide to exercise, you will exercise.

The key is either conserving or restoring your willpower. *She suggests…*

•**Plan in advance.** "This is crucial for people starting an exercise program," she told us. *You need to decide in advance on the following…*

 •Where you will exercise. (Around the neighborhood? At the gym? In the basement?)

- What exercise you will do. (A walk? An aerobics class? A ride on a stationary bike?)
- When you are going to exercise. (First thing in the morning? At lunch? After work?)
- How you will fit that exercise session into your busy day. (Keep your sneakers by the door. Ask your spouse to watch the kids while you go to the gym. Dust off the exercise bike in the basement.)

If you try to do all the planning that produces a workout when you're about to work out, it's likely you'll deplete your willpower and less likely that you'll actually exercise. But if you plan in advance, Dr. Ginis told us, you're more likely to have plenty of willpower when it's time to exercise, and you can just get up and go.

So, at the beginning of every week or every month, get out your calendar and pencil in your exercise sessions. Think through what it will take to make sure they actually happen as planned.

- **Get it done early.** When you roll out of bed, your willpower is as fresh as the proverbial daisy. Exercise right away, before it's depleted!
- **Take a break—and then take a walk.** Any kind of rest—a catnap, a brief meditation— refreshes willpower.
- **Turn on Comedy Central.** It's true: Watching a TV comedy can actually help you exercise. That's because a positive mood helps you summon up your willpower. Do whatever it takes to put a happy or satisfied smile on your face. Read a joke book. Listen to music you like. Pet your cat. Stare at a fishbowl. Whatever works for you.
- **Build up your willpower.** The "limited strength model of self-regulation" says that your willpower is like your muscles. And just like your muscles, if you use your willpower regularly, it becomes stronger. "Using your willpower weakens it for *a while*, but builds more strength for the next time you want to 'exercise' your will," said Dr. Ginis.

Enjoy Your Exercise! (or You Won't Do It Regularly)

"No pain, no gain." You've heard that slogan, of course (and maybe even muttered it under your breath at the gym). It reflects the belief that unless exercise hurts, it's not doing its job.

I have another slogan I want you to say to yourself instead: Pain is insane! At least *deciding* to experience pain is pretty crazy. Pain is your body's way of telling you, "Don't do that." And not only is pain during exercise a bad idea for your health (because it doesn't work, and because you might injure yourself), it is also a bad idea for establishing the habit of regular exercise. Nobody (except a masochist) makes a habit of doing something that hurts!

Exercise should be virtually pain free. And fun filled. And marathons (or half-marathons or quarter-marathons or even one-eighth marathons) are not required.

Going a Little Way Goes a Long Way

A common exercise error: You start a new exercise program by doing way too much, way too soon. People who start a new exercise program by doing a whole lot of exercising right away usually stop exercising fairly quickly because they suffer the consequences of sudden overuse, such as soreness, fatigue, and irritability. The body likes gradual change, so it can easily and comfortably adapt to the new situation. So instead of grunting, groaning, and grinding your teeth through more exercise than your body wants to do, gently recite this motivating mantra: A little movement is better than no movement at all.

"Think of the difference between sitting still and walking up a flight of stairs in your home," Vik Khanna, a clinical exercise specialist certified by the American College of Sports Medicine and the self-described "chief exercise officer" of Galileo Health Partners near Baltimore, told us. "You burn eight times more calories walking up that flight of stairs.

"So if you're sedentary," he continued, "start your 'exercise program' by walking up and down those stairs as many times a day as you can. When you come home with the groceries, make three or four trips bringing them into the house instead of one. There's no minimum when it comes to physical activity—anything is better than nothing."

Like I tell my patients: Window shopping downtown or walking around in the mall is exercise, too! Movement is what matters. Do a little today, and it will feel so good that you'll probably want to do more tomorrow.

Target Heart Rate? Forget About It!

Target heart rate is the percentage of your "maximum heart rate" that many fitness folks say is the true measure of whether or not exercise is doing you any good. (A common formula: Your average maximum heart rate is 220 minus your age, and you want to exercise at 50 percent to 85 percent of maximum.) Do you have to take a refresher course in algebra before you exercise?

"Don't worry about achieving your target heart rate or any other supposed measure of achieving fitness," Khanna told us. "Do whatever is tolerable to you, and do as much of it as feels good to you. Exercise until it doesn't feel fun and comfortable, and then stop. For most people, that's about 45 minutes to an hour a day of any activity they enjoy, whether it's walking, playing tennis, jogging, yoga, Pilates, or working out with weights."

If you experience any chest tightness, chest pain, or worrisome breathlessness when exercising, stop immediately and see a physician. However, just about everybody can start a moderate form of exercise such as walking without a physician's permission, as long as they don't experience the above symptoms.

Find an Exercise You Enjoy

As you know by now, Khanna's advice to choose an exercise that "feels good" jibes with my key advice about health: What feels good *to* you is usually good *for* you.

The exercise expert Dr. Nieman—a 70-year-old who has run dozens of marathons—has the same "feel-good" philosophy about physical activity. "I raced marathons for the thrill and challenge of the activity, but it's no longer a big thing for me," he told us. "Now, I live on 13 acres in the mountains of North Carolina, and I 'work out' by working on my property—putting in trails, chopping cords of wood for the woodstove, preparing terraces for flower gardens, and tending

Exercise in Your Bedroom—Have Sex!

One activity that people often don't think of as exercise is sex. Before orgasm, your exertion level is the same as walking at two miles an hour, playing the piano, or watering plants. During orgasm—when your heart rate rises to about 130 beats per minute, and your systolic blood pressure to about 170 to 180 mm Hg—the exertion level is the same as walking three to four miles an hour, vacuuming, or raking the lawn. (Remember the principle about activity you read earlier in this chapter: Anything is better than nothing. And having sex is a lot better than nothing!)

The health benefits of sex extend beyond a loving workout. In a 20-year study of nearly 1,000 men from Wales, those who had the most sex were 69 percent less likely to suffer a heart attack compared with men who had the least sex. (If you smiled to yourself as you read that statistic, well, so did we. We figure it's a little bit of ribald humor from the universe.) And another study—of Scottish women (are they having more sex in the UK?)—showed that those who had sex an average of three times per week looked 10 years younger than women who had less sex. The researchers suspect the reason is higher levels of sex-sparked human growth hormone (HGH).

Men who exercise regularly are likely to have more sex. Study after study shows that exercise, by improving circulation, dramatically decreases the risk of erectile dysfunction (ED).

to 60 blueberry bushes. That's what I'm *motivated* to do. And, hopefully, I'll do that to the day I die, because I love it."

Similarly, he said, you have to find the activity you love to do—an activity that you look forward to and that fits into your routine. He also urges you to find an activity that builds aerobic capacity (conditioned heart and lungs) and muscular strength, both of which are important for long-term health.

"When I'm splitting wood or hauling stones in a wheelbarrow, I'm getting the benefit of aerobic and muscular activity," he said. "Rowing is that kind of activity. So is swimming. So is walking with one- or two-pound hand weights. You don't have to lift weights—you just have to blend in an activity that increases your muscular workload."

The Pedometer: Step by Step to Better Health

There's one type of exercise that more people choose than any other—probably because it's easy, enjoyable, and low cost, and can fit into your daily schedule without a lot of fuss and muscle.

Walking.

And walking has a lot of fans among health-minded scientists. "Walking is the best way to stay active," James Hill, PhD, a professor at the University of Colorado and coauthor of *The State of Slim*, told us. Dr. Hill is also the cofounder of the National Weight Control Registry (NWCR.ws), a database of lifestyle information about more than 3,000 people who have lost a lot of weight and kept it off. Almost all of those folks have regular physical activity as a weight-maintenance strategy, and for most of them, the physical activity is (you guessed it) walking.

"If I could change one thing in America to improve everyone's health, it would be to get people walking more," said Dr. Hill. And the most reliable way to walk more, he added, is to use a pedometer, a device that counts the number of steps you take.

Dr. Nieman agrees. "Oftentimes, people who have never been motivated to exercise are motivated by a pedometer," he said.

I'll talk in a moment about why a pedometer is so powerfully persuasive. But before I do that, let's take a close look at a fascinating study that proves pedometers can help power you out the door and around the block.

The Best Goal: Steps, Not Minutes

Fifty-eight women who weren't exercising regularly participated in the study, which was conducted by researchers from the Kinesiology, Recreation & Sport Studies at the University of Tennessee. The researchers divided the women into two groups. One group was instructed to take a brisk, 30-minute walk on most days of the week. The other group was instructed to walk 10,000 steps a day.

During the next four weeks, the women told to walk 30 minutes a day walked an average of 8,270 steps a day. However, they didn't walk a lot every day: They walked 9,505 steps on the day they took a walk, and only 5,597 steps on the day they didn't. Meanwhile, the women told to walk 10,000 steps walked an average of 10,159 steps every day.

In other words, the women told to walk 10,000 steps averaged about 2,000 more steps per day—an additional mile's worth of daily physical activity! "The 10,000-step approach gets people more active every single day," Dixie Thompson, PhD, the study leader, told us.

Here's another way to look at these results. Experts in the use of the pedometer say that it takes 9,000 to 10,000 steps, five days a week, to meet the surgeon general's activity recommendation for 30 minutes a day of moderate-intensity exercise most days of the week. That means the women who were told to count their steps using a pedometer met the surgeon general's recommendation, while the women told to take a 30-minute walk didn't meet it! "It is incredible that the pedometer could help sedentary people meet the criteria for the surgeon general's rec-

---

Am I Exercising Too Hard for My Own Good?

There's an easy way to tell if you're exercising harder than is probably good for you: the talk test. "When you're exercising, try to count out loud or recite a verse of a familiar song," explained Vik Khanna, a clinical exercise specialist certified by the American College of Sports Medicine.

If you can talk easily, you're exercising in a comfortable and beneficial range. But if it's hard to talk—if you say (for example), "Mary had a little lamb whose fleece was white as snow," and you can't say the entire phrase without stopping, and have to repeatedly catch your breath (*Mary* BREATH had BREATH *a little lamb* BREATH)—then you're probably exercising too hard.

A simple rule of thumb: If it feels too hard, it is too hard.

---

ommendation, because that goal is so rarely achieved," said Caroline Richardson, MD, a research professor in the Department of Family Medicine at the University of Michigan Medical School, and an expert in using pedometers to help people walk more.

The Convenient Coach

Why is a pedometer so persuasive?

This handy little device helps you do the three things that behavioral scientists say you must do in order to make any positive change:

1. Set a goal.

2. Monitor the goal yourself.

3. Feel the satisfaction of success once you've reached the goal.

Let's take a closer look at how having a pedometer as your literal sidekick—a constant coach and pal—helps you earn three stars from behavioral scientists.

•**Set a goal.** To set and reach a goal, you have to know two things: (1) where you are, and (2) where you want to go. "You can't change your behavior unless you know what your behavior is," explained Dr. Richardson.

If you don't know how many steps you're taking, you can't increase your steps. And without a pedometer, you don't know and can't know. Studies show that non-pedometer step estimates are usually way, way off.

Bottom line: Pedometers show you exactly how much you're walking, so you can set a goal to walk more.

•**Monitor the goal yourself.** The pedometer also allows you to monitor whether or not you've reached your goal—and it does so instantly, since your daily step count is hanging out on your hip, your wrist or in your pocket.

"Pedometers give you instantaneous feedback," Dr. Hill told us. "If my goal is 8,000 steps a day, I can look at my pedometer and know—right away—how I'm doing that day. And that's why it's so powerful. If you can periodically check in to see how you're doing, you're much more likely to achieve your goal."

Compared with a pedometer, other kinds of feedback don't make the grade. "If you're trying to walk 30 minutes a day, what do you do for feedback?" asked Dr. Hill. "Start a stopwatch every time you get up and walk around? That's not going to work. Pedometers provide a simple and instant way to track progress."

•**Feel the satisfaction of success once you've reached the goal.** With a pedometer, it doesn't take very long to feel that satisfaction, said Dr. Richardson. "Say I ask one of my patients to increase her steps by 1,000 a day. She walks down the hall and back, and sees that she's *already* put 100 steps on her pedometer. And she says to herself, 'Wow, I just got 100 steps. I'm going to walk down that hall again.'"

That feel-good experience is quite different from what typically happens when a well-meaning doctor tells you to "get more exercise," said Dr. Richardson. "When you're sedentary and a physician tells you to exercise more, you really don't know where to start."

You might work out too hard and feel lousy afterward. And you might feel like a failure, because you really don't know if you exercised enough. But with a pedometer, you have a concrete goal. You know exactly what you need to do and whether you've done it or not. And when you do it, you feel good about yourself. And that's why it works to wear one!

Buying and Using a Pedometer

There are many types of pedometers on the market. There's the type you clip to your waistband or put in your pocket, with brands such as Omron and Timex. There are devices such as Fitbit and Apple Watch, which you can clip on or wear on your wrist, and which measure steps and many other health parameters, such as calories burned. And there are scores of pedometer apps for your smartphone, such as MyFitnessPal, Google Fit, and Pedometer for Android, and Pacer Pedometer and Step Tracker, Stepz, and Accupedo for the iPhone. Choose the device you like—and get started! (*One caution*: Don't spend less than $10.00 on a clip-on pedometer; cheaper products are usually inaccurate.)

Our pedometer experts recommended this strategy for starting to use your pedometer.

1. Wear the pedometer for three days. At bedtime write down the number of steps you took that day. On the third day, calculate the average: the total number of steps divided by the number of days. (For example, 12,000 steps over three days equals an average of 4,000 steps a day.) That's your baseline.

2. The following week, increase your daily baseline by 2,000 steps. If your baseline was 4,000, for example, try to walk 6,000 steps every day. Two thousand steps is equal to about one mile, or 15 to 20 minutes of walking—an increase just about anybody can do per week, said Dr. Hill.

3. If you want to keep going, add another 2,000 steps to your daily baseline the next week, and add it again the week after that.

4. Set your goal. How many daily steps should you aim for? Ten thousand—about five miles of daily walking—is a common recommendation. But I think your daily goal should be the number of steps you enjoy walking. That might be 6,000, 8,000, or 10,000 (or more!).

Dr. Hill shares my opinion: "I believe people should achieve what they can as individuals, getting in as many steps as possible, given their health and lifestyle."

Don't worry about whether your "intensity" is low, moderate, or high. Exercise recommendations always talk about "low-intensity," "moderate-intensity," and "high-intensity" exercise—with standard recommendations calling for 30 minutes of moderate-intensity exercise most days of the week. Brisk walking is moderate intensity. But you don't have to think twice about your intensity level when you walk.

In a study in the journal *Preventive Medicine*, researchers in Ireland secretly measured the walking speeds of recreational walkers in a park and found they were all walking at moderate intensity, or 55 percent to 69 percent of maximum heart rate.

Making Sense of Official Exercise Recommendations

You may have heard so many different recommendations for how much exercise you need for good health that you're completely confused. After all, there are "official" recommendations (most of which are different from one another) from the following organizations: National Institutes of Health (NIH); U.S Centers for Disease Control and Prevention (CDC); Office of the Surgeon General (OSG); US. Department of Agriculture (USDA); Institute of Medicine (IOM); U.S. Department of Health and Human Services (HHS); and the American College of Sports Medicine (ACSM).

OMG! Fortunately, there's good news (GN) about those recommendations. Guidelines from the HHS and USDA are widely considered to be definitive, said David Nieman, PhD, director of the Human Performance Lab at the North Carolina Research Campus. They're called the Physical Activity Guidelines for Americans (PA Guidelines, for short)—and they're accurate, simple, and practical exercise recommendations for health, fitness, and disease prevention. "The PA Guidelines are a historic and landmark document that goes beyond and supersedes all previous recommendations," Dr. Nieman said.

The first guidelines were issued in 2008, with a 2nd edition in 2018.

Here's what is recommended for adults...

1. **Avoid inactivity.** Some physical activity is better than none at all.

2. **For the most health benefits, do at least 150 minutes a week of moderate-intensity activity** (such as brisk walking), or 75 minutes a week of vigorous-intensity activity (such as jogging). Those 150 minutes are the equivalent of 9,000 to 10,000 steps a day.

3. **More activity is even better.**

4. **You should also do muscle-strengthening exercises, two or more times a week.**

You can find a summary of the guidelines online at https://health.gov/our-work/nutrition-physical-activity/presidents-council

Adding More Steps

The best way to add more steps to your day: Go for a walk. But there are a lot of other ways. In a study on pedometers, researchers in the Department of Sports Medicine at the University of Southern Maine discovered that people relied on 10 basic strategies to increase their steps. *They walked...*

- To a meeting or on a work-related errand
- After work
- Before work
- At lunch
- On the weekend
- While traveling
- With the dog
- To a destination, such as work or a store

- **After parking farther away from a destination**
- **Using the stairs rather than the elevator**

One approach I often recommend is walking with a friend. If you have to meet someone for a walk at a regular time, you're less likely to come up with excuses not to show up. And it's fun to walk with a friend.

Research also shows that walking with a friend—or a couple of friends—is one of the best ways to use a pedometer. "If you give a person a pedometer and tell her to walk 10,000 steps a day, but nobody knows she has a pedometer, and she doesn't know anybody with a pedometer—chances are good she'll throw the thing in a drawer after a week and never look at it again," said Dr. Richardson. "But if you give everybody in the office a pedometer, and there's a chart on the wall recording each person's progress, and every day people are comparing their step counts and planning a walk at lunch—chances are very good that in a year, she'll still be using the pedometer. Social support and group activity have an effect on any kind of physical activity. "And it seems to make a huge difference for pedometer-based walking."

Good Health Starts with a Single Step
(and Continues with a Couple of Thousand More...)

Studies show that the more steps you take, the healthier you're likely to be. In a landmark study in the *Journal of the American Medical Association*, researchers from Stanford University analyzed 26 studies on pedometers involving nearly 3,000 individuals. *They found...*

- **Pedometer use increased steps an average of 2,491 steps per day**—more than one mile. Looked at another way, the average activity level of the participants rose by 30 percent after they started using a pedometer. (And an important predictor of rising activity levels was having a step goal, noted the researchers.)

- **Systolic blood pressure dropped by an average of 3.8 mm Hg.**

- **Weight dropped by 0.4 percent.**

Need some more incentive to get stepping?

- **Reduce your risk of heart disease.** Australian researchers found that people who took more than 5,000 steps a day had the fewest risk factors for heart attack and for dying from heart disease, such as high total cholesterol, low HDL ("good") cholesterol, and high blood pressure, according to a study in the *American Journal of Preventive Medicine*. Even if you already have heart disease, taking more steps can make your heart healthier, concluded researchers from the University of Vermont College of Medicine in a study in the *Journal of Cardiopulmonary Rehabilitation and Prevention*. They found that those walking the most steps had less angina, lower risk of diabetes, less belly fat, and higher HDL cholesterol. In a study in the *American Journal of Cardiology,* researchers found that steps per day was a more accurate indicator than "laboratory-based exercise tests" of whether someone with chronic heart failure would die from the disease.

The Greatest Place to Walk—The Great Outdoors

Walking outdoors is a wonderful way to multitask. You get exercise. And you get sunlight, which triggers the production of health-giving vitamin D. (A study from Australian researchers showed that people with more daily physical activity also had higher blood levels of vitamin D.) But you're getting a third benefit: better mood.

Researchers in England asked people to go for walks either in the country, surrounded by woods, meadows, and lakes; or in a mall, surrounded by shoes, clothes, and appliances. After each walk, they measured the walkers' moods. The outdoor walks decreased mild, everyday depression five times more than the indoor walks did.

"Exercising outdoors in a green environment is a lot more effective in enhancing your mood than an equivalent amount of indoor exercise," concluded the researchers.

•**Lose weight.** Exercise works best for weight-loss maintenance, not for losing weight. It's a matter of metabolic mathematics. Thirty minutes of walking burns 100 calories. You could cut out more than twice that number of calories by not eating a candy bar every day. But those 100 calories a day make a difference. When researchers at the National Academy of Sports Medicine looked at more than 20 studies on pedometer use and weight loss, they found that using pedometers for at least six months was a "better option than a standard weight loss program" for weight loss in middle-aged and older adults.

•**Control diabetes.** Forty people with type 2 diabetes began walking with a pedometer, and after two months had a 37 percent drop in fasting blood sugar levels (measured first thing in the morning) and a 29 percent improvement in "general well-being," reported researchers in the journal *Primary Care Diabetes*.

•**Move easier with arthritis.** In a study in the *Journal of the American Geriatrics Society*, researchers from Johns Hopkins University found that people with knee osteoarthritis who used a pedometer for six months walked 23 percent more per day, walked more easily and faster, and had a 21 percent increase in leg strength. Meanwhile, after six months, a non-pedometer group with knee osteoarthritis was walking less and had weaker legs.

•**Experience less muscle loss with aging.** Sarcopenia is age-related muscle loss—one percent to two percent a year, starting in your fifties. Japanese researchers found that older people who took more than 7,800 steps a day were far less likely to have clinical sarcopenia (muscle loss that creates frailty) than people who walked 5,300 or fewer steps per day, according to their study in the *European Journal of Applied Physiology*.

Well, I hope you're convinced that exercise is a crucial real cure. Now put down this book and go for a walk around the block!

Water Exercise: Perfect for Chronic Illness

Sometimes you might be too ill to move around easily—for example, if you have a severe chronic pain condition. But that doesn't mean you can't exercise.

There's a perfect place for people in chronic pain to exercise and an easy way to do it: a water workout in a heated pool. "In the water, you're lighter and more buoyant, which allows you to do more exercise with less pain," Ruth Sova, president of the Aquatic Therapy and Rehab Institute in Naples, Florida, told us. "Plus, the gentle pressure of the warm water on the body improves circulation."

Studies show water exercise is very effective in soothing chronic pain and improving the lives of people in pain.

●**Fibromyalgia.** Several studies show that water exercise is ideal for people with fibromyalgia. In one reported in the journal *Rheumatology*, 30 women with fibromyalgia were divided into two groups: one participated in warm-water exercise and one didn't. After eight months, the exercisers had less pain, more muscle strength, better daily functioning, fewer physical problems, better balance, more energy, fewer emotional problems, and better general health.

●**Knee replacement.** Fifty women who underwent knee replacement surgery were divided into two groups, with 26 participating in water exercise for three months. After that time, the water exercisers had faster walking speed, climbed stairs faster, and had stronger thighs. Exercise in water has "wide-ranging positive effects on patients after knee replacement surgery," concluded the Finnish researchers in the journal *Archives of Physical Medicine and Rehabilitation*.

●**Lymphedema.** In this common side effect of breast cancer surgery, the arm on the side of the surgery becomes swollen, painful, and tight, with restricted motion. In a study of 48 women with lymphedema, those who participated in water therapy had a significant and immediate reduction in arm swelling and improvement in quality of life.

●**Osteoarthritis.** People with knee or hip osteoarthritis who participated in water exercise for six weeks had less joint pain and stiffness, better ability to function in daily life, and better overall quality of life, reported Danish researchers in the journal *Physical Therapy*.

●**Osteoporosis.** Fifty older women with either pre-osteoporosis (osteopenia) or osteoporosis were divided into two groups: One group participated in regular water exercise and the other group didn't. After 10 weeks, the exercisers had better balance, better everyday functioning, more energy, and a more positive outlook.

Other studies show water exercise improves: pain, balance, mobility, and walking ability in Parkinson's disease; function, balance, and fatigue in multiple sclerosis; pain and disability in chronic low back pain; balance, walking ability, depression, and anxiety after stroke; and falling asleep and staying asleep in people with sleep problems.

If you're interested in water exercise, the Arthritis Foundation Aquatic Program is offered throughout the United States at local YMCAs. You can find a program in your area by visiting YMCA.net or the Arthritis Foundation at Arthritis.org, or by calling the Arthritis Foundation at 800-283-7800.

REAL CAUSE #4

Happiness Deficiency

Joy Is Your Birthright!

You know the kinds of everyday habits that keep you healthy. A whole-foods diet that minimizes processed foods and doesn't overdo it on saturated fat and refined sugars. At least seven hours of sleep a night. Regular exercise. Feeling happy every day...

Feeling happy every day?! Yes, scientific research shows that happiness is next to healthiness. In fact, happiness is so health giving, it can even extend your life. When Dutch researchers analyzed 30 studies on happiness and longevity, they found that happy folks lived 10 percent to 40 percent longer. "The effect of happiness on longevity is remarkably strong," they concluded in the *Journal of Happiness Studies*. And in one study, researchers from the University of North Carolina at Chapel Hill and the University of Colorado at Boulder analyzed 30 years of health data, and found that people who were "not happy" had more than double the risk of death during the study period compared to "very happy" people.

In a similar study, researchers in the Department of Psychology at Carnegie Mellon University in Pittsburgh reviewed a decade of research on emotions and health. Noting that depression, anger, and anxiety have long been linked to an increased risk of disease and death, the researchers decided to look at the effect of positive emotions on health—whether or not people who were consistently joyous, enthusiastic, calm, and content were healthier.

Guess what? They were. They had less pain, fewer symptoms of disease, fewer hospitalizations, and fewer injuries; lived longer if they developed a chronic disease (such as heart disease); lived longer in general—and even caught fewer colds! "We need to take seriously the possibility that positive emotions are a major player in disease risk," said Sheldon Cohen, PhD, the study leader and a professor in the Department of Psychology at Carnegie Mellon University in Pittsburgh.

The modern science of psychoneuroimmunology shows that the mind, nervous system (brain, spine, nerves), and immune system are linked in a complex process: What you think and feel has an immediate effect on your body, for good or ill. *Feeling happy can…*

- **Energize the immune system,** a key defender of health that neutralizes everything from viruses to cancer cells.

- **Prevent overproduction of stress hormones such as adrenaline and cortisol** that, in too-high amounts, can damage every cell in the body.

- **Take a burden off your heart**—people who are hostile, depressed, or anxious have more heart disease, the number-one killer of Americans.

- **Protect your brain**—depression increases your risk of Alzheimer's disease.

In her book *The How of Happiness*, Sonja Lyubomirsky, PhD, professor of psychology at the University of California, Riverside, points out that people who are happier aren't just healthier—research also shows they lead better lives. They're more sociable and energetic, more charitable and cooperative, better liked by others, and more likely to get married and stay married. They have richer networks of friends and social support; have more flexibility and ingenuity in their thinking; are more productive in their jobs; are better leaders and negotiators; earn more money; and are more resilient in the face of hardship. Happy people are happening!

But isn't happiness kind of hit-or-miss? A combination of genes, good luck, and grace, with a grin thrown in. There's no way to *decide* to be happy, is there? I think there is.

As a holistic doctor interested in the well-being of his patients and as a person interested in discovering the fundamental truths of life, I have spent decades investigating the practical science of personal happiness. My conclusion: Happiness is your natural state of being. It is who you are.

This natural state of happiness is obvious when you observe little children—before their light is dimmed by society's happiness-snuffing beliefs, social structures, and fears. Why are little children so easily and spontaneously happy? *Because they feel all their feelings without resistance*—leaving them free to spend most of their time smiling and playful.

Little children don't repress feelings because they think the feeling is somehow "bad" or that they are a "bad" person if they feel it. They don't repress feelings because they're worried about what other people will think of them if they display their emotions. They don't repress feelings in order to present a "nicer" image to the world. They don't repress feelings because they have been taught to regard the feeling as "sinful" or "evil." They don't blame their feelings on somebody else and simmer in resentment. The feeling—be it fear, sorrow, or anger—is simply and completely felt. And once it's felt, the child returns to his or her natural state—happiness.

This fact—that feeling all your feelings allows you to experience a childlike state of joy—is key to rediscovering your innate happiness and all its healthful effects.

Along with this practice of "full feeling," there are two other steps to happiness that I recommend to my patients (and practice myself). Here is a summary of those three steps to happiness.

Step 1: **Feel all your feelings, without resistance.** You don't need to understand them. You don't need to justify them. When you've felt them fully—when it no longer feels good to feel them—let go and move on.

Step 2: **Create a no-blame lifestyle—no fault, no guilt, no judgment, no expectations, no comparisons.** You don't need to find fault with yourself or with anyone else. This step changes you from being a helpless victim to a person in control of your life!

Step 3: **Keep your attention on what feels good.** Life is a massive buffet, with thousands of options. You can choose to keep your attention on the things in your life that feel good. If a problem truly requires your attention, it will feel good to focus on it.

Let's start by looking at the first of these three steps, where happiness truly begins: really feeling all of your feelings.

Feel All Your Feelings Without Resistance

Psyche is a word for the total complexity of mind—thoughts, feelings, desires, and beliefs. On a deep level, your psyche demands honesty. That means you have to truly feel whatever you're feeling. If you don't, two things happen.

•**You get stuck.** A feeling stays with you until you actually feel it. If you don't really feel your anger, you may find yourself simmering for decades. And if you're like most people, you'll think your anger is caused by the stressful situations life delivers every day, from an obnoxious telemarketer to a long line at the supermarket checkout to a plunge in the stock market—but what's actually happening is that your suppressed anger has accumulated into a giant reservoir that spills into your psyche at the slightest provocation.

•**Molehills turn into mountains.** When the body is injured, it usually heals—spontaneously and naturally. You don't have to think about healing or plan it. A cut closes, a muscle mends, an infection is foiled—automatically. Likewise, after a bout of anger or sorrow, your psyche automatically heals itself, regaining its natural state of happiness and ease. When you deny a feeling, however, your psyche magnifies it, to make it bigger and clearer to you, so you'll feel it and be done with it. If you keep denying the feeling, it grows bigger and bigger: The blues turn into chronic depression; anger turns into a constant attitude of hostility, cynicism, and hatred; worry turns into anxiety and panic.

How do you know when you're done feeling a feeling? Well, it actually feels good to fully feel anger or sorrow or fear—that's why we call a session of much-needed, unrestrained sobbing a "good cry." And who hasn't experienced the joy of a good, self-righteous hissy fit? On the other hand, when it no longer feels good to feel sad or angry—which is how you can tell when the feeling has been fully experienced—you're done. Time to move on!

Labeling Not Required

Maybe you don't know why you're feeling the way you're feeling. Not a problem. You may try to jump all over a feeling with your mind, labeling it or trying to figure it out. But that shifts you out of your feelings, paradoxically leaving you stuck in them. You have to *fully* feel a feeling to be done with it. You can't battle it, ignore it, or file it in a box labeled "Angry at Andy."

Are You Resisting?

Your jaw tightens. You cross your arms and legs. You breathe shallowly. These are all signs that you're trying to block your feelings. If you notice this type of resistance, remind yourself to do the opposite. Let your jaw slacken. Uncross your arms and legs. Breathe!

And remember: Resisting a feeling is like trying to stop a cloud because you want it to be sunny again. Letting the cloud pass is the way back to a brighter state of mind.

When your mind attempts to label or explain why you are feeling a feeling, it's okay to just say to your mind, "No, thank you." Then continue to feel the feeling fully, without any resistance and without needing to understand why you are feeling the way you do.

When you're toward the end of feeling the feeling, you may find that you intuitively understand why you're having the feeling. Your psyche may want you to know—but only *after* you've fully felt the feeling! This is because the event that triggered the feeling is just that—a trigger. The actual feeling may reflect an event or, more often, multiple events over your lifetime. Focusing on "understanding" the trigger is like shooting the messenger. You'll never hear the real message!

Chronic Pain—or Chronic Resistance to Feelings?

I got so scared my heart jumped into my throat.

You make me sick to my stomach.

What a pain in the neck!

These are clichés, of course. But they're speaking a profound truth about our emotions: Feelings often have a physical component.

For example, most massage therapists have had a pain-relieving session when tension was released from a client's muscle—and the client burst into tears, recalling feelings and memories from an event that happened decades earlier. The feelings were literally stored in the muscle. When the feelings were released, so was the pain. Why does that happen?

Well, the body has to put your suppressed feelings somewhere—and locks them away in your muscles, which become a kind of "armor" against feeling. Eventually, this chronic muscle tightness can turn into chronic pain.

In many cases, you can relax chronically tight muscles by allowing yourself to feel fully. And feeling your feelings now can prevent chronic pain later. There's another school of thought about muscles and suppressed feelings, championed by the late John Sarno, MD, author of several books including *The Divided Mind: The Epidemic of Mindbody Disorders*. Dr. Sarno described a condition he called tension myositis syndrome. (Myositis means inflamed muscles.) In his view, the brain automatically attempts to protect you from overwhelming unconscious feelings—particularly rage, which is suppressed by perfectionism and what he called "goodism." The brain does this by limiting blood flow to muscles, tendons, and nerves in a particular area, creating low-level chronic pain that distracts you from the feeling.

If you have unexplained and persistent musculoskeletal pain, try this: Every time you feel the pain, tell your mind, "I know you are trying to distract me from becoming aware of uncomfortable feelings. I appreciate what you are trying to do, but I am mature enough to feel all my feelings—and I choose to feel them all."

Then spend 15 minutes or so looking for feelings that are uncomfortable. Simply give your brain a 15-minute "vacation" and allow yourself to feel whatever comes up during that time.

I sometimes ask my patients with persistent, unexplained, localized pain to do this exercise regularly. Often, their chronic pain disappears in about six weeks. (This approach is less effective for the widespread, chronic pain of fibromyalgia. You can find my Real Cure Regimen for that problem in Chronic Fatigue Syndrome and Fibromyalgia on page 189.)

More Ways to Release Your Feelings

There are several specific techniques that I've found helpful for releasing feelings—even ones that are very old and very traumatic. They have been helpful for me and for my patients. My two favorites? Trembling and the Emotional Freedom Technique (EFT).

•**Trembling.** As you feel your feelings, you may find yourself trembling (a kind of all-over shaking), and that's good. It's one of the ways the psyche releases old stresses and traumas stored in the body. If you're in a place where it's safe and comfortable to do so, allow this natural trembling to occur, even if you tremble for quite a while and quite intensely.

Why does trembling help? To find out, let's look at the animal kingdom—keeping in mind that we humans are animals, too (primates, to be exact). When a cheetah chases an impala, and the impala realizes it can't escape, it drops to the ground and "plays possum," appearing to be dead. Physiologists call this the "immobility" or "freezing" response, and many animals do it when death appears imminent.

"Nature has developed the immobility response for two good reasons," writes Peter Levine, PhD, in his excellent book on overcoming trauma, Waking the Tiger. It anesthetizes the animal, making death less painful. And, says Dr. Levine, "It serves as a last-ditch survival strategy. There is the possibility that the cheetah may decide to drag its 'dead' to its lair, where the food can be shared later with its cubs. During this time, the impala could awaken from its frozen state and make a hasty escape in an unguarded moment. When it is out of danger, the animal will literally 'shake off' the residual effects of the immobility response and gain full control of its body. It will then return to normal life as if nothing had happened."

This shaking or trembling is the natural way to release stress and trauma. During periods of stress—when humans feel helpless and have no way to escape—we often go into a similar "freezing" response, during which we are emotionally anesthetized. Think of it as emotional Novocaine—it protects us from trauma in the short term. But if we don't eventually release this energy, we become more and more numb, dulling our feelings, energy, and joy. (This is particularly common in people with post-traumatic stress disorder, or PTSD.) Trembling or shaking can help you release trauma and emotional stress. Unfortunately, when natural trembling occurs, people often feel "stupid" about it and suppress it. Not allowing this natural form of emotional release keeps us stuck in old feelings and is unhealthy.

How to Do the Emotional Freedom Technique (EFT)

Tap on each point about seven times solidly with the tips of three fingers of one hand.

1. **Focus on the issue at hand and feel the feeling as intensely as you can.**

2. **Rate the intensity of the feeling from 1 to 10 (10 being the most intense).**

3. **Correct any "psychological reversals"—self-defeating attitudes (often unconscious) that can get in the way of healing.** Do this by saying the following affirmation three times with conviction while tapping the Karate Chop Point. Affirmation: "Even though I have this (note the feeling), I deeply and completely accept myself."

4. **Tap on each of the 10 points illustrated in the diagram.** Start with point #1 and proceed through point #10. You need to tap on only one side of the body, and it doesn't matter which side of the body you choose. (These points are the end points of the body's acupuncture meridians, and by tapping these points, you are clearing blockages in the meridians.)

5. **How intense is the feeling now (0–10)? If over 1, repeat the process.** (Feelings often release in layers; e.g., anger may turn to sadness. It is important to identify and treat the feeling that is present.)

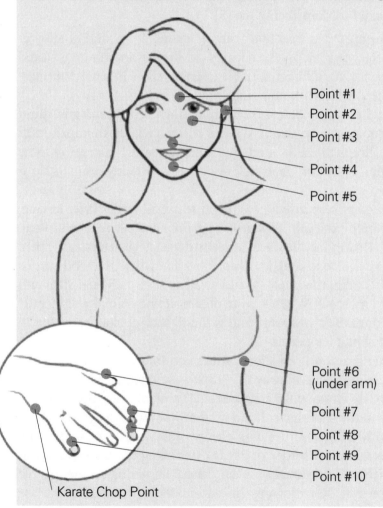

Point #1
Point #2
Point #3
Point #4
Point #5
Point #6 (under arm)
Point #7
Point #8
Point #9
Point #10
Karate Chop Point

Now that you're aware of the significance of trembling, open yourself to it. Just being aware that it's okay to tremble usually allows the process to happen. (For example, you will probably notice that after a time of upset or stress, you are shaky inside. It's the same phenomenon, and it's perfectly okay.) At first, you may want to reserve your trembling experiences for when you're alone, so you don't feel self-conscious.

The trembling can last for a few seconds or a few minutes. Sometimes it continues in waves, stopping and starting. Trembling may recur in the future, as layer after layer of old traumatic feelings presents itself for release. And it's okay for trembling to recur throughout your lifetime, because it's one of the body's natural ways to release you from emotional trauma. Sometimes during trembling, an image or scene may appear in your mind—and it's often the source of the feelings that are being released. Most of the time, however, there won't be an image. What is being released is a collection of feelings from a multitude of old traumas. Either way is fine.

At the end of the trembling session, you will find that you naturally take one or two deep breaths. Trembling is an inexpensive, safe, and effective way to release old traumas. What more could you ask!

●**Emotional Freedom Technique (EFT).** Another simple, straightforward, and powerfully effective technique for releasing old, stored emotions is the Emotional Freedom Technique. It was developed by Gary Craig, who simplified a technique called Thought Field Therapy, developed by psychologist Roger Callahan, PhD, author of *Five Minute Phobia Cure*. Dr. Callahan had found that tapping certain acupressure points could quickly relieve emotional distress. EFT is helpful in dissipating phobias (such as fear of flying), anxieties, traumas, anger, depression, resentment, guilt, low self-esteem, and many other uncomfortable emotions. EFT takes only a few minutes to learn and often produces permanent results. The main ingredient for success is the willingness to use it.

Note: For simple issues, it's fine and effective to do EFT on yourself. But for more severely traumatic, complex, or deep-seated issues (such as child sexual abuse), I find it can be very helpful to work with an EFT practitioner.

To locate one, visit Gary Craig's website (EFTuniverse.com). There are many books on EFT. Two favorites are *Getting Thru to Your Emotions with EFT*, by Phillip and Jane Mountrose, and *The Tapping Cure*, by Roberta Temes, PhD.

The No-Blame Lifestyle

There is a simple attitude that can help you live happily: a willingness to let go of blame.

Yes, blame. Finding fault with yourself and others. Judging yourself and others. Feeling guilty about something you did. Expecting yourself or someone else to do something a certain way—and feeling angry if you or that person fails to do so. Comparing a behavior, person, or experience to another behavior, person, or experience—and finding one lacking.

These are all forms of blame. And they are all emotional and mental habits of unhappiness. Here's why.

The Burden of Expectations

In his wonderful bestseller, *Handbook to Higher Consciousness: The Science of Happiness,* the late Ken Keyes Jr. defined an expectation as a mental/emotional addiction to life being a certain way. The expectation, he wrote, "triggers uncomfortable emotional responses and excites your consciousness if the world does not fit the programmed pattern in your mind, the model of how life should treat you."

"The identifying characteristic" of an expectation, he wrote, "is that if your expectation is not fulfilled, you respond emotionally in a computer-like way and automatically play out a program of anger, worry, anxiety, jealousy, fear, etc."

The need for expectations is based on the illusion that you are dependent on others to meet your needs. Although you may need help from someone else to create what you want, that help can come from many different places—including someone who is happy to meet your needs rather than someone who is resentfully acting in response to your expectations.

Letting go of expectations frees you from being dependent on others to have your needs met. Letting go of expectations frees you from the burden of others' dependency on you.

If you allow others to give only when it feels good to them to do so—rather than when you or they expect it should be done—then giving becomes its own reward, and there is no resentment or "indebtedness" that is created. This allows for more freedom—and freedom is happiness.

You can let go of expectations in the same way you can let go of blame: by "centering" and switching attention to something that feels good. You'll find the instructions to do just that in the rest of this chapter.

How Blame Hurts You

Blame steals your power. When you blame others, you feel like a victim who is powerless to create what you want. When you blame yourself, you feel guilty. But isn't guilt good? Isn't it the core of my conscience? Doesn't it keep me from immoral actions that can harm other people?

No, guilt is one of the most useless emotions. Generally, it doesn't heal or reform you. It simply ties you up in neurotic knots!

Guilt is also irrational. Seeing and experiencing the consequences of an action has always helped me grow and learn much more than wallowing in guilt, which literally "goes nowhere."

To live a full life, you must search for and express who you are: your desires, your creativity, your joys, your satisfactions. To do this requires that you grow. Growth requires experimentation, and experimentation leads to (what seem at the time) mistakes and failure. But when you blame yourself and feel guilty for your supposed "mistakes," you are likely to stop your growth and stifle your life! You're also not likely to change your behavior. Guilt is *not* helpful. Guilt is a waste of time, energy, and emotion. When you let go of guilt, you learn that making mistakes is a natural, normal, healthy part of growing and learning.

You also will find that it is an *incredible* relief—both for you and for the people you love—when you stop pretending that you are perfect and realize that it is totally okay to make mistakes. What I find is "perfect" is not to worry about making mistakes, and simply to grow and learn from them. Accept mistakes graciously, with a sense of humor—which is much easier to do when you let go of blame!

Feeling blame (toward yourself and others) stands between you and your natural way of feeling, which is love (toward yourself and others) and joy.

Blaming Another Is Blaming Yourself

When you blame another person for something, you're actually projecting your own self-blame at them. You're a procrastinator, and you blame others for being late. You're sloppy, and you blame others for not cleaning up. And on and on. So when you stop blaming others, you also begin to end—and to heal—your harsh self-blaming.

There are many tools for becoming conscious of what you dislike about yourself—which is often unconscious, because these disliked qualities are too painful to acknowledge. *My two favorites...*

•**The pointing finger.** The Chinese have an old saying: "When I am pointing at you with one finger, I am pointing at myself with three fingers." Try it and you'll see that it's true. When you point at somebody with your index finger—as if accusingly pointing out to them something they did wrong—your third, fourth, and fifth fingers are pointing back at you. When you blame somebody, visualize pointing at them and remember you're really pointing at yourself!

•**A blame journal.** Yes, keep a journal of the qualities you blame others for. Do you frequently find others to be selfish, greedy, vain, etc.? If so, the qualities you most often dislike in others probably reflect the qualities you (unconsciously) most dislike in yourself.

As you keep the journal, you might say to yourself that these definitely aren't the qualities that you demonstrate in daily life. That's probably because your behavior overemphasizes their opposites, so that the disliked qualities stay unconscious. In other words, if you're selfish, you try to be generous, and if you're vain, you try to be humble. Nevertheless, if you persist in this exercise, you will discover that both qualities—selfishness and generosity, vanity and humility—are within you. And in time, you'll accept both.

Until then, try to keep your sense of humor and not use these tools too seriously, as if you were digging into a pit of personal darkness. You're gently uncovering the full, vibrant, alive *you*—the you that doesn't feel it's necessary to blame yourself or others for anything!

Break the Habit of Blame

Blame isn't a big deal. It's a mental mirage. It's imagination. It's nothing more than an old habit. When you catch yourself playing the "blame game," remember that it is a habit you have chosen to break. Instead, from a centered place, continually and repeatedly drop the blame in mid-thought and shift your attention to something that feels good. (See "How to Center" on page 65.)

How do you do this? Find something in your past, present, or imagined future that feels good. It can be the memory of a positive childhood experience, such as the loving attention of a grandparent. It can be recalling yesterday's satisfying sex. It can be birdsong outside your

> ## Blame Strands You in the Past
>
> When you feel an uncomfortable feeling, such as anger, resentment, or hurt, you are often tapping into vast pools of old, similar feelings that you carry around, some conscious, some unconscious.
>
> By dropping the blame, you can become aware that you are *presently* experiencing pools of old feelings that reflect the past and not the present.
>
> But if you don't let go of the blame, you have to keep amplifying the story of how you were wronged (and what a nasty SOB the other person was to you) to justify why you feel so strongly about an event.

window or the cat napping on the couch. It can be imagining the achievement of a goal that you cherish. There are an infinite number of possibilities. If you look inside yourself, I am sure you can find thoughts and memories that feel good. If you look outside yourself, I am sure you can find something that you enjoy experiencing. Personally, I break the habit of blame by using thoughts of…my children and grandchildren…taking my wife out to lunch…walking around the Hawaiian Botanical Gardens on the Big Island of Hawaii (a delightful experience!)…and my research studies on effective treatments for autism, chronic fatigue syndrome, and fibromyalgia.

Pay Attention to What Feels Good

Here's a simple but profound truth: What you put your attention on tends to create your reality. In the spiritual traditions of the East, this truth is expressed by the ancient saying "What you meditate on, you become." Would you prefer to put your attention on happiness rather than unhappiness, on joy rather than joylessness? You can do so by putting your attention on your soul.

The Natural Happiness of the Soul

Many people today recognize that human beings are more than our limited bodies and the occupations of daily life. Many spiritual traditions teach that a human being is essentially a soul, and the desire of the soul is to fully experience its innate, natural happiness and joy.

When you are in alignment with your soul and its desire for happiness, you feel good. When you aren't, you feel bad. It's really that simple! And the implications are enormous.

(Don't believe in a soul? Abraham Lincoln used to say: "People are about as happy as they choose to be." I think Honest Abe hit the happiness nail on the head!)

Follow Your Bliss, Not Your Brain

When I was a child, my thinking brain was systematically programmed by others—parents, relatives, teachers, clergy, and "authorities" of all kinds. My programming had one main mission: to dictate what I needed to do or to be in order to get approval.

How to Center

You've no doubt experienced a time when you felt particularly connected to life or "in the flow"—walking along the shore, playing with a baby, watching sports, listening to music, praying, doing something you love easily and happily. At those times, you were centered.

I have found that you can focus your attention in a part of your body and stimulate a specific and positive personal reality, a two-part process I call centering.

Center in your heart. I center in my heart (the area right behind the lower half of the breastbone) to create wholeness—a mosaic of compassion, harmony with life, a healing presence, and unconditional love (what a parent typically feels for a newborn child).

To center in your heart, take a deep breath and relax as you exhale. Allow yourself to relax even more with each subsequent breath. Now, put the palm of one hand over the top of the other, so the tips of your thumbs touch (almost like in a butterfly or bird position), and put the centers of both palms over your breastbone, approximately three finger widths above your solar plexus. Next, focus your attention in that area of your chest, while feeling for the four qualities described in the previous paragraph. When you feel them, you are heart centered. While doing this, it may help to think about someone or something you unconditionally love—a spouse, child, friend, pet, favorite place, or spirit (whatever form of God, life, love, or universal power is meaningful to you).

Center in your solar plexus. I center in my solar plexus to check in on my feelings and, if I'm feeling uncomfortable, to allow that feeling to move and pass, like a cloud temporarily passing in front of the constant sun of happiness.

To center in your solar plexus, move your palms and attention down over your solar plexus, the area about one to two inches below the bottom of your breastbone. Now imagine that your eyes are in your solar plexus, and you are looking out from that area. While centered there, allow yourself to gently but fully feel your feelings.

You also can center in either one (or both) of these areas of your body to find out what feels best for you—an important process that I discuss in the next section of this chapter.

"You should obey your parents," said the programmed brain. "You shouldn't play until all your work is done." "You should...you shouldn't...you should...you shouldn't..." and on and on.

As an adult, when I find myself "shoulding" on myself, I know that it is my childhood programming speaking and not my soul (feel free to substitute "authentic self" for "soul"). And since I'm not too impressed by the happiness level of the grown-ups who programmed me, I have given myself permission to stop shoulding on myself with my mind.

My feelings, however, speak in a different voice. If I feel good—if I'm centered and happy and joyful—I know that I am connected to my soul and its desire, and that I am as close to being authentic as I know how to be. If I feel bad, I know that I am not attuned to what my soul prefers. To say this in another way (because it is so important to understand): If, from a centered awareness, what I am doing or paying attention to feels good, then it is what my soul is choosing.

The late Joseph Campbell, the world's most renowned expert on the variety of this planet's different religions, myths, and tribal cultures, summarized what he learned from all these traditions in three words: "Follow your bliss." It's just as accurate to say: Follow your happiness. Happiness is the call and guidance of your soul. But maybe you'd like to ask your soul some questions…

What If Doing Something Bad Feels Good?

I repeatedly advise you to keep your attention on things that feel good from a centered place. If I am angry and very "off center," it may feel good to hurt someone. But from a centered place—when I am connected to my soul—it does not feel good to harm someone.

It may feel good to think about doing something, but not feel good to actually do it. *An example*: Picture hitting someone who is very annoying over the head with a stick. That probably feels good! Doing it would be another story. To be on the safe side, I recommend that you don't do anything to harm anyone else—ever (unless you are in the unlikely situation of having to protect yourself or your loved ones from imminent violence).

But My Responsibilities Don't Always Feel Good—What About Them?

I am not suggesting that you forgo all your responsibilities—just the ones that don't feel good!

Earlier in your life, you may have taken on responsibilities that excited and challenged you. As you grew, you may have forgotten to "shed the old layer," like a snake molts old skin. Or perhaps you felt secure in your job and had too many domestic responsibilities to risk changing careers. Or maybe you were promoted (and accepted the promotions because of the pay) beyond the level of your interest and enthusiasm. (For example, a terrific salesperson is promoted to a manager of salespeople and no longer feels the old spark.)

I'm not recommending that you immediately quit a job that you don't like. From a centered place, that probably wouldn't feel good! On the other hand, it probably would feel very good to make a list of those things about your job that you like (that feel good) and that you don't like (that don't feel good). Then start putting your attention and energy into those items on the list that feel good, and put your attention and energy into those things that feel bad *only* to the degree that it feels better to do so than not to do so.

Of course, there are times when it will feel good to do things that seem very difficult. For example, doing a medical residency and internship can be brutal. It is certainly not how I would like to spend the next three years! But 35 years ago, from a centered perspective, it felt better to do it than not because I knew it would get me where I wanted to go.

Try the as-if technique. As you explore what would feel best to you—at work, at home, in your relationships, in your life altogether—keep an image in mind of the situation that feels best, and feel as *if* it were already happening. If you do this for a few minutes every now and then, I think you will be amazed at the results—as you look back one day and realize that this image has become a reality in your life! For now, knowing these changes are in progress (even if they don't happen overnight) can leave you feeling happier immediately.

Reconciling Inner Conflicts

Each of us is a complex (and ultimately mysterious) assemblage of beliefs and desires and preferences. And some parts of you may be in conflict with other parts!

You want to lose weight; you want to eat a quart of ice cream. You want to exercise every day; you want to sit on the couch and watch TV. You want to be faithful to your spouse; you fantasize about someone else. You think everyone should work hard for what they want; you buy lottery tickets.

It's often the case that the parts of you that don't match your conscious "self-image" are kept unconscious and out of sight—until they barge into the light, much to your chagrin. That's because when you are not conscious of a part of yourself, you lose control of it. You can see this in some public and religious officials who ranted about infidelity and then turned out to be sleeping with a lot of people other than their spouses. Well, we all have parts of ourselves that aren't "ego-enhancing."

But you won't feel whole—or be fully in control of yourself—until you learn to unconditionally accept and love every part of yourself. At that point, there will be no need to judge anything about yourself. Or anyone else. When you are heart centered, it becomes easy to love every part of yourself because you are centered in your soul, which is unconditional love. If you feel inner conflict, or resistance to an aspect of yourself, center in your heart and see what part of you wants to "come to the surface" to be known and loved.

Remember, you aren't trying to fix or rid yourself of those rejected parts. Love them. Hear their voices. Show them compassion. Feel good about every part of yourself. Only then will you be in control of the parts of you that manifest in any given situation.

Worry Doesn't Feel Good—But Won't I Neglect People If I Don't Worry About Them?

There's a big difference between worrying about someone you love and being concerned and caring about them. Worry generally feels bad, and it isn't helpful. Caring and concern generally feel good and may lead you to help the person you love. Feel free to be caring and concerned as long as it feels good to do so. If it doesn't, let go of your care and concern, and allow the other person to go their own way.

Most of the time, you'll find this attitude actually feels good to those you love. And by acting only when *you* feel good, you're much more likely to benefit the other person, rather than contributing to their problems. (How many times does worry-based interference backfire? Many times, in my experience.) For example, the easiest way I know of to tell whether or not unhealthy "codependency" issues are occurring (a form of "caring" that enables another person to continue with self-destructive behavior) is to check with the caregiver to find out if what they are doing to help feels good or not.

If it doesn't feel good, it's not doing any good. If it doesn't feel good, don't do it.

Ask Yourself: Does My Belief Feel Good?

As a child, you asked for directions to find your way.

You asked your parents—and they taught you their beliefs, which they hoped would bring you happiness.

You asked your teachers—and they taught you what they thought was true.

You asked the clergy—and, from a place of spiritual generosity, they may have taught you a system of sin and shame instead of unconditional love and acceptance.

You asked politicians—who may have begun their careers from a desire to help people, but who are now enmeshed in a system that works by forced bribery (so-called campaign contributions and lobbying).

You asked the news media—and journalists who work hard to bring people the truth skewed their reports toward the attention-grabbing and sensational.

As time went on, you adopted these beliefs—and became imprisoned by them.

Now, it's time to realize that those beliefs are optional. Even illusory.

As an adult, you are free to decide on, create, and—if you so desire—continually change your beliefs. Look back on the beliefs you were taught. Perhaps a few succeeded in stirring your soul, giving you a glimpse of joy, inspiration, and happiness. Perhaps others left you feeling bad about yourself and about life.

You can learn from both. Those beliefs that feel good can help you discover your joy and the innocent laughter and smiles you felt as a child. Those beliefs that feel bad can help you learn who you are not and point you in the direction of who you would choose to be.

I have found that when something feels bad, it's usually because I have a false belief about it. Find those false beliefs and let them go. You'll be much happier!

Bottom line: You have a choice in what you believe. There is no absolute right or wrong—simply different beliefs and perspectives. Total freedom is your true nature.

What About Chronic Negative Thinking?

Here's a different way to think about so-called negative thoughts: Sometimes they're the psyche's way of taking care of you. They offer you ideas that are in conflict with your belief system (learned from your parents, teachers, religion, government, etc.) but that actually appeal to you. In other words, the negative thought is a disguised desire that you are afraid to acknowledge, such as wanting to quit your job or leave your spouse. The "negative" thought may be the psyche's way of declaring that you need to stand up for who you are and what you want, forcing you to look at uncomfortable feelings that you need to stop burying. In this situation, it will feel good (although difficult and uncomfortable) to stay with the thought. A negative thought can also help you understand yourself by providing you with a clear view of what you don't like.

Bottom line: Don't struggle with negative thoughts. It's like struggling in quicksand—the more you struggle, the more you get stuck. Instead, take a moment to feel the negative thought without any guilt or reactivity.

What If You Died Tomorrow?

One of the most freedom-giving realizations I've ever had was this:

If I died tomorrow, the world would go on just fine without me.

My family would miss me, of course. And those I help would have to find help elsewhere. And it would take a while for people to carry on the scientific research that I have been conducting into the cures for chronic fatigue syndrome, fibromyalgia, and other diseases. Nonetheless, everyone would eventually get on just fine. The world would continue—even if I totally ceased to exist.

As I said, this realization was incredibly freeing. If the world would go on just fine without me, this meant there was truly nothing that I absolutely had to do. There is nothing that you absolutely have to do, either. Which means you can do only those things that feel good to you.

What if I am wrong about focusing on what feels good? Then the downside is that you will have spent a life feeling great! I can live with that.

If it doesn't feel good, simply recognize (with a smile) that the thought is *not* who you are. It's a kind of mental gremlin, a mean-sounding (but somewhat comical) creature scampering across your mind. Thank the gremlin for showing you who you aren't and who you are. Then simply let it go, perhaps with a simple "No, thank you."

For example, say you find yourself thinking one of those "gremlin" thoughts: You're listening to a man loudly talking on his cell phone in front of you on the bus, and you want to yank it out of his hand. (I know, I know—an upstanding person such as yourself would *never* have such a thought. But humor me.) Instead of battling the thought or trying to run away from it, take a moment to be with it gently, without reacting to it—an approach called mindfulness.

As you observe the thought, if it feels good to stay with it, then stay with it. Soon, you may become aware of something that you are angry about that is underlying the thought. Maybe you want to "yank" a toxic person out of your life! Often, that anger will be from a situation in which you didn't care for or stand up for yourself. This is important to discover. When you recognize the real cause of your anger and you decide to stand up for yourself, the number and intensity of these types of thoughts will decrease.

See—a negative thought can actually serve and enhance your well-being and authenticity!

On the other hand, you may feel into the thought—and notice that it simply feels bad. In that case, realize that someone who acts aggressively toward a stranger on a bus is not who you are. Tell the thought "thank you" for helping you recognize who you are and who you aren't.

To summarize your two options...

- **Feel into the negative thought and realize its underlying cause and motive.**

- **Feel into the negative thought and realize it's not you.**

For more information about happiness, I recommend my short e-book *Three Steps to Happiness—Healing Through Joy*! It's available at Amazon.com and on my website, EndFatigue.com.

Prescription Medications

Don't Let Pills Make You Ill

To put prescription medications into perspective as a real cause of ill health, let's start by talking about the worst health of all: death.

In a study in the *Journal of the American Medical Association*, researchers from the University of Toronto estimated that "adverse drug reactions" kill 106,000 people yearly in American hospitals—and harm hundreds of thousands more. I think that is a very conservative estimate of the total number of deaths from prescription drugs, with the actual number probably double that. Many deaths from prescription drugs aren't reported or are mistakenly ascribed to the disease for which the person was taking the drug.

How do prescription drugs kill people? Overdosing at hospitals, severe liver damage, kidney failure, bleeding ulcers, allergic reactions, strokes from brain bleeding—to name a few causes. Plus, the slow causes, such as acid-blocking drugs causing fractures that lead to hospitalization, pneumonia, and death, or those dying in nursing homes who have been diagnosed with Alzheimer's disease but are actually suffering severe confusion from taking multiple medications.

Why don't you hear more about this medical tragedy? Because multinational drug companies readily spend billions of dollars in advertising and in helping politicians get elected. Supplement companies don't. So while you might hear a lot about the supposed dangers and drawbacks of supplements, the fact that several hundred Americans a day are killed by prescription drugs never becomes an important item—in the headlines or on the agendas of government officials. Why do prescription medications hurt so many people? Because most drugs work by slowing enzyme systems—proteins that spark biochemical processes throughout the body. When you control a runaway train (the symptom or disease) by derailing it (the drug action), you injure a lot of passengers.

For example, cholesterol-lowering statin drugs block the action of an enzyme that helps create cholesterol, thereby lowering cholesterol levels. But statins also block the production of coenzyme Q10, which supports the function of the mitochondria, tiny energy factories in every cell. The compromised mitochondria contribute to muscle pain (weakened muscle cells), memory loss (weakened brain cells), and a host of other side effects from statins. People on statins often develop heart failure, which is then blamed on the high cholesterol. I suspect that much of this heart failure is actually caused by coenzyme Q10 deficiency from the statins. This "side effect" is largely preventable by simply giving coenzyme Q10 with the medications. Sadly, this option is often ignored.

Or consider nonsteroidal anti-inflammatory drugs (NSAIDs), such as aspirin, *ibuprofen* (Advil, Motrin), and *naproxen* (Aleve). They block the action of *cyclooxygenase* (COX), an enzyme that helps manufacture prostaglandins, hormonelike compounds that play a key role in inflammation and pain. But prostaglandins play a key role in a lot of other functions, too—including maintaining the protective mucous lining of your stomach. Millions of people with arthritis regularly take NSAIDs that knock out COX. And every year, about 16,500 of those folks die from bleeding ulcers caused by the erosion of their stomach linings. Another 200,000 are hospitalized.

But there's more bad news about NSAIDs: Massive studies, called meta-analyses, show that these medications increase heart attack and stroke risk by 35 percent. In the U.S., this translates to 50,000 unnecessary deaths a year! (And those deaths are doubly unnecessary—because herbal mixes for pain relief, such as Curamin, which I discuss throughout the book, have been shown in published studies to be *more* effective than NSAIDs in relieving pain.)

The Natural Difference

In contrast to prescription medications, natural remedies such as nutrients and herbs work *with* bodily systems to help the body heal. In fact, most vitamins and minerals work by activating rather than blocking enzymes. Plus, many herbal formulas contain several gentle compounds that work in harmony, rather than one super-powerful active ingredient—thereby reducing the risk of side effects. For example, the herb red yeast rice is a natural source of monacolins, which are synthesized to create statins. But when people who develop muscle pain from taking a statin switch to red yeast rice, their muscle pain typically goes away while their cholesterol stays low. That's probably because red yeast rice contains several monacolins at low dosages rather than (as is the case with cholesterol-lowering prescription medicine) one monacolin at a high dose. It's a therapeutic caress with five fingers rather than a knockout punch with a fist.

Unfortunately, fearing that red yeast rice would cut into pharmaceutical profits, the drug companies petitioned the FDA to make red yeast rice illegal, to which the FDA responded by banning forms of the supplement containing lovastatin (one of the monacolins)—not because of risk to the public, but because of risk to corporate profits.

If nutrients and herbs are so wonderful, why aren't they promoted as aggressively as drugs? Simple: It's hard to patent natural products because they're natural. You can't patent air, water, vitamin C, glucosamine, or chamomile because they've been around a long time. And if you can't patent it, you can't create an exclusive product that makes billions of dollars for your company. Unfortunately, it's profit—not effectiveness or safety—that drives the culture of 21st-century American medicine. And as you'll read in a moment, the fact that profit is paramount is the main reason why bad news about medications—the side effects, the secrecy about side effects, the scandals when the secrets are revealed—is nearly constant.

"Marketing Machines Selling Drugs of Dubious Benefits"

That's a statement by Marcia Angell, MD, former editor-in-chief of the prestigious *New England Journal of Medicine*, a faculty member at Harvard Medical School, and author of *The Truth about the Drug Companies: How They Deceive Us and What to Do About It*. "Doctors and consumers believe drugs are a lot better than they are and have fewer side effects than they do," she writes. And she's hardly alone in her opinions. In his book *Overdosed America: The Broken Promise of American Medicine*, John Abramson, MD, a lecturer at Harvard Medical School, describes why he decided to give up his family practice to spend several years researching what he calls "the commercial takeover of medical knowledge."

"Many of my patients were being drawn in by the growing number of drug ads, and when I tried to refocus patients on interventions proved to be safe and effective, many were reacting as if I were purposely trying to withhold the best treatment," he wrote.

His conclusion: There is "a scandal in medical science that is at least the equivalent of any of the corporate scandals that have shaken Americans' confidence in the integrity of the corporate and financial worlds." For example, studies run by the pharmaceutical industry are 70 percent more likely to produce a positive result than government-funded studies. And 35 out of 36 positive studies about antidepressants have been published—compared to three out of 36 negative studies!

Something to think about the next time your doctor takes out his prescription pad.

The Responsible Use of Medications

After reading all the above, it may surprise you to learn that I am *not* opposed to the appropriate use of prescription drugs, and in this book (and my previous books) I recommend drugs I consider uniquely effective. For example, I think the use of sleeping medications is critical for chronic fatigue and fibromyalgia, which are fueled and worsened by chronic insomnia. But I always advise that a patient use a prescription medication judiciously—in the smallest possible dosage, for the shortest possible time, and when effective nondrug alternatives have failed to work after a reasonable trial. I base my recommendations on what is safest, not what is most expensive.

If you need to take a prescription medication, it is often useful to also take supportive natural remedies that can help you…

•**Take less of the drug** (such as taking a migraine medication and headache-easing magnesium and riboflavin supplements)

•**Decrease its side effects** (such as taking a statin and coenzyme Q10)

That being said, the rest of this chapter focuses on several classes of drugs that I consider the riskiest on the market. For each class, there are safe and effective natural alternatives.

Statins: Low Cholesterol, High Side Effects

Heart disease is the number-one killer of Americans, so it's no surprise that one of the most prescribed class of drugs in America are the statins, which lower cholesterol by blocking the action of an enzyme involved in its production. The three most prescribed statins are *simvastatin* (Zocor), *atorvastatin* (Lipitor), and *pravastatin* (Pravachol). There are more than 235 million yearly prescriptions for these and other statins, putting more than $17 billion into the coffers of drug companies. In fact, many doctors now recommend statins even when you don't have high cholesterol but do have high levels of C-reactive protein, a biomarker for artery-hurting inflammation.

When they came on the market in 1987, statins were immediately touted as a "miracle medicine" that could prevent heart attacks and strokes, with nary a side effect. Well, maybe the drug didn't produce many serious side effects in the original clinical trials, which lasted a couple of months. But as the years passed, the reported side effects piled up.

Unfortunately, it's taken most doctors decades to catch on to the fact that statins aren't perfectly safe—and many doctors still haven't gotten the news. In one study, published in the journal *Drug Safety,* 50 percent of doctors dismissed the possibility that a statin could have caused the side effect reported by a patient who recently started the drug. Twenty-five percent said the statin might be the cause, and 25 percent wouldn't commit either way. In another study, in the journal *Drug Safety—Case Reports*, five doctors (yes, *doctors!*) who took statins and had side effects experienced "dismissive attitudes" from the prescribing physicians.

But Beatrice Golomb, MD, PhD, and her colleagues of University of California, San Diego, know all about statin side effects. They conducted the Statins Side Effects Study—collecting anecdotal reports from more than 5,000 people who had one or more side effects after starting a statin. *They found that the following side effects were very commonly reported…*

- **Muscle pain** (myalgia)
- **Fatigue**
- **Exercise intolerance** (muscles too painful and weak to exercise)
- **Memory loss**
- **Peripheral neuropathy** (tingling, numbness, or burning pain in the hands, arms, feet, or legs)
- **Irritability**
- **Sleep problems**
- **Sexual dysfunction,** such as erectile dysfunction (ED)

Intrigued by these reports, Dr. Golomb and a colleague reviewed 880 scientific studies on statin side effects, publishing their findings and conclusions in the *American Journal of Cardiovascular Drugs*. Here are the side effects you need to watch out for. Remember, it's very likely your doctor doesn't know or won't acknowledge that statins can cause them.

●**Cognitive problems.** Memory loss, poor concentration, and slower reaction time "are second only to muscle problems among reports of statin adverse effects," wrote Dr. Golomb. In one study, people who took statins after open-heart surgery had much less recovery of lost cognitive function (a common side effect of the operation) than did people who didn't take a statin.

●**Diabetes.** In a review of 20 studies on the link between statins and diabetes, Italian researchers at the University of Milan found that the drug raised diabetes risk by 44 percent.

●**Digestive problems.** "Gastrointestinal adverse effects" were the most common side effect in an analysis of clinical trials of the drug, notes Dr. Golomb. Other studies link statins to serious digestive diseases, such as ulcerative colitis and stomach ulcers.

●**Dry mouth.** In a study from Spanish researchers, 23 of 26 patients on statins reported dry mouth (a common drug side effect). Others had oral itching, a bitter taste, and coughing. When statins were discontinued, these oral symptoms usually went away.

●**Headaches.** Several reports link statins to tension headaches and migraines.

●**Insomnia.** One study shows "significant reductions in average sleep quality" in people taking statins, compared with those taking a placebo.

●**Personality changes.** Dr. Golomb notes that there are many reports of "severe irritability" and "aggression" among statin takers. Her study, published in the *Journal of Psychiatric Research*, that showed that people with very low cholesterol were twice as likely to commit violent crimes.

The possible cause: Cholesterol helps form healthy brain cells and is the main building block of many key mood-influencing hormones. Other "personality changes" that have been shown to start when statin use starts and stop when it stops: depression, anxiety, and paranoia.

●**Kidney disease.** Studies show that statin use can nearly triple the risk of decreased kidney function.

●**Muscle pain, fatigue, and weakness.** These are the problems from statins "most reported" in the scientific literature and in patients, wrote Dr. Golomb. She's not talking about a little soreness. She's talking about pain, cramps, stiffness, tendinitis, pain when exercising, even difficulty walking. She points out that these muscle problems don't necessarily stop when you stop the statin. If enough damage has been done, they can be persistent. The most extreme muscle problem is rhabdomyolysis, in which muscle breakdown in the body becomes so extreme and rapid the kidneys are overwhelmed by discarded muscle cells. The statin Baycor was taken off the market in 2001 after it was linked to more than 400 cases of rhabdomyolysis, 31 of them fatal.

●**Peripheral neuropathy.** A study by Danish researchers in the journal *Neurology* showed a 16-times-greater risk of developing this painful nerve disorder among people taking statins.

●**Sexual dysfunction in men.** There are at least five case studies in the scientific literature of erectile dysfunction and other sexual problems after taking a statin. (There are even three case studies of gynecomastia—abnormal breast development—in men on statins.) And one study, from the Johns Hopkins University School of Medicine, and published in the *Journal of Clinical Lipidology*, found that men who took a statin had a "significant decrease" in their "erectile function." Dr. Golomb points out that cholesterol is a precursor for testosterone and that "statins reduce testosterone in men."

•**Stroke.** Statin use is linked to lower risk of ischemic stroke (83 percent of strokes, caused by a blood clot) in middle-aged people. But studies also link the drug to a 66 percent increased risk of hemorrhagic stroke (17 percent of strokes, caused by a burst blood vessel).

•**Weight gain.** People who take statins eat more calories and fat and gain more weight than people not taking the drug, according to Japanese researchers in *JAMA: Internal Medicine.*

How can one drug cause so many problems? Your body makes cholesterol for an important purpose: producing many of the hormones in your body. Block cholesterol and interfere with hormone production, and you create a body-wide disaster. In addition, blame the toxicity of statins on the loss of one crucial nutrient: coenzyme Q10, or CoQ10.

CoQ10—a biochemical sparkplug and antioxidant—is found in every cell of the body except red blood cells. Its key role is protecting and nourishing mitochondria, the tiny factories in every cell that manufacture cellular energy. Each heart cell, for example, is 40 percent mitochondria, because the heart requires so much energy to beat constantly and regularly.

Statins work by inhibiting the enzyme HMG-CoA reductase, which plays an important role in creating cholesterol *and* CoQ10. In other words, statins can and routinely do cause a CoQ10 deficiency. And when a drug interferes with a process so basic to cellular well-being, it can cause side effects in just about every system in the body. Statins do just that.

That's the risk of statins. The benefits are exaggerated. Statins are effective in lowering cholesterol levels in just about everybody—the young and the old, men and women. But they only effectively decrease the risk of heart attacks, strokes, and death from cardiovascular disease in people with a known history of heart disease (angina or heart attack). In this population, they can be lifesaving and I recommend them.

But in those without a history of heart disease who take statins—a use called primary prevention—the drug lowers death rates by less than two percent. *To put that result in perspective…*

•**Having thyroid hormone levels in the high versus the low part of the normal range is linked to a 69 percent lower risk of death from heart disease.**

•**Taking the arthritis supplement glucosamine is linked to a 22 percent lower risk of death from heart disease.**

•**Owning a cat is linked to a 30 percent lower risk of death from heart disease.**

Basically, in my humble opinion, I consider the use of statins in most people without demonstrated heart disease to be a 17-billion-dollars-a-year scam.

Protecting Yourself

There are many ways to protect yourself from the side effects of statins.

•**Talk to your doctor—now!** If you develop a side effect after taking a statin, talk to your doctor *immediately*—because the longer the side effect lasts, the longer it may take to go away.

My advice: Ask to go off the medication for three months to see if the side effect abates, and consider natural cholesterol-lowering alternatives.

•**Lower the dose.** If you develop a side effect but do need a statin, talk to your doctor about lowering the dose. A study published in the *Annals of Internal Medicine* shows that people with

Preventing Drug Interactions

Medical research on drugs typically focuses on one medication. Is the medication effective or isn't it? Does it cause side effects? If so, what are they?

But most people don't take only one drug. Fifty-five percent of Americans take prescription medications—and most take an average of four drugs! And an estimated 15 percent of side effects aren't caused by taking one drug, but by taking two or more at the same time. Those side effects are often caused by the two drugs interacting.

Drugs can interact in lots of ways, but the most common is that both drugs are metabolized (broken down) by the same limited supply of enzymes; neither is broken down sufficiently, and higher levels of the drugs circulate in the body, making a side effect more likely.

Don't rely on your doctor to protect you. Your doctor has about six minutes to treat you. That's enough time to write a prescription. But it's not nearly enough time to stop a medication, which requires that the doctor review all the medications you're taking. Plus, the doctor incurs a legal risk unless he can virtually guarantee that stopping the drug won't cause any problems. And insurance isn't likely to pay for stopping the medication—there's no diagnostic code for that.

All these factors have led to an increasingly common problem, particularly among the senior set, who take the most drugs and are the most vulnerable to side effects—fatigue, depression, or confusion caused by multiple medications. If you're 50 or older, taking multiple drugs, and suffering from any of those three symptoms, talk to your doctor about the possibility of safely and carefully weaning you off all noncritical medications, to see if your energy and mental clarity are restored. (Amazingly, it's not uncommon to see what has mistakenly been diagnosed as Alzheimer's disease clear up when the medications are stopped.)

If you feel better after the drugs are stopped, you need to work with your physician and pharmacist to find different drugs or nondrug ways to protect your health. As you are weaned off your medications, I suspect you and your doctor will find you no longer really need them.

one or more side effects from a statin are less likely to experience the problem when put on a lower, but still effective, dose of the drug.

•**Take coenzyme Q10.** If you take a statin, I strongly urge you to talk to your doctor about taking a coenzyme Q10 supplement, which can help protect you from side effects and which is available in most health food stores and retail outlets that sell dietary supplements. I recommend 200 milligrams daily. Get a brand made by a well-established supplement company.

If you stop the medication (only with your physician's approval), I recommend continuing to take coenzyme Q10 for three months for optimal mitochondrial repair.

•**Watch out if you're taking more than one drug.** Be extra cautious when taking a statin and another drug, such as a blood pressure medication or antifungal. Those drugs and many others are broken down by the same set of liver enzymes that break down statins. When you take two drugs at the same time, less of the statin is broken down—in effect, you're taking a higher dose of the statin, with a greater risk of side effects.

•**Consider switching to red yeast rice.** If you develop a side effect (particularly muscle pain), talk to your doctor about using cholesterol-lowering red yeast rice, the natural product from which synthetic statins were developed. Studies by doctors at the University of Pennsylvania, published in the *Archives of Internal Medicine*, show that this natural remedy is just as effective as statins, but much less likely to cause myalgia. The study doctors used a red yeast rice manufactured by Sylvan Bio, which is available at GNC's online or retail stores, as Red Yeast Rice, from Traditional Supplements.

•**Think about a nondrug approach.** Consider a healthful diet, supplements, exercise, and other powerful LDL-lowering methods as an alternative to statins. I talk about these in Heart Disease on page 239. If your physician isn't open to these types of natural alternatives, consider seeing a doctor who is board certified in holistic medicine. You can find organizations that provide lists and contact information for such doctors in Resources on page 360.

Heartburn Drugs: Are You Addicted to Antacids?

There's a reason that acid-blocking proton pump inhibitors such as *esomeprazole* (Nexium, aka "the purple pill") are one of the best-selling classes of drugs in the United States, with nearly 141 million yearly prescriptions, innumerable over-the-counter purchases, and billions in yearly sales: The drugs douse heartburn—sour stomach acid splashing into the esophagus and throat, painful post-meal burning, and belching—a problem suffered by more than 60 million Americans. Fifteen million experience heartburn symptoms every day.

Heartburn has many names. Acid indigestion. Acid reflux. Gastroesophageal reflux disease (GERD). But no matter the name, the mechanism behind heartburn is basically the same: Powerful digestive acid irritates your stomach lining or "refluxes" out of the stomach and up into the esophagus, the food tube that is meant to be a one-way road into the stomach.

Many classes of drugs have been developed to battle heartburn. First, there were the standard antacids, such as Maalox and Tums, which work by neutralizing the acid with alkaline minerals such as calcium, aluminum, and magnesium.

Then there were the H_2 receptor antagonists, such as *cimetidine* (Tagamet), *ranitidine* (Zantac), and *famotidine* (Pepcid AC), which work by blocking histamine, a compound that sparks the action of the stomach's acid-producing cells. But "H_2 blockers" only reduced stomach acid. The next generation of heartburn drugs—the proton pump inhibitors, or PPIs (such as Nexium, Prevacid, and Prilosec)—halted the production of stomach acid by blocking an enzyme system in the acid-producing cell. PPIs are used with the rationale of stopping Barrett's esophagus (damage to the lining of the esophagus) from turning into esophageal cancer. But newer research is showing that those benefits are overrated. And with chronic PPIs now being associated with a greater risk of premature death (which I'll talk about it a moment), I suspect these medications are far more likely to kill you than Barrett's esophagus.

Yes, PPIs can help you heal from a stomach ulcer. But stomach acid is a key part of the digestive process, and when it isn't produced—day after day, year after year—something's gotta give. Like your health.

PPIs came on the market in 2003. Studies of their long-term use are now showing that acid-blocking is health-blocking, too. *PPIs...*

•**Increase the risk of heart attack and stroke.** A meta-analysis of dozens of studies on the risk of PPIs, published in *Heart, Lung and Circulation*, found they increased the risk of "major cardiovascular events"—heart attack, stroke, death from cardiovascular disease—by 57 percent.

•**Increase the risk of dementia.** A study from Germany involving more than 70,000 people showed that using PPIs increased the risk of dementia by 44 percent.

•**Double the risk of hip fractures.** A study in the *Journal of the American Medical Association* showed that daily use of PPIs for four years or longer can more than double the risk of hip fractures. In fact, the longer people took PPIs, the greater the risk of fractures—41 percent higher after two years, 54 percent higher after three years, and 59 percent higher after four years. For those on the highest doses, the risk was 265 percent higher, or nearly triple. "The general perception among physicians and the public is that PPIs are relatively harmless, but that may not be the case," concluded the researchers, from the University of Pennsylvania. School of Medicine. And in a study from the Women's Health Initiative, involving more than 130,000 women, PPIs increased fracture risk by 25 percent.

The theory: Stomach acid helps you digest and absorb calcium, which builds bones. No stomach acid leads to less calcium, which leads to weaker bones. Of course, bone building is more complicated than that, involving many other nutrients, but you get the picture.

•**Double the risk of colds and flu.** Stomach acid doesn't just digest your food; it also kills viruses and bacteria. PPIs give those bugs a reprieve, and they settle down in your respiratory tract, where they can cause colds and flu.

•**Increase by 89 percent the risk of developing "community-acquired" (outside the hospital) pneumonia.** PPIs increase your risk of pneumonia for the same reason they increase your risk of colds and flu. The drugs also increase by 30 percent the risk of developing pneumonia in the hospital, where an estimated 40 percent of hospital patients are given PPIs—even if they don't have heartburn!

•**Triple the risk of a hospital-acquired infection with *Clostridium difficile*.** *C. diff.* (as it's known) is increasingly common, striking 500,000 Americans every year, causing everything from diarrhea and abdominal cramping to life-threatening inflammatory bowel disease.

•**Increase your risk of dying—from any cause.** Given all the above risks, it's not surprising that a review study published in the journal *Heart, Lung and Circulation*—which looked at 37 other studies on PPIs—found that the drugs increased the risk of "all-cause mortality" (death from any cause) by a shocking 68 percent. For comparison, a study from scientists at the Centers for Disease Control and Prevention showed that people who don't smoke, exercise regularly, eat a healthy diet, and drink alcohol moderately lower their risk of all-cause mortality by 38 percent—in other words, doing all those things and taking PPIs would completely wipe out the advantages of a healthy lifestyle!

•**Double the risk of B$_{12}$ deficiency.** The body needs stomach acid to digest vitamin B$_{12}$. Low levels of the vitamin can cause or contribute to fatigue, memory problems, confusion ("brain fog"), indigestion, and cardiovascular disease (heart attack and stroke).

•**May not be as effective as advertised.** Studies show that 40 percent of people who take prescription PPIs continue to suffer heartburn and also take over-the-counter antacids.

•**Addict you to PPIs.** Yes, research shows that PPIs aren't only bad for you, they're also addictive! Researchers in Denmark gave Nexium for two months to 120 people without heartburn. Within two weeks of stopping the drug, 44 percent of the study participants developed heartburn and indigestion. In 22 percent, those symptoms continued for the next four weeks.

Why did healthy people stopping the drug develop heartburn? Because of the phenomenon the researchers call "rebound acid hypersection." It's natural for the stomach to produce stomach acid; if you foil that function and then allow it to resume, it returns with a vengeance, generating huge amounts of stomach acid that cause heartburn and indigestion. "The observation that 40 percent of the volunteers—who had never been bothered by heartburn, acid regurgitation or dyspepsia [indigestion]—developed such symptoms in the weeks after cessation of PPIs is remarkable," said the study leader.

The lesson of this study: If you start taking a PPI and stop the drug, your heartburn symptoms may intensify, forcing you to start taking the drug again. In other words, heartburn medication can be addictive!

PPIs are not intended for long-term use. Prescribing guidelines instruct doctors to put patients on the drug for no longer than one month. But about one-third of people who start PPIs continue to take them, month after month. Are they addicted? Quite possibly, said the study researchers. "Our results justify the speculation that PPI dependency could be one of the explanations for the rapidly and continuously increasing use of PPIs," they wrote in *Gastroenterology*, a leading medical journal.

PPI use is rapidly increasing because they aren't just prescribed for ulcers anymore. They're also routinely prescribed for indigestion and other upper gastrointestinal symptoms. In fact, 70 percent of people prescribed PPIs don't have ulcers! (Plus, the PPIs such as *omeprazole* [Prilosec OTC] and *lansoprazole* [Prevacid] are now available over-the-counter, making them far more available.) In thinking about this developing pattern of prescribing, and the fact that the drugs cause the very symptoms they're meant to treat, digestive experts had this to say in the pages of *Gastroenterology*: "The current finding that these drugs induce symptoms means that such liberal prescribing is likely to be creating the disease the drugs are designed to treat, and causing patients with no previous need for such therapy to require intermittent or long-term treatment." PPI therapy, he concluded, "should be reserved for those with clear symptoms of heartburn or acid reflux."

The bottom line? PPI medications are likely responsible for over 30,000 U.S. deaths yearly. Using the medications Zantac and Tagamet were significantly safer. Much safer yet is to simply improve digestion using the approach we will discuss in upcoming chapters on digestive upsets and diseases.

Antidepressants: The Sad Fact About Effectiveness

The people who manufacture and sell antidepressant drugs probably aren't depressed. In fact, they're laughing—all the way to the bank. Antidepressants are one of the top three most-prescribed class of drugs in the United States, with more than 250 million prescriptions yearly. Astoundingly, *one in eight* Americans over the age of 12 are taking these drugs.

The main class of antidepressants—selective serotonin reuptake inhibitors, or SSRIs—work by increasing levels of serotonin, a brain chemical linked to better mood. It includes drugs such as *citalopram* (Celexa), *escitalopram* (Lexapro), *fluvoxamine* (Luvox), *paroxetine* (Paxil), *fluoxetine* (Prozac), and *sertraline* (Zoloft).

But here's a very sad fact about SSRIs. Four out of five times, they don't work. A study from researchers at the University of Pennsylvania, published in the *Journal of the American Medical Association*, analyzed data from antidepressant studies involving more than 700 people. It found that results from the drugs were "nonexistent to negligible" for people with mild or moderate depression—and that's four out of five people who are diagnosed with depression!

The results were similarly dismal for many with severe depression. Only people with extremely severe depression benefited from antidepressants. (Taken in this type of situation, the drugs can be literally lifesaving, preventing suicide.) The study authors pointed out that all the research used by drug companies to support their claim that antidepressants work involved severe depression—a fact you're unlikely to know, because it's almost never mentioned by the drug companies or by the doctors who write those 250 million prescriptions.

"What this and other studies show is that the majority of people on antidepressants—the four out of five depressed people with mild or moderate depression—are essentially taking an expensive placebo with nasty side effects," Stephen Ilardi, PhD, associate professor of clinical psychology at the University of Kansas and author of *The Depression Cure: The 6-Step Program to Beat Depression without Drugs*, told us.

What are some of those nasty (and common) side effects?

- Anxiety
- Bruxism (tooth grinding)
- Constipation
- Diarrhea
- Dizziness
- Dry mouth
- Fatigue and drowsiness
- Headaches
- Insomnia
- Loss of ability to orgasm
- Loss of libido
- Nausea
- Photosensitivity (sensitivity to light)
- Restlessness
- Tremors
- Weight gain

Other side effects can include thinking a lot about committing suicide in children and adolescents who take the drug; difficulty withdrawing from the drug (depression returns, and with greater intensity); and increased risk of bone fractures.

If antidepressants aren't truly anti-, what is? For mild to moderate depression, natural cures work—such as walking in the sunshine, eating more fatty fish, and feeling your feelings instead of burying them. You'll find my Real Cure Regimen in Depression on page 207.

NSAIDs: Side Effects That Are Hard to Stomach

There are more than 20 NSAIDs and over 100 NSAID-containing products. Some of the most common are aspirin, *celecoxib* (Celebrex), *ibuprofen* (Motrin, Advil), *indomethacin* (Indocin), and *piroxicam* (Feldene). Thirty million Americans take these drugs regularly, usually to relieve arthritis pain—and one in three suffer digestive disturbances as a result. For the most unfortunate, the disturbance is terminal: a sudden, massive, and deadly bleeding ulcer.

As study after study shows, NSAIDs can also hurt your heart, boosting blood pressure and doubling the risk of a heart attack or stroke. High blood pressure is also a leading cause of chronic kidney disease.

NSAIDs may even be counterproductive. While relieving arthritis pain, they may simultaneously destroy cartilage, the cushioning at the end of bones, thereby worsening arthritis in the long run. Arthritis specialists (rheumatologists) also point out that NSAIDs effectively relieve pain only about 30 percent to 40 percent of the time.

And there's more bad news for men and their sexual partners: NSAIDs double the risk of erectile dysfunction.

Bottom line: NSAIDs are responsible for about 50,000 excess U.S. deaths yearly. That risk is often worth the pain relief. But the vast majority of the time—using the information in this book—you'll be able to get pain free *without* NSAIDs.

In most cases, NSAIDs aren't necessary or can be used short term (though you should never stop any drug without the supervision and approval of your physician). A study sponsored by the National Institutes of Health showed that after three months of treatment for arthritis pain with either a prescription or natural remedy, pain relief persists.

As you'll read in Arthritis on page 155, there are many safe and effective natural alternatives to this class of drugs.

Antibiotics: More Drugs, More Bugs

Antibiotics were a true wonder drug, countering the infections that plagued humankind, such as tuberculosis and pneumonia.

But we've overdone it with antibiotics, using them so widely (in treating humans and in raising cattle, pigs, and chicken for food) that bacteria have evolved to resist them—an increasingly common condition called antibiotic resistance. "Virtually all important bacterial infections in the U.S. and throughout the world are becoming resistant to antibiotics," concluded experts at a symposium on "The Global Problem of Antimicrobial Resistance" at Columbia University.

Urinary tract infections. Sinusitis. Pneumonia. Staph infections. Tuberculosis. You name the bacterial infection, and bacteria have outflanked the antibiotic used to treat it. For example,

Antibiotics Don't Work for Sinusitis

You've got acute sinusitis—a viral, bacterial, or fungal infection of the sinus cavities that followed a cold. If you're like 20 million other Americans, you see a doctor. And if the physician is like nine out of 10 physicians, he prescribes an antibiotic.

Wrong choice.

Research shows that antibiotics don't work for sinusitis. They don't reduce the severity of symptoms, and they don't shorten the length of the infection. They also trigger the overgrowth of yeast that is the cause of sinusitis becoming chronic.

See Sinusitis on page 315 for natural remedies for acute and chronic sinusitis.

you've probably read about the flesh-eating bacteria that are resistant to all treatment. Those are antibiotic-resistant *Staphylococcus aureus*. Aside from feasting on flesh, they're also causing an epidemic of antibiotic-resistant pneumonia and sepsis in hospitals.

In the past, new generations of antibiotics came to the rescue, beating back the resistant bugs. Not now. There are more and more types of resistant bacteria and a dearth of new antibiotics. They are contributing to the rise in antibiotic-resistant bacteria and conditions.

The more antibiotics you take, the more likely that you (and others) will be infected by resistant bacteria. The good news is that there are many natural antibacterial remedies that you can use instead of antibiotics. You can read about them in Colds and Flu on page 202.

Osteoporosis Drugs: Building or Wrecking Bones?

If you want to find out the latest news about osteoporosis, talk to Susan Brown, PhD, director of the Better Bones Foundation and author of *Better Bones, Better Body*. (Her website is Better Bones.com.) Dr. Brown, a nutritionist and medical anthropologist, has deep insights into the causes and cures of osteoporosis—insights contrary to the myths that dominate the medical establishment's perspective, such as the all-importance of calcium in combating the disease. She favors a natural approach to preventing, slowing, and reversing the disease.

If you're diagnosed with eroding bone (the early stage, osteopenia, which affects 48 million Americans, or the more advanced stage, osteoporosis, which affects about 10 million), the key question is: Should you take a bisphosphonate, the most commonly prescribed class of bone-building drugs?

Many women decide, at the urging of their doctors, to take these drugs—at their own risk. There are billions of dollars' worth of yearly prescriptions for these drugs, which include *alendronate* (Fosamax), *ibandronate* (Boniva), *risedronate* (Actonel), and *zoledronate* (Zometa, Aclasta). Dr. Brown points out that there are certain conditions of rapid, sustained bone loss in which bone-building drugs can be lifesavers. They include cancer treatment; taking high doses of the bone-robbing anti-inflammatory drug *prednisone* over a long period of time; and Paget's disease, a genetic condition that destroys bone.

But for everyone else, bone-building drugs are probably a bad idea, Dr. Brown told us. In fact, research now shows that long-term use of these drugs may actually destroy bone!

"These medications dramatically reduce bone loss by bringing premature death to osteoclasts, the cells that break down and recycle old, worn-out segments of bone," explained Dr. Brown. "However," she continued, "bone breakdown and bone buildup are closely linked." As Fosamax and other bisphosphonates effectively reduce bone breakdown, they also decrease new bone formation. Studies show that Fosamax suppresses bone forming by 60 percent to 90 percent.

Yes, said Dr. Brown, studies show Fosamax increases bone density, the standard measurement of osteoporosis. But Susan Ott, MD, a professor of medicine at the University of Washington and another critic of these drugs, said, "This is because the bone is no longer remodeling and there is not much new bone. The older bone is denser than the newer bone. There is less water and more mineral in the bone, and the radiographic techniques thus measure the higher density." In other words, what *looks* like added bone tissue is *not*. "Many people believe that these drugs are bone builders," said Dr. Ott. "But the evidence shows they are actually bone hardeners."

Dr. Brown told us that her main objection to the drugs is when they're used to address low bone density without any effort to identify the reason for the bone loss. "It's not uncommon for physicians to simply hand out a prescription when they see a bone scan that indicates osteoporosis—or even osteopenia—without taking any steps to determine *why* bone is being lost, or even *if* bone is being lost!"

No real cause—no real cure.

"Treating the symptom with a drug doesn't cure the disease—it simply masks the problem," she added. "And most physicians don't mention that these are very powerful medications with a profound impact on the body's most fundamental processes."

For example, there are now many case histories of women who took bisphosphonates for years and ended up with spontaneous and serious fractures. That's because, as Dr. Brown explained, the drugs actually weaken bone, stopping both bone breakdown and bone formation, and creating bone that isn't capable of renewing and healing itself.

The data is clear: These medications cause more harm than good after five years of use. "In almost all cases, taking a prescription drug is not needed," Dr. Brown told us. "Osteoporosis and osteopenia medications are big business, but despite all the hype and marketing from drug companies, there is a safer, more effective and natural approach to bone health available to you." Needless to say, I recommend a natural regimen that is proven to be nearly twice as effective as the medications. You'll find my Real Cure Regimen in Osteoporosis on page 302.

Hormonal Imbalances

Rev Up Your Glands

I remember my delight the first time I paged through an anatomy book, with its series of clear plastic overlays showing the body's systems one by one.

There was the circulatory system—the heart propelling blood through (the book told me) tens of thousands of miles of arteries and veins. The respiratory system—the spongy bellows of the lungs, filling and emptying. The nervous system—the brain and spine, with their branching circuitry. And the skeletal, muscular, digestive, reproductive, urinary, and immune systems—I was amazed that there was enough room in the body to fit them all in!

But then there's that other system, the endocrine system—the glands and the hormones they manufacture. Uh, what are the names of those seven (or is it eight) glands? And what hormones do they manufacture? And what functions do those hormones perform, exactly?

Well, the answers to *those* questions might help you answer *these*…

Why are so many Americans fatigued, fat, and frazzled? Why do we sleep so poorly? Why do we get colds and other infections so easily and find them hard to kick? Why are so many of us depressed, anxious, and irritable? Why is our collective sex drive stalled? Why do so many postmenopausal women feel like they're also post-health? Why does pain claw at our bodies like a cat playing with a mouse? Why do so many of us die of heart attacks?

Every one of these health problems (and many more) can be caused by a problem with the endocrine system—usually an underproduction of one or more of the powerful hormones that regulate every system of the body.

Understanding hormonal deficiencies as a real cause (a cause that is usually undetected and therefore rarely cured) is crucial to your health and well-being. Most conventional doctors don't accurately diagnose or treat hormonal imbalances and deficiencies, particularly common but little-recognized deficiencies in thyroid, adrenal, and reproductive hormones.

And because undetected hormonal problems are so common in my new patients, I'm willing to bet that if you're tired, anxious, overweight, or in pain, you, too, are likely to be deficient in one or more of the hormones manufactured by the thyroid, adrenal, or reproductive glands (the three most common deficiencies). In this book, I provide the information you need to make sure that you are accurately tested and effectively treated. These deficiencies can be diagnosed easily and corrected safely, even though standard testing is unreliable. You can feel great again.

Understanding Your Endocrine System

Hormones are like bosses on a business trip—they travel throughout the body via the bloodstream, telling organs and cells what to do. Some control growth (the explosion of puberty is set off by hormones). Some control your metabolism—your energy level, heart rate, speed of digestion, and body temperature. They all function via feedback: If you're overheated, they tell your body to cool down; if you're freezing, they order up more fuel for the internal fire. This feedback mechanism sometimes works like a set of biochemical dominoes, with one hormone telling another to get busy and then *that* hormone issuing its own instructions. To understand the endocrine system better, let's take a quick look at the various glands and the hormones they produce.

•**Hypothalamus.** How much you want to eat and drink. Whether you sweat or shiver. How fast your heart beats. Whether your sleep is deep or shallow. All these functions are supervised by hormones from the hypothalamus, an almond-size gland just above the brain stem. Much of the work the hypothalamus does is through releasing hormones that tell the pituitary to release its hormones, which stimulate other endocrine glands.

•**Pituitary gland.** This pea-size gland underneath the hypothalamus is a big performer in spite of its size. *The hormones it generates include...*

•Human growth hormone (HGH). For tissue growth in kids and tissue repair and muscle building in adults.

•Thyroid-stimulating hormone (TSH). Triggers the thyroid to produce its hormones. (As I'll discuss in a minute, the underproduction of thyroid hormones—hypothyroidism—is an unrecognized and untreated American epidemic, with terrible consequences for health.)

•Luteinizing hormone (LH) *and* follicle-stimulating hormone (FSH). These two hormones influence the sex and reproductive organs (gonads), playing a role in the production of estrogen and progesterone in women and testosterone in men.

•Prolactin. Breastfeeding doesn't happen without it.

•Antidiuretic hormone (*vasopressin*). Regulates kidney function (how much you urinate) and the volume of blood.

•Oxytocin. In women, it tells the uterus to contract during childbirth and also plays a role in milk production. It's called "the hormone of love" because it may stimulate the positive feelings that help a new mother bond with her baby. It also plays a key role in a woman's ability to have an orgasm and the "afterglow" of sex. In men, oxytocin is produced during orgasm, aiding sperm release, and it may help keep the prostate gland healthy. Studies also show the hormone may help men bond with children and spouses.

•**Pineal gland.** This is a small (and to scientists still somewhat mysterious) gland in the middle of the brain. It manufactures melatonin, the hormone that regulates your sleep-wake cycle.

•**Thyroid gland.** Located in the neck, this gland is the body's gas pedal—it controls how fast or slow just about every part of you goes. And when you're slow, you feel low. If your metabolism is sluggish, you gain weight easily and lose it with difficulty. If your digestion is pokey, you become constipated. If your body temperature is set too low, you're cold all the time. If your brain is plodding, you can't think clearly. These are just some of the symptoms of hypothyroidism. (There are many more, as I'll talk about in a minute.)

•**Parathyroid glands.** These two small glands on either side of the thyroid generate parathyroid hormone. This hormone controls calcium levels in the blood. Without enough calcium in your circulation, hormones couldn't travel from spot to spot, your heart couldn't beat, your blood couldn't clot, and your nerves couldn't transmit their electrical signals.

•**Thymus gland.** This often-ignored gland in your midchest helps regulate the immune system. It creates thymulin, a hormone that helps T-cells (a type of infection-fighting white blood cell) multiply and also energizes the immune system's natural killer cells. Thymulin requires zinc to function optimally. Unfortunately, zinc is depleted in chronic infections, leading to weaker thymulin and more infections.

•**Adrenal glands.** Famous for producing adrenaline—the hormone that puts the "fight" in the fight-or-flight response—these two glands sit atop your kidneys. The adrenals have an outer section (the adrenal cortex) and an inner section (the adrenal medulla). The cortex makes corticosteroids, which help regulate your response to stress, your immune system, and the functioning of your sex organs. The medulla kicks out catecholamines (including adrenaline in the form of epinephrine and norepinephrine), and they ready you to respond to sudden stress.

•**Testicles and ovaries.** The testicles make testosterone, and it does more than turn a boy from a soprano into a tenor. Too-low levels (a common problem among my middle-aged and older patients) can drain your enthusiasm and energy, lower your libido to half-mast, muddle your moods, and install a spare tire. Men produce much more testosterone than women do, but women do produce the hormone (in their ovaries and adrenal glands). Low levels in women also can pull the plug on vitality, optimism, and sex drive.

Produced mainly by the ovaries, estrogen and progesterone are involved in every aspect of sexual development and reproduction in women. An imbalance in estrogen and progesterone levels—with progesterone being too low—can trigger symptoms of PMS (premenstrual syndrome). This menstrual difficulty affects more than 75 percent of reproductive-age women, with 20 percent to 40 percent saying the symptoms (such as irritability, depression, food cravings, back pain, headache, pelvic cramps, bloated abdomen, and tender breasts) interfere with daily life. The decrease of estrogen in later life can serve up a second round of distressing symptoms, such as hot flashes, insomnia, brain fog, muscle pain, and loss of libido. In men estrogen and progesterone are produced by the adrenal gland, and imbalanced levels (too low or too high) can depress libido, cause erectile difficulty, and reduce sperm production.

•**Pancreas.** Located behind the stomach, this organ pumps out digestive enzymes and two hormones that control blood sugar (glucose). The one you've probably heard a lot about, insulin, helps glucose move out of the bloodstream and into muscle and fat cells for energy or storage. The condition called insulin resistance—when the "locks" of insulin receptors on cells are clogged with fat and can't use the "key" of insulin—is the prologue to prediabetes. But it also makes glucagon, which boosts blood sugar if it's too low.

Hypothyroidism: Millions of Missed Diagnoses

Do these symptoms sound familiar to you?

•**You're tired most of the time**—and you have trouble falling asleep.

•**Your muscles and joints ache, seemingly for no reason.**

•**Your mood pendulums between anxiety and depression.**

•**You're forgetful and also find it hard to focus.**

•**Your sex drive can't even get into first gear.**

•**You've gained a lot of weight and can't seem to shed it,** even when you don't eat much.

•**You're trying to have a baby but can't.**

•**Menopause has put your health on pause,** with hot flashes so frequent and intense it feels like somebody installed a sauna inside you.

•**Your skin and hair are so dry they feel like they were imported from the Sahara.**

•**You're so constipated that you've started to regard laxatives as dessert.**

•**Even your feet bother you**—cold as bricks in winter, and you always wear socks to bed.

Those are some of the many symptoms of hypothyroidism, an underactive thyroid that doesn't manufacture enough T4 (the storage form of the thyroid hormone) and/or T3 (the active form). Low production of thyroid hormones can limit the full functioning of just about every part of the body. The disease may also underlie many cases of chronic pain, osteoporosis, miscarriages, and learning disabilities in children born to women with low thyroid. But like most diseases that mainly affect women, hypothyroidism has been dramatically underdiagnosed.

My favorite thyroid specialists—Richard L. Shames, MD, and Karilee Shames, RN, PhD, authors of *Thyroid Mind Power* and *Feeling Fat, Fuzzy, or Frazzled?*—estimate that 50 million Americans may have low levels of thyroid hormone. The cause of this hidden epidemic? The Shameses think it's the flood of 80,000-plus artificial chemicals in our environment, many with a molecular structure similar to that of thyroid hormones. The chemicals confuse the immune system, which attacks the thyroid.

Why aren't thyroid hormone levels as easy to test for and detect as, say, your cholesterol level? A couple of reasons. Doctors don't routinely think of hypothyroidism when seeing a patient and

Your Thyroid and Your Heart

The obvious symptoms of hypothyroidism—such as fatigue, depression, and overweight—are bad enough. But hypothyroidism can cause more than everyday suffering. It can end your life.

Women with untreated hypothyroidism are more than twice as likely to suffer a heart attack, reported a team of Norwegian researchers in an issue of the *Archives of Internal Medicine*. In their eight-year study of more than 25,000 people, they found that women with somewhat low thyroid levels (considered normal by most doctors) had a 69 percent higher risk of dying from heart disease. "These results indicate that relatively low but clinically normal thyroid function may increase the risk of fatal coronary heart disease," they wrote.

A 69 percent higher risk means that hypothyroidism could cause more heart attacks in women than smoking, elevated cholesterol, high blood pressure, or diabetes. Another way to look at it: Detecting and treating those cases of hypothyroidism could save 30,000 lives a year—one of which may be yours!

---

instead treat (or try to treat) the symptoms of hypothyroidism—the constipation, depression, overweight, whatever. And even if your doctor does test for low thyroid, the test is routinely misinterpreted, with too-low thyroid levels designated "normal."

Unreliable Thyroid Tests

Most doctors don't know about research showing that the TSH (thyroid- stimulating hormone) test—the test typically used to check your thyroid—is very unreliable, failing to spot most of the people who need to take extra thyroid hormone. And the test for "free T4"—one form of stored thyroid—is considered "abnormal" only if you have outright thyroid failure! Why do standard tests fail to identify such a common problem?

Well, most labs establish a "normal" range for test results using a statistical formula called "2 standard deviations": Out of every 100 people tested, those with the two highest and the two lowest scores are abnormal, and everybody else is normal. Imagine applying the same medical standard to determine a "healthy" shoe size. Any size between 4 and 13 would be "normal"—and if a man was fitted with a too-small size 5 shoe or a woman with a too-large size 12, the doctor would say the shoes were perfectly okay! That approach is wrong. Human beings aren't statistics; they're individuals. Thyroid tests within the so-called normal range may be abnormal for you, producing symptoms that are never solved because conventional medicine can't find their cause.

Here's another problem with thyroid tests. Over the decades, they have been continually updated, with ever-expanding definitions of who is and isn't hypothyroid. There's no reason to believe that the current test effectively detects every case of hypothyroidism—because none of the previous tests did!

Some history about this situation: When I was in medical school, doctors diagnosed hypothyroidism by measuring the metabolic rate during a treadmill test. A decade or so later, a new, more accurate test used protein-bound iodide (PBI) as a measure of thyroid function. After that, there was the T4-level thyroid test, outdating the PBI test and detecting even more cases of hypothyroidism. That test was followed by the new and improved T7 test. And then the T7 test was replaced by the TSH test. Are we accurate yet? No.

In one of the most recent changes, the American Association of Clinical Endocrinologists (AACE) revised the "normal" range for the TSH test (0.5 to 5.0), stating that anyone with a TSH over 3.0 was hypothyroid. That means over 10 million Americans with ranges from 3.1 to 5.0 had *not* been treated for hypothyroidism because their lab results had been previously regarded as normal.

Here's what the press release stated: "…doctors had relied on a normal TSH level ranging from 0.5 to 5.0 to diagnose and treat patients with a thyroid disorder who tested outside the boundaries of that range. Now, AACE encourages doctors to consider treatment for patients who test outside the boundaries of a narrow margin based on a target TSH level of 0.3 to 3.0. AACE believes the new range will result in proper diagnosis for millions of Americans who suffer from a mild thyroid disorder, but have gone untreated until now."

Bravo for the AACE. But apparently that press release wasn't read by a lot of medical professionals. Most labs (and doctors) still use the old criteria, considering TSH up to 5.5 to be normal—resulting in more than 10 million American women having their low thyroid levels missed by standard testing. And that isn't the only way hypothyroidism is missed.

Your thyroid also could be underactive because of an underactive hypothalamus, so you can suffer the hypothyroidism and have a normal TSH.

Case in point: Dr. G. R. Skinner, of the United Kingdom, and his colleagues tested thyroid hormone levels of 80 "clinically hypothyroid patients" (people with symptoms of hypothyroidism) and found their TSH was "well within" the normal range. When Dr. Skinner treated those patients with 100 to 120 micrograms a day of thyroid hormone (Synthroid), the large majority of them improved. Ignoring thyroid-caused symptoms in people with "normal" lab results can "condemn many patients to years of hypothyroidism with its pathological complications and poor quality of life," said Dr. Skinner and his colleagues in the *British Medical Journal.*

Yet another study shows that only three percent of those tested for low thyroid have tests that confirm their hypothyroidism. In other words, the doctor suspected it, tested for it, but didn't find it.

To me, there is an obvious conclusion: Current thyroid testing misses diagnosing most people who are hypothyroid, which I define as having significant health problems that improve when treated with thyroid hormone. I say: Treat the patient and not the test!

If you have just one or two of the possible symptoms of hypothyroidism—unexplained fatigue, persistent depression, achy muscles and joints, miscarriages, infertility, heavy periods, constipation, easy weight gain, cold intolerance, dry skin, thin hair, and a body temperature that tends to be on the low side of normal—you deserve to be treated for hypothyroidism. You'll find my Real Cure Regimen—the best way to test for and treat this—in Hypothyroidism on page 254.

The Armpit Test

If you have several of the symptoms of hypothyroidism and suspect that you have the problem, self-tests using a thermometer can provide more evidence.

One self-test recommended by many holistic physicians is to check your axilla (armpit) temperature for several days in the morning when you wake up. Before you get out of bed, put the thermometer in your armpit. Lie quietly for 10 minutes. If your temperature is under 97.4°F on two repeat measurements, you and your doctor should consider treatment with thyroid hormone, no matter what your blood tests show.

In my own practice, I ask patients with thyroid symptoms to take an oral temperature between 11:00 a.m. and 7:00 p.m. on two different days. If it's below 98.1°F on both days, it's reasonable to treat the person for hypothyroidism.

One caution: Fatigue, anxiety, and muscle pain also can be caused by an overactive thyroid. This problem shouldn't be diagnosed using just the TSH test. If free T4 is elevated or high-normal, your doctor should consider the possibility that you have an overactive thyroid.

Adrenal Burnout: The Stress Disease

The adrenal medulla pumps out adrenaline, speeding your heart and breathing, boosting your blood pressure, and shunting blood from your guts to your muscles. You're ready for action! And that's fine if you're dealing with a temporary emergency, like running away from a mugger. But what if you're being mugged day after day by unemployment? What if the stress doesn't stop? Then your endocrine system takes its anti-stress action plan to the next level. Your hypothalamus pumps out corticotropin-releasing hormone (CRH)…which tells your adrenal cortex to release cortisol…which triggers the release of glucagon from your pancreas…which raises your blood sugar, giving your brain and muscles more energy to cope with extended stress.

But there's a problem with that plan: Your body wasn't built to endure the excessive, everyday stress of the 21st century. It was built to flee from a saber-toothed tiger and then chill out for a couple of weeks. So after hours and days and weeks and months and years of constant stress, the adrenal cortex is literally exhausted, and chronically high cortisol levels (bad for you) give way to chronically low ones (worse for you). I call this condition adrenal burnout, or adrenal exhaustion. *Adrenal burnout usually has one or more of the following symptoms…*

•**You're tired all the time.** Cortisol is a must for energy. When levels are low, you're leveled.

•**You're intensely irritable whenever you feel hungry—and maybe all the time.** Your exhausted adrenal gland can't pump out enough cortisol to trigger the production of glucagon—a compound that converts stored blood sugar (glycogen) into active blood sugar (glucose)—and your blood sugar is often too low. That low level of glucose also starves your brain, resulting in irritability (and anxiety and depression). In fact, this condition—called hypoglycemia—can cause ongoing irritability and anxiety.

In my book *Beat Sugar Addiction Now!*, I discuss adrenal fatigue as one of four leading caus-es of sugar addiction. If you have hypoglycemia from adrenal exhaustion, you feel better after eating sweets, which boosts your energy and mood—for a little while. Sweets launch your blood sugar level into the stratosphere, but then it plummets and crashes, causing you to crave more sweets (and coffee and other stimulants).

(I've noticed that adrenal exhaustion can cause havoc in a relationship, because a partner becomes repeatedly irritable from low blood sugar—what I call the "Feed me now or I'll kill you!" syndrome, and what is now commonly referred to as being "hangry." Instead of *arguing* with your spouse, *feed* him or her. If you're the irritable person, feed yourself!)

•**You have frequent infections** (such as a sore throat and colds), and the infections take quite a while to clear up. Both high and low cortisol levels diminish the power of your immune system.

•**You have allergies.** Another sign of impaired immunity.

•**You ache all over.** Widely fluctuating blood sugar levels keep your muscles tense.

•**You feel dizzy when standing.** Cortisol controls blood pressure; a shortfall can cause this symptom.

•**You're crashing from stress.** Even the littlest problem leaves you feeling overwhelmed.

•**You have chronic health problems.** Cortisol interferes with insulin, the hormone that helps control blood sugar. After a while, your cells develop insulin resistance, and insulin resis-tance is a setup for chronic disease, such as type 2 diabetes and heart disease.

"The body starts to break down from the effects of elevated cortisol," Charles Moss, MD, an instructor at the UCLA School of Medicine, and author of *The Adaptation Diet*, told us. The re-sult, he said, is not only insulin resistance, but also "immune system suppression, poor wound healing, thinning bones, loss of muscle mass, weight gain around the midsection, depression and anxiety, poor sleep, and elevated blood pressure—all courtesy of elevated levels of cortisol and epinephrine." And, Dr. Moss continued, depleted cortisol "leads to fatigue, anxiety, poor resis-tance, and an inability to recover from life's challenges." In other words: adrenal burnout.

More Adrenal Deficits

Adrenal burnout can cause low levels of several other adrenal hormones, adding to your woes.

•**DHEA (dehydroepiandrosterone).** The adrenal glands produce more of this hormone than any other, and low levels can cause fatigue and just plain old "feeling poorly." (Some studies link higher DHEA levels to longer life.) My patients often have a dramatic boost of energy and well-being when their DHEA level is optimized to midrange for a normal 29-year-old.

•**Aldosterone.** This hormone supervises the balance of salt and water in your body. Low levels can cause blood pressure problems.

•**Estrogen and testosterone.** The ovaries and testicles specialize in these hormones, but the adrenal gland chips in. I discuss the downside of low estrogen and testosterone in the next two sections.

Are you under constant stress and experiencing one or more of the symptoms we've been discussing? If so, you're a candidate for adrenal support: an eating pattern that keeps your blood sugar on an even keel, plus supplements that revitalize your adrenal gland. For the Real Cure Regimen for this problem, please see Adrenal Exhaustion on page 138.

Low Testosterone

If there was a top-10 all-time bestseller list for self-help books bought by middle-aged and older men (or their wives), it might look something like this (the following are all titles of real books)...

1. *Testosterone for Life*
2. *The Testosterone Advantage Plan*
3. *The Testosterone Syndrome*
4. *The Testosterone Factor*
5. *Natural Remedies for Low Testosterone*
6. *Super "T"*
7. *The Testosterone Revolution*
8. *The Testosterone Edge*
9. *Testosterone Deficiency: The Hidden Disease*
10. *Testosterone Is Your Friend*

The subtitles of these books make a lot of promises. With more testosterone, they claim, you'll also have more energy (including more sexual energy), more muscle, less fat, better moods, and fewer illnesses.

In my experience with my patients, supplemental testosterone—natural bioidentical testosterone, that is—keeps its promises. (Please don't confuse the synthetic, high-potency, and very toxic testosterone used illegally by some athletes with bioidentical natural testosterone in safe doses.)

Testosterone is, of course, the quintessential male hormone, manufactured by the testes. (Women also generate a small but important health-giving amount of the hormone in their adrenal gland.) Every cell in a man's body has testosterone receptors, and the hormone endows males with muscles, strength, erections, a beard, a deep voice, and the "desire to take charge and take on the world," said Shafiq Qaadri, MD, author of *The Testosterone Factor*. Optimal testosterone levels also decrease the risk of heart disease, hypertension, and type 2 diabetes, and can help slow or stop the progress of those diseases in men who already have them.

But time takes its toll on testosterone. Production of the hormone begins to decline around the age of 30, and that drop can become a plummet around 50—with levels bottoming out as a medical condition called late-onset hypogonadism, in which testosterone is scarce. (Testosterone in women also decreases with age, causing or contributing to problems similar to those found in men with low T—fatigue, depression, poor stamina, osteoporosis, muscle wasting, diabetes, high cholesterol, weight gain and poor libido.)

Maybe you don't have late-onset hypogonadism. But just because you don't have a diagnosable medical problem doesn't mean you don't have a problem. Testosterone levels that are clinically "normal" but lower than ideal are very common. (One study shows that men's average testosterone levels have dropped by 16 percent in the past 15 years, with many possible factors underlying the change, such as excess weight and environmental toxins.)

Testosterone Doesn't Increase the Risk of Prostate Cancer

You may have heard that testosterone therapy (TT) increases the risk of prostate cancer. And that was the nearly universal opinion among medical professionals, based on decades-old research indicating testosterone fueled the disease. That opinion is probably wrong.

"The notion that pathological prostate growth, benign or malignant, can be stimulated by testosterone is a commonly held belief without scientific basis," Abraham Morgentaler, MD, associate clinical professor of urology at Harvard Medical School and author of *Testosterone for Life*, wrote in an issue of the journal *European Urology*. "The available evidence strongly suggests that TT neither increases the risk of prostate cancer diagnosis in normal men nor causes cancer recurrence in men who were successfully treated for prostate cancer."

That "available evidence" includes a study in the *International Journal of Impotence Research* by researchers from the Department of Urology at Maimonides Medical Center in Brooklyn, New York. They looked at 44 studies on TT and prostate cancer, including four studies of men with a history of the disease. None of the studies showed that TT increased the risk of prostate cancer. In fact, testosterone may *protect* the prostate.

"There is mounting evidence that low testosterone is associated with greater prostate cancer risk," wrote Dr. Morgentaler in another scientific paper. For example, in a study of 156 men with newly diagnosed prostate cancer, those with the most aggressive and advanced form of the disease also had the lowest testosterone levels, reported researchers from the University of Vienna in the journal *The Prostate*.

Bottom line: There is no clear evidence of a link between TT and the development of prostate cancer, and low testosterone may actually increase your risk of the disease.

However, I also recommend taking the most conservative and responsible approach. If you begin TT, ask your doctor to do a yearly digital rectal exam, to make sure you're not developing the disease. And if you've been diagnosed with prostate cancer, don't take testosterone.

The low-normal level of testosterone can produce a range of symptoms in middle-aged and older guys, including fatigue, irritability, poor concentration, memory loss, vague aches and pains, extra fat around the middle, and erectile dysfunction. And while you can inspire an uncooperative penis with Viagra, there's no sex life without *life*—a five-year study in the *American Journal of Cardiology* of more than 18,000 men showed that those with the lowest testosterone levels were 48 percent more likely to die than those with the highest levels. About 70 percent of my male and female patients with chronic fatigue syndrome and fibromyalgia (the two diseases I specialize in) are low in testosterone (in the lowest 30 percent of the population). My own clinical findings and scientific studies show that testosterone therapy (TT) in these patients can decrease fatigue and pain (the primary symptoms), increase red blood cell levels (to help oxygenate a tired, aching body), improve heart function, and revitalize libido.

I advocate detecting and treating low testosterone in a way that's somewhat different from what some medical doctors advise—a way that's more accurate, safer, and more effective.

The Real Test

Most physicians check only for "total" testosterone (the amount of the hormone in storage and not available for immediate use). But I think it's important to check for total testosterone *and* "free" testosterone (the amount that's available for immediate use).

Labs also sometimes make the mistake of presenting "normal" ranges that combine all age groups, rather than breaking them down into 10-year age groups—31 to 40, 41 to 50, etc. If you're 28, it's meaningless to have a normal range that includes an 80-year-old. Ask your doctor to make sure your lab isn't using this method.

Another mistake: Labs define "abnormal" as only the lowest two percent of the population. I think that's far too rigid a definition, telling many people their levels are normal when they're not.

And be especially careful of so-called normal ranges if you're a woman. Some labs have ranges that begin at zero. That's like having a normal range for women's heights that ranges from 0 to 72 inches!

If total testosterone is below normal (or even in the lowest 30 percent of normal range) and you have symptoms suggesting low testosterone, I urge you to talk to your doctor about trying TT. Ditto if your free testosterone is below the upper one-third of the normal range and you have high cholesterol or high blood pressure. (If your doctor ignores you and says, "The test is normal," see a holistic physician instead.)

Some doctors who research the benefits of TT favor a slightly different approach for measuring testosterone that they (and I) think is more reliable: They check the total testosterone, check the level of proteins that transport testosterone (sex hormone binding globulin, or SHBG), and calculate the free testosterone on that basis. If you're intrigued by this approach, ask your doctor to use a lab that is willing to do it. (You can find organizations of holistic physicians in Resources on page 360.)

Please see Male Menopause (Testosterone Deficiency) on page 287 for my Real Cure Regimen for this problem.

Low Estrogen and Progesterone

More than 37 million American women are menopausal, a condition characterized by low estrogen. *And that means tens of millions of Americans may be experiencing symptoms like these…*

- **Hot flashes**
- **Insomnia**
- **Fatigue**
- **Thinner, drier vaginal tissues,** with painful intercourse and more vaginal infections
- **Bladder problems,** such as recurrent infections and urinary incontinence
- **Headaches**
- **Muscle pain**
- **Dry skin, eyes, and mouth**
- **Dimmer memory, poorer concentration, and less mental clarity**

- **Mood swings,** with more anxiety and depression
- **Diminished sex drive**
- **Irregular bleeding during perimenopause,** the years before menopause, when the length and frequency of the menstrual cycle start to change

Low estrogen has such wide-ranging effects because there are estrogen receptors throughout the body. But estrogen (a general term for several estrogens, including estradiol, estriol, and estrone) doesn't act alone. Before menopause, it teams up with its sister hormone progesterone to keep reproductive organs healthy, regulate the menstrual cycle, and prepare the body for pregnancy. In fact, throughout the body, estrogen is the "see" to progesterone's "saw." Estrogen attracts fat; progesterone burns it. Estrogen retains fluid; progesterone drains it. Estrogen excites emotions; progesterone calms. But a toxic combination of unnatural estrogen (derived from horse urine) and synthetic progesterone (from chemicals)—a combination dubbed hormone replacement therapy (HRT)—might kill you.

The Hormone Horror Story—With a Happy, Natural Ending

That was the 2002 finding from the Women's Health Initiative (WHI) study of more than 16,000 healthy postmenopausal women who for five years or more took HRT: a combination of estrogen from horse urine (Premarin) and the synthetic and very unnatural progestin *medroxyprogesterone* (Provera). The combo increased the risk of breast cancer by 26 percent, the risk of heart attack by 29 percent, and the risk of stroke by 41 percent. (Up to that point, HRT was touted as a way to *prevent* heart disease.)

A study published in the *New England Journal of Medicine* confirmed the findings on breast cancer. Researchers at Stanford School of Medicine looked at data from more than 56,000 women, including 15,000 in the original WHI study.

They found: (1) that women who stayed on HRT for five years doubled their risk of breast cancer; (2) that a 50 percent decrease in HRT between 2002 and 2003 was linked to a 43 percent reduction in breast cancer rates; and (3) that among women who stopped taking HRT, rates of breast cancer dropped by 28 percent.

No wonder that since the WHI results, the use of HRT has fallen by more than 60 percent. But menopausal women don't have to forgo the advantages of estrogen and progesterone.

There's a safer form of HRT: Replacement therapy with bioidentical, or natural, hormones, which have been recommended by holistic doctors for decades.

The Beauty of Bioidentical Hormones

Conventional HRT uses hormones that aren't chemically similar to those produced by your body, and in many cases those hormones are synthetic—a concoction of lab-invented chemicals. Those hormones are used for one reason and one reason only: Companies can patent them and profit from them.

Natural bioidentical hormones are not patentable because they're exact replicas of the chemical structure of your own hormones, and they're derived from plants (such as soybeans).

Natural vs. Synthetic: Science Says Natural Is Better

Many scientific studies—particularly those comparing bioidentical progesterone with the synthetic version (medroxyprogesterone acetate, or MPA)—show that natural hormones are superior to synthetic. *A sampling of research findings…*

•**More relief from menopausal symptoms.** In a study of 176 postmenopausal women by doctors at the Mayo Clinic published in the *Journal of Women's Health & Gender-Based Medicine*, those who switched from using synthetic progesterone to natural progesterone reported more relief from hot flashes, insomnia, anxiety, and depression.

•**Healthier HDL levels.** In a study of 26 postmenopausal women, those on synthetic hormones had a drop of 15 percent in levels of good HDL (high-density lipoprotein) cholesterol, including a 25 percent drop in a "fraction" of HDL known to be particularly protective against heart disease. Meanwhile, those on natural hormones had little or no change in HDL. "As regards the effects on the lipoproteins," natural hormones "might be more suitable" than synthetic hormones, concluded the researchers in the *European Journal of Clinical Investigation.*

•**Less risk for women with heart disease.** In a study of 18 postmenopausal women with heart disease or a previous heart attack, those taking natural hormones had more blood flow to the heart during exercise than those taking synthetic hormones, reported Italian researchers in the *Journal of the American College of Cardiology.* "These results imply the choice of progestin [synthetic progesterone] in women at higher cardiovascular risk requires careful consideration," the researchers write. I'd say that's true of everybody who is treated with hormones!

•**Fewer menstrual problems, better memory.** In a study by Canadian researchers of 182 perimenopausal and menopausal women 45 to 65 years old, only those taking bioidentical progesterone had improvements in menstrual problems and in memory, concentration, and mental clarity. Therapy with bioidentical hormones "is a clinically effective, well-tolerated and cost-comparable alternative" to HRT, concluded the researchers in the journal *Clinical Therapeutics.*

•**Less vaginal bleeding and breast tenderness.** In a study of 10 postmenopausal women, those taking MPA had more vaginal bleeding and breast tenderness than those taking bioidentical progesterone. "These lesser side effects" of the bioidentical hormone "suggest that some women may prefer it to an MPA-containing regimen," concluded the researchers from the University of California, San Francisco, in the journal *Menopause.*

An interesting aside from the researchers: "In contrast with the widely held belief among psychiatrists that progesterone depresses mood, neither of the progesterones we used in normal, non-depressed and non-anxious women showed this effect."

All of this positive research led the FDA to recently approve the bioidentical estrogen/progesterone drug Bijuva—with a study from the Eastern Virginia Medical School showing that it safely relieved unwanted symptoms of menopause, such as hot flashes and poor sleep.

Bottom line: The science clearly shows that bioidentical hormones are better and safer. But synthetics are more profitable. So which do you think physicians have learned about?

Synthetic hormones are dangerous, with potentially deadly side effects. Natural hormones are safe. In fact, synthetic hormones and natural hormones probably have completely opposite effects on cells, said the late Joel Hargrove, MD, who was a professor in the Department of Obstetrics and Gynecology at Vanderbilt University School of Medicine in Nashville, and a leading proponent of bioidentical hormones. *He theorized that synthetic hormones...*

- **Damage genes within cells, much like an environmental toxin**
- **Are toxic to estrogen-sensitive tissues**
- **Blunt the liver's ability to detoxify carcinogens**
- **Bind differently to estrogen receptors**
- **Alter the way other hormones bind to those receptors**

"It is this distinction and potential difference in metabolic consequences, as well as the shorter half-life of bioidentical hormones, that motivates me to almost exclusively use bioidentical hormones," Tori Hudson, ND, an adjunct clinical professor at several naturopathic medical schools, medical director of A Woman's Time Clinic, and author of *Women's Encyclopedia of Natural Medicine*, told us about the findings of Dr. Hargrove.

It's so important that you understand this point that I'll summarize it again: Natural hormones do not have the same negative side effects as synthetic hormones. They are a safe and reasonable approach to hormone replacement therapy that doesn't carry the risk of Premarin and Provera.

In my own practice, I prescribe bioidentical hormones taken in a balance of estrogen and progesterone that duplicates that found in a young woman. The form of estrogen I use is called Biest, and in the past, 1.25 milligrams to 2.5 milligrams daily, containing 0.5 milligram of estradiol and 2 milligrams of estriol, was considered a good dose for most women. The good news? I am starting to believe that much lower dosing may be even better, with 0.10 milligram to 0.50 milligram a day being plenty.

If you take supplemental estrogen, you must also take natural progesterone to prevent uterine cancer. (Estrogen can mutate uterine cells in postmenopausal women.) I usually add natural progesterone even in women who have had a hysterectomy, because progesterone also improves sleep and decreases anxiety. You'll probably find that a dose of 30 milligrams for topical creams or 100 milligrams a day by mouth, taken at bedtime, is best.

Progesterone also can be used to treat PMS, and bioidentical progesterone—usually in the form of a topical cream—is a superb option for that problem. "As a practitioner, when using the progesterone creams, I largely use the creams that have at least 400 mg progesterone per ounce because they yield the best results for most women suffering from PMS," said Dr. Hudson.

See my Real Cure Regimen for Menopausal Problems on page 290.

Digestive Difficulties

It Takes Guts to Feel Good

"You are what you eat" goes the famous saying about food and health. But a more accurate version might be "You are what you digest." The digestive tract—a 20- to 30-foot-long pipe extending from mouth to anus—turns the food you eat into, well, into *you. And that manufacturing process requires an assembly line of organs…*

•**In your mouth,** chewing and saliva start to break down food before you swallow it. (Even before you take a bite, the sight and smell of food prompt your brain to rev up your salivary glands and pump out digestive juices.)

•**In your esophagus,** the tube from the mouth to the stomach, peristalsis begins its rhythmic action—the waves of muscular contractions that push food along the length of your digestive tract. A few seconds after you swallow a bite of food, peristalsis has accomplished its first task, and at the bottom of the esophagus a miniature door of muscle—the lower esophageal sphincter—opens to admit the food into your stomach.

•**In your stomach,** millions of specialized parietal cells in the lining produce hydrochloric acid (HCl), which further breaks down food (and mercilessly dissolves any nasty bacteria and viruses that have piggybacked on your lunch). Your stomach also produces pepsin, a digestive enzyme that breaks down protein; lipase, an enzyme that breaks down fat; and intrinsic factor, a compound that is critical for the absorption of B_{12}, a nutrient essential for the health of your blood, nerves, muscles, brain, and overall energy. The end product of all that action: chyme, a soup-like slurry that exits at the bottom of the stomach through the pyloric valve.

•**In your small intestine,** the chyme travels down the 20-foot stretch of the digestive tract. It's here that the food is reduced to its respective nutrients. These mealtime molecules are absorbed into the bloodstream via the villi, a microscopic mob of thumb-shaped structures that line the small intestine. The villi also pump out digestive enzymes and block the absorption of germs, toxins, and other undesirables. Digestion in the small intestine (and in other sections of the digestive tract) is aided by several other organs outside of, but connected to, the digestive tract: your pancreas, which produces digestive enzymes and bicarbonates to reduce the acidity of the chyme; your liver, which (among its many functions) manufactures bile to digest fat; and your gallbladder, a storage tank for bile.

•**In your large intestine,** or colon, the last of the nutrients and water are absorbed, and stool is formed. This task is aided by microscopic creatures that have taken a liking to your tract: trillions of friendly bacteria called microflora, microbiota, and (when they're packed into a supplement) probiotics. They keep bad bacteria in check, manufacture vitamins, aid peristalsis, strengthen the immune system, and regulate blood fats.

•**In your rectum,** stool is stored until there's enough for a bowel movement, when a ring of muscle called the internal sphincter relaxes, signaling the brain it's time to find a toilet.

Digestive Diseases

What we just described is Digestive Utopia—your digestive tract when all is literally going well. But most of us don't live in Wellville. An estimated 65 million Americans have digestive problems. And as we discuss later in the chapter, digestive diseases can cause and complicate many other chronic health problems. *Here's a quick review of the most common digestive problems, from the merely discomforting to the potentially deadly...*

•**Heartburn.** Instead of staying in the stomach where it belongs, hydrochloric acid "refluxes" up through the esophageal sphincter, burning the vulnerable lining of the esophagus and throat. (This problem is called by various names, including acid reflux and gastroesophageal reflux disease, or GERD.) Sixty percent of Americans have regular bouts of heartburn, and we spend billions of dollars a year on heartburn drugs to prevent and stop the pain.

•**Ulcers and gastritis.** The chances are about one in seven that sometime in your life you'll suffer a peptic ulcer—a painful hole in the lining of the stomach (gastric ulcer) or in the lining of the section between the small intestine and the stomach (duodenal ulcer). In milder cases, called gastritis, the stomach lining is irritated. A very common cause of ulcers: aspirin and other nonsteroidal anti-inflammatory (NSAID) medications, estimated to cause up to 16,500 deaths per year due to bleeding ulcers. Other ulcers are caused by stomach infections with *H. pylori* bacteria.

•**Indigestion.** You feel uncomfortably full after a meal and your stomach aches. Doctors call indigestion *dyspepsia*. If dyspepsia doesn't have a diagnosable cause (such as GERD, an ulcer, or stomach cancer, to name three possible causes), they call it *functional dyspepsia*. (*Functional* is a term doctors like to use when they can't figure out the cause of an ongoing problem.)

●**Food poisoning.** Noxious bacteria such as salmonella—hiding out in meat, greens, nuts, and other foods—sicken approximately 48 million Americans every year. (Most think they have the stomach flu and never figure out the food that caused it.)

●**Irritable bowel syndrome (IBS), or spastic colon.** An estimated 45 million American adults—two-thirds of them women—struggle with this so-called functional disease (conventional doctors don't have a clue what causes it). Symptoms can include abdominal pain, abdominal cramping and bloating, straining with constipation, or rushing to the bathroom with diarrhea. In some cases, constipation and diarrhea take turns. But IBS does have treatable causes, such as an undiagnosed bowel infection, a thyroid disorder, inadequate digestive enzymes, or stress.

●**Inflammatory bowel disease (IBD).** Three million Americans suffer with this inflammation of the lining of the intestine. It's called *Crohn's disease* when the inflammation is in patches in the small or large intestine, and called *colitis* when it's a sheet of inflammation in the colon or rectum. IBD typically flares up and then quiets down. Its short- and long-term symptoms can include fever, bloody stools, abdominal pain and cramping, thickening of the intestinal lining, and fistulas—tunneling growths out of the intestinal tract that may require surgery.

●**Food allergies.** We're not talking about a "classic" allergy to a food like peanuts, which produces acute allergic symptoms such as hives and swelling. We're talking about a type of food allergy also called *food intolerance* or *food sensitivity*. In this case, the small intestine doesn't adequately digest a food component (typically a protein), and the immune system attacks the remnant. The result is a dizzying array of possible symptoms, including digestive upsets of all kinds, headaches, fatigue, depression, joint and muscle pain, and rashes. Two very common forms of food intolerance are gluten intolerance (gluten is a protein component of wheat, barley, rye, and several other grains) and lactose intolerance (caused by a deficiency of the enzyme that digests lactose, the natural sugar found in dairy products). In the most serious form of gluten intolerance, an individual has celiac disease: Gluten triggers the immune system to attack and damage the villi, thread-like extensions on the digestive wall that aid digestion.

●**Gallstones.** Every year, 1.2 million Americans have their gallbladders removed to stop gallbladder attacks—caused by a gallbladder filled with gallstones, which can be microscopic shards or as big as a golf ball, and usually consist of congealed cholesterol.

●**Flatulence.** Passing gas is normal—everybody does it, about a dozen times a day. But if you're passing gas a lot more than that, and it's really smelly, you've got a digestive problem.

●**Constipation.** Most doctors consider it normal for their patients to have a bowel movement every three days. I don't. One movement a day is what's healthy. Otherwise, your stool is sitting in your digestive tract for too long, releasing toxins. A truly healthy transit time (the time it takes food to travel from mouth to anus) is 12 hours to 30 hours. A normal stool is large, relatively soft, and easy to pass, not small, hard, and difficult to dispose of.

●**Hemorrhoids.** Fifty percent of Americans over age 50 have hemorrhoids, damage to the blood vessels around the anus, with possible itching, pain, and bleeding. A common cause is constipation and straining at stool.

Chilled Drinks Stop Enzymes Cold

The digestive enzymes in your mouth and stomach and the enzymes in food work best at body temperature. A 40°F drink literally stops those enzymes cold. If your digestion is fine, you're cool to enjoy your iced drinks with meals.

But if indigestion is your plight, take a tip from traditional Chinese medicine, which emphasizes the relationship of food and health: Drink warm liquids during meals, to aid digestion. Tea is delightful, as is warm water with a squirt of lemon. Save those iced drinks for between meals.

Why Your Digestion Doesn't Work

To conventional doctors—including most gastroenterologists—the underlying causes of bad digestion remain a mystery. That's why medicine's so-called cures are usually nothing more than a pill to quiet symptoms or surgery to remove the offending organ.

But there *are* real causes of digestive problems, even if conventional doctors don't acknowledge them. *Here are the main culprits...*

The Case of the Disappearing Enzymes

Ask a conventional digestive expert what role enzymes play in your digestion, and he'll talk about the digestive enzymes that your body manufactures: the amylase from the salivary glands that digests carbohydrate; the pepsin from the stomach that digests protein; the lipase from the small intestine that digests fat (not to mention the trypsin, the lactase, and many more).

But here's a crucial fact about digestive enzymes that doctors aren't taught: They play a secondary role in digestion to another set of enzymes—the enzymes in food. The most important enzymes for digestion are those normally found in foods, such as the enzymes that ripen an apple or tomato. "You've seen the brown spots that appear on fruit when it's been bruised. The brown shows the work of enzymes beginning to digest the fruit. When we chew these foods, these same enzymes are released and go right to work on the food substance," we were told by Martie Whittekin, CCN, a certified nutritionist, host of the *Healthy By Nature Radio Show*, and author of *Natural Alternatives to Nexium, Maalox, Tagamet, Prilosec & Other Acid Blockers*.

But food manufacturers learned long ago that removing enzymes lengthens shelf life (and increases profitability). So that's just what they did, using chemicals, gassing, and other processing techniques to strip out the natural enzymes. The upside: The food doesn't rot on the shelf. The downside: It becomes hard to digest, causing indigestion.

Failing the Acid Test

The burning sensation and sour taste of acid indigestion are extremely unpleasant. But those symptoms are usually easy to clear up. One-half teaspoon of alkaline bicarbonate of soda in four ounces of water can quickly neutralize the acid and relieve the pain. Over-the-counter antacids with alkalinizing minerals (which use calcium combined with magnesium; see page 103) also work, and as little as ¼ tablet can squelch the pain of heartburn when it acts up. But Americans no longer rely on those old-time yet effective antacids.

Instead, we've become enamored of the newest class of heartburn drugs: the proton pump inhibitors (PPIs), which shut down the stomach's acid-producing parietal cells. Those drugs include *esomeprazole* (Nexium), *lansoprazole* (Prevacid), and *omeprazole* (Prilosec), which are available both over the counter and by prescription—with more than 140 million prescriptions written a year. What happens when you regularly take a drug that cuts the production of stomach acid by 80 percent so that the two quarts of stomach acid your body naturally produces every day is reduced to a trickle?

You may not have acid indigestion, but you also won't have enough acid to thoroughly break down nutrients to prepare them for absorption in the small intestine. For example, you probably won't absorb a normal amount of calcium, which is why studies are showing that taking PPIs can double your risk of bone fractures. PPIs also can double your risk of a vitamin B_{12} deficiency. That's because B_{12} digestion requires both stomach acid and the intrinsic factor produced by your parietal cells—cells that have been virtually paralyzed by the drug. Low blood levels of B_{12} can cause a host of problems, from nerve damage to dementia.

Those are the science-proven nutritional deficiencies linked to PPIs. I think it's likely that taking the drug generates many other vitamin and mineral deficiencies, including critical nutrients such as zinc, magnesium, and folate. And while PPIs are stealing your nutrients, they're also hustling bad guys into your body. Stomach acid kills nasty bacteria and viruses. That's why people who take acid-blocking PPIs have a higher risk of viral, bacterial, yeast, and parasitic infections. And those bad bacteria not only cause respiratory infections. They also overwhelm the friendly bacteria in the colon, causing all kinds of digestive and health problems.

But PPIs aren't finished with you yet. If you have heart disease, PPIs increase your risk of dying from a heart attack. (Talk about heartburn!) Nobody knows why this happens, but when you mess with the fundamentals of digestion, you mess with the fundamentals of health.

Finally, PPIs are addictive. That's right, addictive, like cigarettes.

Here's what happens: When you stop the drug, your parietal cells start to party (like a binge after a diet), generating huge amounts of stomach acid. This phenomenon—called rebound acid hypersecretion—causes the very heartburn symptoms the drug is intended to prevent. In one study, 60 healthy people were given PPIs for two months, and 44 percent had heartburn when they stopped the medication. And the heartburn can take one month to three months to go away.

Needless to say, if you've been taking the drug to prevent heartburn or indigestion (70 percent of PPIs are prescribed for digestive problems other than heartburn), and you stop the drug and the symptoms return, you're not going to tough it out. You're going to start taking the drug again. In other words, you're addicted.

Calcium Antacids—Weapons of Mass Destruction?

Sometimes, it's the small things that sneak up on us. With food processing triggering widespread indigestion, there are millions of people using chewable calcium antacids (e.g., Tums). With a research review in the *British Medical Journal* (*BMJ*) (reviewing about 12,000 women in 11 studies) showing a 41 percent increased risk of heart attack in women taking plain calcium (without vitamin D or magnesium) for osteoporosis, major red flags were raised.

Consider this: The "tolerable upper intake" of daily calcium has been set at 2,500 milligrams a day by the Food and Nutrition Board. Tums and most chewable antacids have as much as 1,000 milligrams of calcium per chewable tab. With many people chewing five to 10 antacids a day, this is not how I would spell relief.

The good news? There is a simple solution! Though taking plain calcium raised concerns, when it was taken along with vitamin D (e.g., in the Women's Health Initiative study with 36,000 women), there was no increased risk. In addition, I suspect that adding magnesium to the calcium will likely not only cancel out the risk, but actually be heart healthy. So when you need a chewable antacid to put out the fire, use one that includes both magnesium and vitamin D to protect your heart. Better yet, add plant-based digestive enzymes to help improve digestion.

Also: Try Heartburn Rescue (D-limonene and sea buckthorne oil by Terry Naturally) to help heal your stomach.

Now, it's fine to take a PPI a few times a month, if you really think you need it. But regular use of this type of drug is a big mistake. When heartburn hits, try a chewable antacid instead. Avoid antacids containing only calcium (like Tums). Plain calcium is associated with a 31 percent higher risk of heart attack, so change to an antacid that includes magnesium. (For more on this, see "Calcium Antacids—Weapons of Mass Destruction?" above.)

Here's another little-known fact about heartburn that makes taking PPIs all the more problematic: Chronic heartburn is often caused not by too much stomach acid, but by too little. This condition is called hypochlorhydria. "I've observed that nine out of ten of us who suffer from so-called 'acid indigestion' actually have *lack-of-acid indigestion*," observes Jonathan Wright, MD, a nutritionally oriented doctor and medical director of the Tahoma Clinic in Tukwila, Washington, in his book *Why Stomach Acid Is Good for You.*

How can an underproduction of stomach acid cause the problem most everyone thinks is due to acid overload? Simple. Meals and heartburn-causing acid hang around in the stomach longer than nature intended because you don't have enough concentrated stomach acid to turn the food into the soupy chyme that is ready for the small intestine. After a couple of hours, your body says to itself, "This meal isn't working out. Maybe we should send the undigested food back the way it came." And an HCl-loaded slurry sloshes out of your stomach into your esophagus.

The Chew-Chew Train of Good Digestion

You might not think of your mouth as part of your digestive tract, just as you don't think of the ticket booth at the theater as part of the movie—but it's the entrance.

Nature intended one-third of digestion to take place at the entrance to the digestive tract, before food descends to the stomach. You chew food, of course, breaking it down. And chewing generates saliva, which contains enzymes that start to digest carbohydrates.

Chewing, however, is out of style. We eat in our cars, hardly noticing we're eating. Or we eat while watching TV—more attentive to advertisements for antacids, gas reducers, and diarrhea stoppers than to our meals. And we eat massive portions, wolfing down our Biggie Burger, Gigantic Fries, and Colossal Cola so fast that it's more like inhaling than chewing.

Savoring our food with slow, sensuous chewing that allows us to enjoy every bite? Not a chance. The result of too little chewing is poor digestion. And packing on extra weight—because research shows that when you don't chew, you mindlessly consume more calories. When scientists instructed a group of study participants to chew each bite of a meal 15 to 20 times (and put down their utensils between bites), they ate fewer calories. They also said they enjoyed the meal more.

And enjoyment is crucial for good digestion. A low-stress mind-set sends calming messages to your digestive tract to keep food moving along. On the other hand, stressed-out, high-speed eating triggers the fight-or-flight response, which tenses our digestive muscles.

The moral of this story: Slow down and chew, enjoying your meal and better digestion.

Other problems caused by low levels of HCl can include…

•**The esophageal sphincter that keeps acid in the stomach doesn't get a signal to close**—another reason why low levels of acid can cause acid reflux.

•**Protein digestion doesn't begin in the stomach, as it should.**

•**The small intestine isn't signaled to start generating its protein-digesting enzymes.**

•**Similarly, the small intestine isn't signaled to generate acid-neutralizing bicarbonate.**

"In short," says Whittekin, "low digestive acid breaks the digestive chain." Low stomach acid is often the real cause of heartburn—and you can find my Real Cure Regimen for the problem in Heartburn and Indigestion on page 250.

100 Trillion Bacteria Gone Bad

Let's start this section with an astonishing statistic: There are more bacteria in your digestive tract than there are cells in your body—as many as 100 trillion, 10 times the number of cells.

But if all is right in your digestive world, most of those bacteria aren't there to infect you. They're so-called friendly bacteria, there to lend your health a helping hand (or maybe some helping fimbriae, the little extensions that allow bacteria to stick to surfaces). The vast majority of these friendly bacteria live in your colon. In terms of total volume, half the colon is bacteria.

What are they doing there, exactly? Nutritionist and digestive expert Elizabeth Lipski, PhD, provided us with a long list. It may not have a trillion items, but it's still impressive. *Friendly bacteria…*

- **Acidify the colon,** keeping bad bacteria in check (including the bacteria that cause food poisoning)
- **Stop disease-causing fungi from setting up shop**
- **Hold down the production of toxins**
- **Protect against environmental toxins,** such as pesticides
- **Keep peristalsis normal**
- **Regulate transit time,** preventing constipation and diarrhea
- **Break down bile**
- **Manufacture B vitamins and vitamin K**
- **Increase the absorption of minerals such as magnesium and calcium**
- **Manufacture essential fatty acids**
- **Break protein into amino acids**
- **Convert flavonoids** (plant compounds that calm inflammation and oxidation) into forms the body can use
- **Strengthen the immune system,** by manufacturing natural antibiotics and boosting the production of immune cells
- **Limit the side effects of antibiotic drugs**
- **Break down and rebuild hormones, such as estrogen**
- **Regulate cholesterol and triglycerides, blood fats that can hurt the heart**
- **Kill cancer cells or stop them from dividing**

Now think about what might happen if all those functions of good bacteria were drastically reduced. You'd be sick! And that's just what is happening to tens of millions of Americans, who have a problem called *dysbiosis*.

Good bacteria continually have to hold their own against bad bacteria, stopping the bad guys from gaining too big a foothold (or fimbria-hold). But many factors of modern life defeat the good guys, producing dysbiosis—too big a population of bad bacteria.

In fact, a scientific study from Italian researchers showed that Italian children who ate a Western diet—high in red meat, fat, sugar, and other refined carbohydrates, and low in fiber—had many more bad bacteria and fewer good bacteria in their intestines than African children who ate a high-fiber, low-fat, vegetable-rich diet. The study researchers theorize that the predominance of bad bacteria is a key cause of the higher rate of allergy, autoimmune disease, and inflammatory bowel disease among people who eat a Western diet.

"The intestine is the site where the immune system meets the microbiota," said Italian gastro-enterologist Paolo Lionetti, MD, PhD, the study leader. "If we change our diets, then we change our microbiota—and then we can improve our health."

Eating more vegetables, fruits, and fiber-rich whole grains and less processed food is key to preventing and correcting dysbiosis. But you have to do a little more. You have to stop taking PPIs (not suddenly, though; see Heartburn and Indigestion on page 250). These drugs block the production of stomach acid, letting bad bacteria into the digestive tract—kind of like having an open border in a totally hostile environment.

Similarly, you have to limit your use of antibiotics to when they are absolutely necessary, because every time you take an antibiotic, you commit bacterial genocide in your colon. Perhaps you're hoping that friendly bacteria will recolonize. Maybe they will, maybe they won't. Many people who take antibiotics end up with colons overrun by *Clostridium difficile*, an antibiotic-resistant bacteria that causes diarrhea. And sometimes those *C. difficile* run amok, causing *Clostridium difficile* disease (CDD), with high fever, bloody stools, nausea, abdominal pain, dehydration, and, in a few cases, death.

You can read more about the problems with antibiotics—and how to minimize their use—in the chapter titled Prescription Medications on page 81.

But bad bacteria don't only bother the colon. They can also cause a condition called small intestine bacterial overgrowth (SIBO), in which the relatively "sterile" small intestine (with billions rather than trillions of intestinal bacteria) is overgrown with 10 times the normal amount. And most of that overgrowth consists of bad guys. The symptoms of SIBO are similar to those of irritable bowel syndrome: abdominal pain and bloating, diarrhea and/or constipation, and excess gas. (Some digestive experts assert that IBS is caused by SIBO, but I think there are many more factors involved, and they differ from person to person.)

How to distinguish SIBO from irritable bowel? It can be very easy! Although most doctors will do a Hydrogen Breath Test, I prefer a more low-tech approach. In SIBO, bacteria in the small intestine start feasting on amino acids before they're completely absorbed. When the bacteria eat these proteins, they release their sulfur—which causes a rotten egg smell. Remember the kid in

SIBO and Your Thyroid

An Italian study of 90 people showed that 54 percent of those with hypothyroidism also had small intestine bacterial overgrowth (SIBO), compared with five percent of those without the thyroid problem.

The researchers noted that low thyroid function slows peristalsis, the contraction of the intestinal muscles that moves food through the digestive tract. When food is stalled, bad bacteria can thrive, and you can end up with SIBO. You'll find the real causes of hypothyroidism discussed in Hormonal Imbalances on page 84 and the real cures in Hypothyroidism on page 254.

elementary school who would pass those "silent but deadlies?" If your gas smells like that, you probably have SIBO. Achy muscles, fatigue, and hypothyroidism are also common among people with chronic SIBO.

Sugar Feeds the Yeast Beast

How much sugar do you eat every year? 10 pounds? 20? Keep going...

If you're an average American, you eat 57 pounds of sugar a year. And you ate more this year than last year: In the last several decades, our consumption of sugar has increased dramatically to 17 teaspoons a day, according to the Centers for Disease Control and Prevention. And you might consume significantly more than that if you regularly drink sweetened beverages such as soda or bottled teas.

What happens to all that sugar when it hits the warm, moist gut? It ferments. It churns. It bubbles. It produces gas. It creates exactly the type of intestinal action that produces the symptoms of digestive discomfort, such as bloating and flatulence.

Fermenting sugar is also the preferred diet of one type of microbiota: the yeast (or fungus) *Candida albicans*. It's fine for there to be *some* fungus in your intestines, but you don't want that fungus to multiply and take over. With a daily diet rich in sugar, the yeast do just that, pushing aside good bacteria, pumping out toxins, sparking inflammation, and generally causing ill health.

An overgrowth of candida can cause many problems conventional doctors don't link to yeast, such as chronic sinusitis, allergies, skin rashes, susceptibility to infections—and sugar cravings, as the yeast "channel" their desire for more sugar into your body and nervous system.

You can find my Real Cure Regimen in Candida Overgrowth on page 181.

Leaky Gut, Sinking Health

But the yeast aren't finished with you yet. During their growth period, yeast produce mycelia, threadlike structures that burrow into the intestinal wall—and poke holes through it!

This problem is called leaky gut syndrome. And it can sink your health. Here's what happens. A protein is a chainlike structure made up of links called amino acids. To digest a protein, the small intestine splits it up and allows single links through the intestinal wall into the bloodstream. But when the intestinal wall has holes in it, several links can slip into the bloodstream before they're broken down. And your immune system thinks those oversize links—such as chunks of the gluten from wheat or the casein from dairy—are foreign invaders.

So why is this a problem, exactly? Picture someone infected with cold or flu viruses every day, day after day. Think how worn out their immune system would become...how the weakened immune system would leave them vulnerable to all kinds of other infections and health problems...how the constant activity of the immune system would create chronic inflammation. You get the picture.

As you've probably surmised, that's exactly what can and does happen when people develop leaky gut syndrome, albeit in a milder form. The good news? It's very treatable.

Poor Digestion, Poor Health

By now, we bet you've gotten the main point of this chapter: When your digestion is poor, your health suffers the consequences. You develop not only digestive diseases, but diseases of all kinds. *Let's take a final look at the core factors that make digestive problems a real cause of disease...*

●**Poor nutrition.** When digestion is second rate, you absorb fewer nutrients—and nutritional deficiencies are a real cause of many diseases, including heart disease, cancer, and stroke, the leading killers of Americans. You can read more in Nutritional Deficiencies on page 3.

●**Taking more prescription drugs.** If you have heartburn, you're likely taking PPIs. These drugs increase your risk of nutritional deficiencies, bone fractures, infections, and dying from heart disease. You also have less stomach acid, which hobbles digestion, causing who knows what other problems. You can read more about PPIs as a real cause of disease in Prescription Medications on page 70.

●**More inflammation.** Poor nutrition means that there are fewer circulating antioxidants sweeping up cell-damaging free radicals—and those free radicals are a leading factor in heart disease, cancer, Alzheimer's, and other diseases. Poor digestion also causes leaky gut syndrome, which leads to inflammation, a risk factor for dozens of diseases. You can read more about this as a real cause in Chronic Inflammation on page 118.

●**More toxicity.** Think of a hamburger sitting out on a sidewalk in the heat for a couple of days. Kind of disgusting, right? Now think of that hamburger sitting in your body—a steamy 98.6°F—for a couple of days. That's the ugly reality if digestion is disabled and your transit time is slow. And slow transit time is very common among us digestively challenged Americans. You can read more about toxicity in Cellular Toxicity on page 109.

●**Poor immunity.** The lack of nutrients, the candida invasion, and the dysbiosis all weaken immunity, setting you up for colds; flu; and other respiratory diseases such as chronic sinusitis, asthma, and allergies (which often go hand in hand); autoimmune diseases such as rheumatoid arthritis and multiple sclerosis; and even cancer.

The Solutions Are Surprisingly Simple

In the chapters ahead, you'll find many other simple but effective solutions for digestive problems. After you read these chapters, we have a gut feeling that you'll be feeling a lot better!

Cellular Toxicity

Stay Clean in a Dirty World

t's a basic and natural part of the process of being alive: You take in what you need, and you get rid of what you don't.

You take in oxygen and get rid of carbon monoxide. You take in food and get rid of feces. You take in water and get rid of urine. And for the most part, what you get rid of are toxins, stuff that your body can't use and that can cause disease if it hangs around and damages cells.

Toxins include formerly good stuff (such as hormones) that has done its job and been broken down for disposal, and bad stuff (such as pollutants and pesticides) that in an ideal world wouldn't have ended up in your body in the first place.

Detoxification 101

The body detoxifies in a couple of different ways.

The liver. This football-size organ sits under your ribs on the right side of your abdomen. If it suddenly stopped working, you'd be dead in a day. Among its many metabolic chores, the liver detoxifies, using what are called phase I and phase II detoxification pathways. In phase I, liver enzymes (proteins that spark biochemical activity) dismantle toxins. In phase II, the liver shunts the tidied toxins into various channels of chemical action for disposal through the kidneys (in the form of urine) or the bile (via the feces). *Speaking of which...*

Bile. From Hippocrates in ancient Greece to the physicians of the 19th century, Western doctors thought health was determined by a balance of four "humors." Two of the four were bile—yellow and black—and one idea was that too much bile could make you ill-tempered or depressed. Well, it's hard not to regard bile as a bit vile. The liver produces the brown fluid and then deposits toxins in it, like a chemical company dumping waste into a stream. The bile is stored in the gallbladder and then squirted into the intestinal tract, where it performs double duty: disposing of those toxins via the feces and breaking down fats for absorption.

Urine. Among their many tasks, the kidneys filter blood, removing toxins to the urine for disposal. The kidneys also rid the body of excess urea and other toxins produced by normal metabolism.

Sweat. Your skin has *millions* of sweat glands, which squeeze out sweat to not only cool the body but also to send toxins on their way.

Breathing. This moment-to-moment process is the epitome of natural detoxification. You inhale life-giving oxygen and exhale a poisonous gas. And breathing demonstrates another basic fact about detoxification: The body does it automatically. No worries!

But modern life has added some plot twists to that simple story.

The Toxic 21st

Creative chemists have cooked up more than 80,000 synthetic compounds that industry enthusiastically employs—and that end up polluting our environment.

A good example is the polychlorinated biphenyls, or PCBs. This nearly indestructible class of chemicals are perfect conductors, and are widely used as coolants and insulators in the generation and flow of electricity. Unfortunately, PCBs are as toxic as they are handy: They can damage the skin, liver, immune system, and reproductive system. And at this point in human history, there's nowhere on Earth that PCBs are not. You can find them in the soil in New York's Central Park, in the ice cap at the North Pole, and in your body fat.

But in spite of the presence of PCBs and those 80,000-or-so other chemicals that are dumped into our environment, I'm in favor of the attitude expressed in the slogan made famous by the bestselling (and very humorous) book *The Hitchhiker's Guide to the Galaxy*:

Don't Panic!

There has never been a time on Earth when we humans didn't have to deal with a set of pressing problems. But in my experience, problems come packaged with their solutions. The healthiest approach does not include fearfully focusing on the problem. (That fearful state is itself a toxin for the body and mind.) Instead, ask yourself this problem-solving question: How can I support my body in its natural process of eliminating the toxins that are an inevitable part of 21st-century life?

Good news, fellow Earthlings: There are many easy ways to do just that.

If You Can't Read It, Don't Eat It

I used to give a yearly lecture on nutrition to third-graders in a local school. And at least one of my recommendations to those kids is relevant for everybody, from kindergarteners to postdocs to AARP members…*If you can't read it, don't eat it.*

You know what I'm talking about: ingredients on food labels that are virtually unreadable, such as…

•**Butylated hydroxytoluene** (the preservative BHT)

- **Sodium stearoyl lactylate** (a "whipping agent" that whips white bread into fluffier shapes)

- **2-methoxyacetophenone** (a flavoring favorite, in everything from frostings to fried chicken)

- **Acetaldehyde phenethyl propyl acetal** (a "fruit" flavoring found in ice cream, candy, cookies, and sodas)

- **2-hexyl-S-keto-1,4-dioxane** (tastes like cream)

These are just a few examples of the literally thousands of lab-concocted chemical additives used to process, preserve, and flavor our food. I don't think I need to do much more convincing on this point, because not eating a lot of food with ingredients you can't even read is common sense. Why barrage your body with toxic chemicals if you don't have to?

So if it's not exactly a food—if it's a foodlike substance of some kind—put it back on the shelf. Even if you can read the ingredients, you should still ask yourself these kinds of questions: Does it contain blueberries, or is it just blue? Is it naturally tasty, or has some clever food chemist conned me? If it wasn't propped up by preservatives, would it be rotting on the shelf right now?

Sum it up in this way: Choose whole foods whenever you can! At breakfast, sprinkle some strawberries, blueberries, or banana slices on whole grain, low-sugar oatmeal or cereal (such as Life or Cheerios). At lunch, have a tuna salad sandwich on whole grain bread, with a green salad and tomatoes. At dinner, enjoy a side dish of steamed vegetables with butter. After all, it's easy to pronounce *banana* and *tuna* and *lettuce* and *peas*...

Supplementing Detoxification

Various aspects of phase II liver detoxification require specific nutritional compounds to do their work. For example, glutathione—a protein-like antioxidant—is a must for detoxifying various pharmaceutical drugs, a wide range of pollutants, alcohol, and fungus found in food. To make glutathione, your body needs three key amino acids (components of protein): glycine, cysteine, and glutamine, along with vitamin C.

How can you make sure you're getting those nutrients? The multivitamin/mineral supplement I formulated—the Energy Revitalization System powder, from Nature's Way—supplies all those amino acids, vitamin C, and many other nutrients that support detoxification. It's one of the easiest ways to purify! Another good multivitamin mineral is Clinical Essentials, from Terry Naturally.

Drink Up!

Water plays a key role in daily detoxification. In fact, drinking enough water is probably the best action you can take to support your kidneys as they clean up your blood.

Water is also a key part of daily nutrition—a beverage that is as essential for your body as essential fatty acids, essential amino acids, and other basics that your body doesn't make on its own and that you must regularly consume. For example (and what follows is a very short list

Is Acid Raining on Your Health's Parade?

To stay alive, the body monitors and maintains a delicate balance between two basic types of compounds: alkalies and acids. Your cells prefer a slightly alkaline environment, but metabolic activities (from breathing to digesting) generate acids. To keep the pH value on the alkaline side, just above 7, the body detoxifies itself of the acids it's constantly producing, via the kidneys, skin, and lungs. But many Americans suffer from an internal environment that is too acidic, a condition called chronic low-grade metabolic acidosis. *That's because so many factors of modern life raise the body's acidity, such as...*

- **Too few alkalinizing vegetables, fruits, nuts, and seeds in the diet**
- **Too much acidifying meat, sugar, white flour, and other refined grains in the diet**
- **Too much acidifying alcohol and coffee in the diet**

Maybe you noticed a trend here, as in diet, diet, and diet? That diet-generated excess acid can play a role in causing and complicating a lot of health problems, including...

Osteoporosis (as alkaline minerals are pulled out of bones to counter the acidity)

High blood pressure (as pressure-lowering alkaline minerals such as potassium and magnesium are depleted)

Urinary and bladder problems (the bladder and urinary tract are irritated by the excess acid)

Kidney stones (which form more easily in an acidic environment)

Dysbiosis (the imbalance of good and bad bacteria in the colon, with bad bacteria thriving in an acidic setting)

Gum disease and dental decay (acids eat away at teeth and gums)

Rapid aging (because cells don't thrive in an acidic environment)

You might also have weaker immunity, fatigue, and chronic inflammation. In other words, excess acid burns your health! But as with most toxins, acid is surprisingly easy to neutralize.

Two smart tips: Eat more alkalinizing fresh vegetables and fruits; and when you drink water (an important detoxification method that we'll discuss in a second), add a slice of lemon—that extra acid paradoxically works to make bodily fluids more alkaline!

To see whether your system is alkaline or acid, measure the pH of your saliva or urine first thing in the morning using a strip of pH paper. Simple instructions come with the test strips, which you can purchase at BetterBones.com/shop and in many other online and retail stores.

of functions), water is critical for energy production, protects your DNA, transports compounds around the body, and is the solvent that helps the body break food into nutrients.

How much water should you drink every day? Well, if I imagine a hellish eternity, it includes spending eternity counting how many glasses of water to drink every day. Was that eight 8-ounce glasses a day, or six 6-ounce glasses, or half your body weight in ounces, or—arrgghh!

There's a saner, easier, and more natural way of making sure you're drinking enough water: Just check your lips and mouth. If they're dry, you need to drink more water. It's that simple!

Another simple method: Take a look at the color of your urine. If it's a dull yellow color, there's not enough water diluting it, so you should drink more water. (Urine can also turn bright yellow from B vitamins, but that's different from the murky yellow of overly concentrated urine.)

A third and interesting method: When you feel tired, drink a glass of water and see if your energy improves in a couple of minutes. If it does, you were dehydrated.

And yet another method, which I like to use: When I'm thirsty, I can easily chug a whole glass of water; when I'm not thirsty, I prefer to sip it.

The Importance of Pure Water

All tap water is not created equal. It can come from surface water (a river, lake, or reservoir), groundwater (an underground aquifer), or a well. It might be filtered by your municipality, or it might not. (Cities with so-called protected watersheds, such as New York and San Francisco, don't filter their water.) And as the *New York Times* reported in a series of articles called "Toxic Waters," it's very likely your tap water is filled with toxins. Consider these facts uncovered by the reporters and confirmed for us by Robert Morris, MD, PhD, an expert on drinking water and health, a visiting scholar at the University of Washington School of Public Health, and author of *The Blue Death: The Intriguing Past and Present Danger of the Water You Drink.*

●**During the past decade, an estimated 63 million Americans** have been exposed to drinking water that didn't meet governmental health guidelines.

●**Contaminated drinking water** sickens more than about 7.2 million Americans annually (according to the Centers for Disease Control and Prevention)—illnesses range from digestive upset to cancer.

●**The Safe Drinking Water Act regulates 91 chemicals,** but there are more than 60,000 chemicals in our drinking water.

You probably figure your local water treatment plant is protecting you from those chemicals and other contaminants. Don't count on it. Like the federal and state governments, local governments are hard-pressed to find funds to maintain and repair aging infrastructure. Treatment plants—and the pipes that bring tap water to your house—are getting on in years, putting you at risk. *What are some of the toxins that might be sneaking into your drinking water?*

●**Disease-causing germs,** such as *Cryptosporidium, Giardia,* and viruses

●**Metals and minerals,** such as lead and arsenic (Flint, Michigan, and Newark, New Jersey, are two glaring examples of cities where drinking water was and is polluted by lead)

●**Agricultural chemicals,** such as fertilizers and pesticides

●**Industrial chemicals** linked to cancer, such as the gasoline additive MTBE (methyl tert-butyl ether)

●**Chlorine by-products**—probably the most toxic of all—generated in the process of purifying water

●**Pharmaceutical drugs.** Yes, our drinking water is dosed with prescription drugs. A study by the U.S. Geological Survey and the Associated Press national investigation team showed that the drinking water of at least 46 million Americans contains traces of drugs for pain, infection, heart disease, high cholesterol, asthma, depression, and hormonal problems—a pharmacopoeia of pollutants from drug residue in urine and old drugs flushed down the toilet.

Knowing about the pollutants in tap water, perhaps you've decided to drink bottled water instead. Surveys show that more than half of us Americans think bottled water is safer and healthier than tap water, and we back up our opinion by drinking more than 14 billion gallons a year, or more than 40 gallons per person. But research shows that some of those bottles are contaminated with one of the chemicals used to produce them: bisphenol A (BPA), which studies link to poorer brain development and behavior problems in children, and reproductive problems in adults. (Although a lot of bottled water companies now offer BPA-free bottles, these bottles often contain a similar chemical—BPS, or bisphenol S—that may be just as harmful.)

A study published in the journal *Human Reproduction* linked male occupational exposure to BPA to a four-times-greater risk of erectile dysfunction, a seven-times-greater risk of ejaculation difficulty, a three-times-greater risk of reduced sexual desire, and a four-times-greater risk of "reduced satisfaction with sex life." The study also found the higher the exposure to BPA, the greater the risk of sexual difficulties—and the risk started to climb after only one year of BPA exposure.

Have you been exposed to BPA or BPS? Probably. A study by the government's Centers for Disease Control and Prevention showed that 93 percent of those tested had detectable amounts of BPA in their bodies. Another study showed that 80 percent of participants had detectable BPS.

It's not only the bottle that puts you at risk. Bottled water is sometimes less safe than tap water, according to tests conducted by the Environmental Working Group (EWG). "The bottled water industry is not required to disclose the results of any contaminant testing that it conducts," they said in a report. "Our tests strongly indicate the purity of bottled water cannot be trusted." (By the way, the EWG says the cities with the cleanest tap water include Boston, Honolulu, St. Louis, Minneapolis, and Austin. Cities at the bottom of the list include San Diego, Houston, Reno, Las Vegas, and Omaha.) I favor filtered tap water. Problem is, a lot of home filters don't work all that well. The most reliable types have either solid carbon block filters and/or reverse osmosis filters. A solid carbon block filter works by doing what its name says: The carbon blocks the contaminants. Reverse osmosis works in a different way, by applying pressure to the water and literally squeezing out the toxins.

I've found that the company Multipure makes excellent home water filters, which you can easily install at the faucet or below the sink. For more information, see Multipure.com.

Having said all this, it's also important to say that drinking tap water or bottled water is far better than being dehydrated.

But remember: Expensive is not superior. Over time, we will be much better off for having been weaned off disposable plastic bottles.

Sweat It Out in a Sauna

Sweating for health is a worldwide tradition. In Ayurveda, the ancient natural healing system of India, sweating therapy is one of the methods of detoxification. The ancient Slavic (Russian) tribes used a sauna-like structure called a *banya*. For millennia, Native Americans have used sweat lodges for physical purification and ceremonies to contact and receive direction from spirit ancestors. The Turkish hammam—a steam bath—was often attached to mosques as a place of purification. And the Finns, of course, have made the sauna famous worldwide.

All these traditions have one thing in common: They cause you to sweat, detoxifying through the skin. I think regular "sweat therapy" is a great way to aid detoxification, and a lot of scientists agree with me. *Here are some studies on sweating therapy and health…*

• **Type 2 diabetes.** People with type 2 diabetes who took 20-minute saunas three times a week, for three months, had an improvement in their health and well-being, reported Canadian researchers in the *Journal of Alternative and Complementary Medicine.* (The study participants used a far infrared sauna, which is the type I use for myself and recommend. You can read more about far infrared saunas—what they are and how to buy one—in "Sauna Suggestions" on page 116.)

• **Heart failure and peripheral artery disease.** Japanese researchers reviewed the benefits of Waon therapy, or "soothing warm therapy" (a type of Japanese sauna in which temperatures are kept at about 140°F, compared to a typical sauna, with temperatures ranging from 160° to 190°F). They noted that it helps patients with congestive heart failure and with peripheral artery disease, or PAD (clogged arteries in the legs, with painful walking). In patients with heart failure, it can increase circulation, normalize heart rhythm, and improve symptoms. In patients with PAD, it improves circulation, decreases pain, and speeds the healing of leg ulcers (a common symptom).

• **High blood pressure.** In a review of the health benefits of far infrared saunas, Canadian researchers note that these saunas have been shown to lower high blood pressure and improve congestive heart failure, as well as possibly easing chronic pain and aiding weight loss.

• **Rheumatoid arthritis.** Seven people with rheumatoid arthritis (an autoimmune disease that attacks and inflames the joints) took two far infrared saunas a week for four weeks. At the end of the study, they had less pain, stiffness, and fatigue, reported Dutch researchers in the medical journal *Clinical Rheumatology.*

• **Emotional well-being.** In a study of 45 people, mood was measured before and after a sauna. Afterward, the participants had less anxiety, depression, and anger, reported Japanese researchers in the journal *Complementary Therapies in Clinical Practice.*

• **Healthy skin.** People who regularly use saunas have stronger and moister skin than people who don't, found German researchers.

• **Fibromyalgia.** In a study published in the journal *Internal Medicine,* Japanese researchers found that 10 treatments with Waon therapy improved the painful symptoms of fibromyalgia (near-constant muscle pain, usually all over the body) by as much as 78 percent.

• **Chronic fatigue syndrome.** Japanese researchers treated 11 patients with chronic fatigue syndrome—severe, unrelenting fatigue—with far infrared sauna therapy. Symptoms improved in all 11 patients, including two for whom fatigue levels "dramatically improved." The patients also felt more relaxed and had better appetites and less depression.

Speed Up Transit Time

To make a particular point, we'd like to start this section with a rather unappetizing description (repeated from our Digestive Difficulties chapter). Imagine chewing up a hamburger and then putting it out in the sun on a 98.6°F sidewalk. After about three days, that hamburger would be

Sauna Suggestions

A couple of tips will help make your sauna experience optimally effective and pleasant.

•**Don't overdo.** As with exercise, many people try to do too much too fast. Start with a lower temperature (about 115° F) and gradually work your way up (a max of 135° F), from sauna to sauna. Start out with a sauna of only a few minutes, lengthening the time as you feel comfortable.

•**Listen to your body.** Your body tells you whether something is good for you or not. If your body feels good, the experience is probably good for you. If you're feeling lightheaded or otherwise strained in a sauna, it's time to come out.

•**To prevent dehydration,** take drinking water into the sauna with you and sip throughout.

•**Rinse off after the sauna** so that the toxins won't be reabsorbed.

For home use, I favor far infrared saunas from High Tech Health. Far infrared rays warm up the sauna without the need for moisture, so the air is warm and dry, as compared with the humid air found in traditional saunas. You can find more information about these saunas at the website HighTechHealth.com.

If you don't have space for a home sauna, or it's too expensive, you can use a sauna at a local health club, gym, or Y. For the same purification benefits without a sauna, look to any activity that makes you sweat, such as a brisk walk or any other type of body-heating workout. However you build up a sweat, it helps to rinse off soon after, to wash toxins in the sweat off your skin and down the drain.

For relaxation (but not purification), a hot shower or bath can have the same benefits as a sauna. Throw a cup of Epsom salts in the bath to relax your muscles even more.

---

toxic—so gnarly that most animals wouldn't even eat it, except for vultures. And you certainly wouldn't want it in your body.

But that rotting hamburger might be in your body right now if you have slow transit time. *Transit time* is the term for the hours and days it takes for a meal to move from mouth to rectum—the transit from one end of your digestive tract to the other. A healthy transit time is about one day, although conventional docs assert that three days is fine. (They can join the vultures eating that hamburger on the sidewalk.)

Faster than 12 hours, and your body doesn't have enough time to pull all the nutrients out of the food. Slower than 24 hours, and the digesting food starts to turn toxic—and those loitering toxins are reabsorbed into your system, causing and contributing to disease.

In a landmark study a couple of decades ago, the late Denis Burkitt, MD—the first scientific champion of high-fiber diets—compared the transit times of Africans who lived in cities and ate a typical low-fiber Western diet with the transit times of Africans who lived in rural areas and ate a high-fiber diet. He found that the Africans in the cities had transit times that were four times slower. They also had more heart disease, diabetes, colon cancer, obesity, gallstones, hemorrhoids, and varicose veins.

To discover your personal transit time, eat some corn-on-the-cob or a can of corn. The yellow outer hulls are indigestible and will show up in your stool. The time from eating the corn to a hull-containing bowel movement is your transit time.

Advanced Detoxification

Some diseases, such as cancer, may require intense detoxification. Holistic-minded practitioners have devised techniques to help with this process, such as a gallbladder flush (a treatment in which you drink a combination of apple juice, Epsom salts, olive oil, and lemon juice to cleanse the gallbladder) and coffee enemas (yes, an enema with coffee, which quickly delivers compounds directly into the digestive tract that stimulate the liver to release toxins).

Another intensive type of detoxification—used anciently for physical, mental, and emotional purification—is fasting, in which you only drink fluids rather than eat. Fasting can vary in intensity (from water-only to liberal use of vegetable and fruit juices) and in length (from one day to several weeks).

If you decide to undergo any form of intensive detoxification, I recommend doing so only under the guidance and supervision of a qualified health practitioner experienced in the method, such as a naturopathic physician. For help locating such a practitioner, please see "Finding a Holistic Health Practitioner" in Resources on page 360.

If it's slower than a day, here are a few tips to help you speed it up.

●**Eat more fiber.** Eating more whole grains—rich in the fiber that bulks up stool—is probably the easiest way to speed up transit time. Have whole grain cereal every morning for breakfast—oatmeal, Cheerios and Life cereal are tasty, low-sugar choices. Add a slice or two of whole grain toast, and you'll have the transit time of your life! Five or so servings of vegetables and fruits help contribute fiber, too.

●**Take magnesium.** Magnesium is a must for healthy muscles and nerves, including those responsible for peristalsis, the rhythmic muscle contractions that move food through the digestive tract. But more than half of Americans don't get the RDA for the mineral. There are 200 milligrams of magnesium in the Energy Revitalization System powder made by Nature's Way (the vitamin/mineral supplement I recommend on page 30). You can add another 300-milligram magnesium supplement for greater effect. Magnesium-rich foods include black beans, pumpkin seeds, cooked spinach, and halibut.

●**Drink more water.** Without enough water, your stools tend to be small and hard, slowing transit time. Follow earlier recommendations in this chapter to know if you need to drink more.

●**Take vitamin C.** Vitamin C attracts water into the colon, softening stool and helping speed transit time. Between 500 milligrams and 1,000 milligrams a day is a good level for most people.

●**Optimize thyroid function.** An underactive thyroid slows down everything in the body, including transit time. For more on optimizing thyroid function, see the Real Cure Regimen for Hypothyroidism on page 254.

●**Exercise regularly.** It provides a kind of internal massage to the intestinal tract that can speed transit time. Move your feet and you'll move your bowels.

Chronic Inflammation

You Can Cool Down Disease

"-$\blacksquare$tis" diseases can set up shop in every part of your body. In your bones and muscles—as arthritis, bursitis, or tendinitis. In your digestive tract—as gastritis, diverticulitis, or colitis. On your skin—as dermatitis or folliculitis. And then there's gingivitis (your gums), cystitis (your bladder), plantar fasciitis (your feet)—and dozens more "-itis" diseases, from acanthamoeba keratitis (an infection of the cornea by an amoeba) to yeast vaginitis.

Those conditions share the suffix "-itis" because they share a single symptom: inflammation.

What Is Inflammation?

To understand inflammation—both the acute variety, from an infection or an injury; and the chronic variety, which can be a hidden cause of disease—you need to understand a bit about your immune system. Think of it as a military organization, with the sole purpose of protecting you from outside invaders called antigens. And just as the U.S. military has branches so does your immune system.

There's the infantry: white blood cells (lymphocytes) such as the aptly named natural killer cells that swarm and attack antigens.

There's military intelligence: antibodies, a type of protein that detects invaders and labels them "foreign" so that other immune cells can recognize and kill them. *There are five types of antibodies, or immunoglobulins…*

•**IgM are like the Marines.** They go in first, figure out the weak points of the enemy—the best way to attack and kill them—and then teach the other troops what to do.

•**IgA are like scouts,** patrolling the linings body in the nose, mouth, digestive tract, and other areas.

•**IgG are sentries that have signed up for life.** After IgM have identified an invader, IgG recognize an antigen whenever it shows up again and sound the alarm.

•**IgE are special forces that respond to environmental challenges such as excessive dust.** But these combative proteins can overreact, causing allergic reactions to substances such as pollen and dander that don't have any evil intentions.

There's a fifth antibody—IgD—but, like the National Security Agency, nobody quite knows how it works or what it does. Other immune cells include...B-cells, which produce antibodies; T-cells, white blood cells that check for antibodies and attack anything labeled an invader; helper T-cells, which instruct B-cells to produce antibodies; suppressor T-cells, which let the troops know the battle has been won and they can go back to base; neutrophils, bloblike battlers that patrol the bloodstream and literally engulf, kill, and dissolve invaders; and macrophages, killing cousins to the neutrophils, with some assigned to protect specific organs, such as the liver.

Although there are many players, the immune system is engaged in one essential activity, a kind of ID check in which everything is interrogated with the same basic question: Are you self or other? If the answer is self, it's sent on its way. If the answer is other, the battle begins.

Instigating Inflammation

Inflammation occurs when an "other" is detected, war is declared, and your immune system rushes troops to the battlefield—anywhere on or in your body, from your scalp to your big toe.

In acute inflammation, millions of white blood cells charge to the area of injury, maybe a bite, burn, scrape, or cut. As the battle rages, the area becomes swollen, red, hot, and painful—all signs that the immune system is on the job, making sure the injury doesn't become infected. But if inflammation goes on too long—if it becomes chronic rather than acute—all that healing hyperactivity can eventually damage the tissues of your body. It's like your immune army never heard the order to stand down. Troops are running all over the place, attacking everything in sight, but there's no real threat. In fact, it's supposed to be peacetime! What happens when a temporary state of emergency turns into a perpetual state of war? A few examples tell the tale.

Can You Pass the Paper Cut Challenge?

There's an easy way to tell if your immune system is in overdrive and your troops are out of control: See if you notice your next paper cut.

Ordinarily, these minuscule slices of skin are so insignificant that you don't notice them a few minutes after they happen. But if the cut becomes red and painful—in other words, inflamed—it's a sign that your immune system is responding with way too much might. Then it's time to put into practice some of the immune-calming real cures discussed in this chapter, such as increasing your intake of the anti-inflammatory omega-3 fatty acids in fatty fish and in fish oil supplements.

In your mouth, a long-term buildup of bacteria can stimulate constant inflammation of your gums (gingivitis)—chronic, cell-damaging inflammation that studies show is a risk factor for heart disease, diabetes, rheumatoid arthritis, kidney disease, pregnancy complications, Alzheimer's disease, and pancreatic cancer.

In the respiratory tract, chronic inflammation can become asthma or chronic obstructive pulmonary disease (COPD), easily inflamed airways that swell and clog with mucus.

In your intestinal tract, chronic inflammation can take the form of the aptly named inflammatory bowel disease (Crohn's disease and ulcerative colitis).

And in your arteries, your immune system responds to cholesterol as a foreign invader. White blood cells not only rush to the scene, they stick to the scene, inflaming the arterial lining and forming plaque. (You can read more about inflammation and how it leads to heart disease in "Your Overheated Heart" on page 121.)

What causes all this chronic inflammation? Many of the real causes have already been discussed in this book. *Those real causes include...*

●**Nutritional Deficiencies** (page 3). An optimal level of nutrients is a must for healthy immunity. For example, an imbalance of fatty acids (too little omega-3 and too much omega-6) can create inflammation. And low levels of zinc can weaken the immune system.

●**Poor Sleep** (page 33). Laboratory scientists know that one of the best ways to suppress an experimental animal's immune system is to deprive it of sleep. Same goes for us humans participating in the 24/7 "experiment" of modern life, with insomnia an epidemic.

●**Happiness Deficiency** (page 55). Studies show that stress can even hamper your white blood cells.

●**Hormonal Imbalances** (page 84). Levels of adrenal hormones that are too low or too high can imbalance immunity.

●**Digestive Difficulties** (page 98). Dysbiosis (too many bad gut bacteria and too few good ones) injures immunity. Leaky gut syndrome (often from an infestation by the candida fungus) allows incompletely digested proteins into the bloodstream, putting the immune system into overdrive.

●**Cellular Toxicity** (page 109). Environmental toxins of all kinds pollute the immune system.

By addressing these real causes with real cures, you can optimize the functioning of your immune system, prevent it from overreacting, and stop chronic inflammation from undermining your health. You'll find those real cures throughout the book. In the rest of this chapter, we'll highlight a few ways to start optimizing immune function immediately.

The Anti-Inflammatory Diet

A major cause of inflammation in the American diet is the skewed proportion of bad fats to good fats. Yes, dietary fat isn't *always* a dietary villain. *In fact, it's a must for good health...*

The outer coverings of your cells—including your brain cells—are made from fat. Many hormones require fat for their manufacture. Eating fat triggers the release of a hormone (cholecystokinin) in the GI tract that signals your brain that it's time to stop eating. Plus, fat tastes good!

Your Overheated Heart

Chronic inflammation is now widely understood to be a key underlying process behind the plaque buildup that causes heart disease and stroke (cardiovascular disease, or CVD)—the number-one and number-five killers of Americans. In fact, high levels of C-reactive protein (CRP)—an inflammatory biomarker—are linked to five-times-greater risk of CVD.

How does chronic inflammation overheat your heart?

To get the clearest possible picture of the details, we talked with preventive cardiologist Stephen Sinatra, MD, an integrative cardiologist, and coauthor of *Reverse Heart Disease Now.* Dr. Sinatra describes the process in several basic stages.

Stage 1: The smooth lining of the artery—the delicate endothelium, one cell thick—becomes damaged. Maybe from high blood pressure, which stresses the arteries. Or cigarette smoke, toxic chemicals, a sugary diet, scads of saturated fat, or unrelenting stress. (Modern life can be heartless!) Droplets of circulating LDL cholesterol become wedged into the damaged lining and oxidize.

Stage 2: Oxidation—ouch! The injured cells in the endothelium release chemicals alerting the immune system that something is amiss, and troops are rushed to the scene. Some of them— clever white blood cells called monocytes that can morph into macrophages—stick to the endothelium.

Stage 3: The damaged endothelial cells release more distress signals, motivating the monocytes to turn into macrophages, which engulf the LDL. But instead of dissolving the LDL, the macrophages get stuck in it. The mired macrophages send out an SOS, more soldiers arrive on the scene, and they get stuck, too! And they perish en masse.

The result: The beginning of arterial plaque, a fatty layering of oxidized LDL and dead macrophages. Yuck!

Stage 4: Immune factors called cytokines send out messages that attract even more inflammatory immune cells, increasing the buildup of plaque. The proliferating plaque attracts other substances that are typically sent to sites of infection, such as fibrinogen (a protein that helps clot blood) and CRP. "Think of plaque progression in terms of the body's responding to a growing internal infection," said Dr. Sinatra. "The immune system's natural reactions feed on itself, creating a general state of inflammatory alert."

Stage 5: The body concocts a sturdy batch of proteins from connective tissue (collagen and elastin) and seals the inflamed area with a hard, fibrous cap. Underneath the cap, dead cells decay and pus builds up. This boil-like lump is plaque. And plaque begets plaque, points out Dr. Sinatra. The inflamed area agitates nearby cells, starting the plaque-producing process in new spots.

Stage 6: One type of plaque is stable: the hard, fibrous cap stays in place. But plaque can also be unstable: Inflammation continues inside and outside the plaque, until the cap ruptures and spills its noxious contents into the artery—possibly triggering the artery-plugging blood clots that cause most heart attacks and strokes. "Inflammation causes the plaque to rupture, and the rupture is what kills most of the time," said Dr. Sinatra.

He summarized the situation: "When inflammation becomes chronic and goes into constant overdrive, it can cause heart disease."

The problem isn't fat, per se. It's a diet with the wrong mix of fats—too many inflammatory omega-6 fatty acids and too few inflammation-calming omega-3 fatty acids—causes chronic inflammation. What are fatty acids, exactly?

The Omega Mix-Up

Protein is composed of tinier units called amino acids. Similarly, fat is composed of fatty acids. Fat from beef, pork, and chicken contains more arachidonic acid (AA), a so-called omega-6 fatty acid. (Omega-6 is a chemical designation based on the arrangement of carbon atoms in the fatty acid molecule.) AA and some other omega-6s are pro-inflammatory—they stimulate inflammation.

Fat from oily fish such as salmon contains eicosapentaenoic acid (EPA) and docosahexaenoic acid (DHA), omega-3 fatty acids. EPA, DHA, and other omega-3s are anti-inflammatory—they calm inflammation.

Our hunter-gatherer ancestors consumed a diet with a very healthy omega-6–to–omega-3 ratio of less than 2:1. Fast-forward 1,000 generations to the Industrial Revolution. We started (and continue) to eat a lot more foods loaded with omega-6s, such as certain cooking oils (corn, soybean, cottonseed), trans fats (in many store-bought baked goods, chips, and other processed products), and margarine.

We also started (and continue) to eat feedlot-raised meat. And the grain-based diets of these cattle, pigs, and chickens give their meat an omega-6–to–omega-3 ratio of 4:1, compared with grass-fed meat or free-range chicken with a ratio of 2:1. (These numbers are courtesy of a conversation with Floyd Chilton, PhD, formerly a professor in the Department of Nutritional Science at Wake Forest University in Winston-Salem, North Carolina, and currently a professor of nutritional sciences at the University of Arizona. He's an expert in inflammatory diseases and omega-3s, and author of *Inflammation Nation*.)

What happened to our omega-6–to–omega-3 ratio with this increase in omega-6s? The ratio of the average American is now at 16:1. Add to that imbalance the fact that the overload of sugar, white flour, and other refined carbohydrates in our diet—about 36 percent of our total calories—increases the production of pro-inflammatory hormones.

That's a lot of fuel for the inflammatory fire. No wonder heart disease and stroke—diseases of chronic inflammation—are leading causes of death in America. Fortunately, there are simple ways to put more omega-3s in your diet and decrease the levels of the wrong kinds of omega-6s…

•**Eat mostly whole, fresh foods.** Avoiding processed foods is one of the best ways to reduce omega-6 fatty acids and improve your overall health.

As for which fresh foods are best: In general, the more colorful a fresh fruit or vegetable, the healthier it is. For example, sweet potatoes are a lot better for you than white potatoes.

•**Buy grass-fed and free-range meat.** Grass-fed beef and free-range chicken are much richer in omega-3s. They're available at natural supermarkets such as Whole Foods Market and Sprouts. Although this type of meat is a bit more expensive, it also tastes better, helps prevent weight gain, and will save you a fortune on doctor bills!

•**Favor healthy snacks,** such as nuts. You can cut your intake of omega-6s by passing on the chips and sweet snacks and favoring walnuts, almonds, cashews, and other nuts rich in monounsaturated fatty acids. Walnuts also contain a goodly dose of alpha-linolenic acid (ALA), an omega-3. (ALA may have the added benefit of helping with weight loss!)

•**Substitute olive oil for other vegetable oils.** Olive oil contains healthful monounsaturated fat and is also rich in anti-inflammatory oleic acid (an omega-9 fatty acid). You can use it for frying and cooking, and instead of butter on your bread. (Butter is fine for occasional use and way healthier than deadly margarines.) I recommend extra-virgin, which indicates a higher-quality oil. Flaxseed oil and canola oil are also rich in ALA.

•**Eat three to four weekly servings of omega-3–rich fish.** In a study conducted at the University of Washington, women who ate one or two servings of fish a week were 22 percent less likely to develop rheumatoid arthritis, an inflammatory disease. Those who ate more than two servings reduced risk by 43 percent. But remember, not all fish are beneficial. The women who ate more deep-fried fish (usually fried in omega-6 fats) were more likely to develop the disease.

The richest sources, Dr. Chilton told us, contain more than 500 milligrams of omega-3s per 3.5-ounce serving. They include salmon (wild is richest, including canned wild salmon), mackerel, tuna, sardines, and trout. Choosing canned tuna? The solid white albacore has three times as much omega-3 as the chunk light tuna. The second-best fish for omega-3s contain 150 milligrams to 500 milligrams per serving. They include haddock, cod, halibut, shrimp, sole, flounder, perch, black bass, and farmed Atlantic salmon. (Oysters are good, too.)

•**Take a fish oil supplement.** For my patients who don't want to or can't manage to eat fatty fish a couple of times a week, I recommend omega-3 supplements. I favor a unique form of omega-3s from fish, called Vectomega (from Terry Naturally). It has a chemical structure identical to that found in salmon, which increases absorption dramatically—50 times as much as other fish oils. One to two tablets a day deliver all the EPA and DHA you need. Other good brands of fish oil include Nordic Naturals. Follow the dosage recommendations on the label.

The anti-inflammatory benefits of fatty fish and fish oil are remarkable. And in a study from Scotland, 64 people with rheumatoid arthritis who took fish oil reduced their use of anti-inflammatory medication by 40 percent. As we discussed in Nutritional Deficiencies on page 28, fish oil can also help prevent and control cardiovascular disease.

For an Agreeable Immune System, Think Zinc

You can read a lot about the immune-defending power of zinc in Nutritional Deficiencies on page 21. Zinc performs such an important role in optimizing immune function and keeping chronic inflammation at bay. It...

•**Helps you make T-cells,** which identify antigens

•**Helps thymulin**—a hormone that regulates immune function and helps turn baby T-cells into adults—work properly

•**Powers your antigen-slaying macrophages and natural killer cells**—too little of the nutrient and they're weakened

Two Tests for Inflammation

If you want to find out for sure whether you have an overactive immune system and excess inflammation, talk to your doctor about taking one of two medical tests...

•**C-reactive protein (CRP) test.** C-reactive protein is a biochemical produced by an overactive immune system and is a sign of excess inflammation. (The cost of the test is covered by most insurers, including Medicare.) *Here's what the results mean...*

  •1.0 milligrams per liter (mg/L) or lower: Normal

  •Between 1.0 mg/L and 2.0 mg/L: Mildly elevated

  •Higher than 2.0 mg/L: Very elevated

One precaution: Don't have the test right after an event that excites acute inflammation, such as an infection, injury, surgery, or high-intensity exercise (such as running a marathon).

High CRP is not necessarily a cause of disease (and not everyone with high CRP will develop health problems), but studies have shown a link between elevated levels and many conditions. Reducing CRP (inflammation) may help control those diseases and lessen their impacts. *They include*...Alzheimer's disease, atrial fibrillation, autoimmune disease, rheumatoid arthritis, cancer, colitis, depression, diabetes (type 2), high blood pressure, high cholesterol, hypothyroidism, insulin resistance (prediabetes), macular degeneration (a leading cause of blindness), overweight, and stroke.

•**Sed rate (erythrocyte sedimentation rate, or ESR) test.** This blood test costs about $15 to $20, and also can detect an overactive immune system. It measures how fast red blood cells settle to the bottom of a test tube. The faster they settle, the more active your immune system. That's because an overactive immune system generates proteins that cause red blood cells to stick together; a clump of red blood cells is heavier and falls faster than individual cells.

  •Normal, men: 0 to 15 millimeters per hour

  •Normal, women: 0 to 20 millimeters per hour

If these tests are high, consider the anti-inflammatory strategies in this chapter, particularly eating more fish rich in omega-3s. Better yet, skip the tests and just eat more fish!

•**Can reduce levels of two inflammatory cytokines** (factors that keep your entire immune system on high alert): TNF-alpha and IL-1 beta

In clinical studies, zinc supplements have helped treat a wide range of infections, including colds and other upper respiratory tract infections, dandruff, pneumonia, chronic hepatitis C (a viral infection of the liver), Helicobacter pylori (a stomach infection that causes ulcers), tuberculosis, shigellosis (a bacterial infection of the intestinal lining), HIV, and leprosy.

When I was in medical school, I noticed that many of the symptoms of AIDS mirrored the symptoms of acrodermatitis enteropathica (AE), a genetic disease that causes severe zinc deficiency and secondary severe immune deficiency. Later, it was discovered that people with AIDS have levels of zinc that are as low as those found in AE.

What is happening in AIDS (and other chronic infections, such as those commonly found in people with fibromyalgia and chronic fatigue syndrome)? Chronic infections and inflammation cause you to urinate a lot of zinc, leaving you zinc deficient and weakening your immune system, which results in more infections and more zinc losses. In fact, a study showed that people with heart disease lose one-third more zinc in their urine than people without heart disease. Modern medicine ignores this phenomenon, because the remedy—zinc—is dirt cheap.

To end this vicious cycle is to make sure your diet and daily nutritional supplement contain plenty of zinc. How much is enough? An optimal level of zinc in a nutritional supplement is 15 milligrams to 20 milligrams a day. (And that's *every* day—your body doesn't store zinc very well.) More than that, and zinc can cause a drop in levels of "good" HDL cholesterol and also push you toward a copper deficiency. (Zinc is yang to copper's yin—more of one means less of the other.)

For zinc-rich foods, look to oysters. They supply nine times more than any other food. Canned smoked oysters on whole wheat crackers are a delicious snack. Lobster and Alaskan king crab are also tasty ways to get zinc. Generally, high-protein foods are rich in zinc. Red meat—grass-fed, preferably—is a good source of the mineral. Among nonmeat sources, look to fortified breakfast cereals, beans and legumes (such as chickpeas and peas), nuts, and dairy products.

Hey, Inflammation—Chill Out!

If you're happy, your immune system is probably healthy. *A couple of scientific studies help prove this simple but very important point…*

•**More negative thoughts, fewer natural killer cells.** When researchers from Denmark studied 510 people, they found that those with the most negative thinking—or what psychologists call rumination—had lower levels of natural killer cells and T-cells.

•**More happiness, less immune hypersensitivity.** One way to test the state of the immune system is to "challenge" the skin with toxic substances and measure the resulting inflammation—a so-called hypersensitivity test. When researchers at the University of Kentucky tested 124 people, they found that those with the most "positive affect"—that is, the happiest people—had the least hypersensitivity.

•**More optimism, more helper T-cells.** In a study by psychologists at UCLA, those who were the most optimistic and had better moods had higher levels of helper T-cells, and their natural killer cells were better at slaying antigens.

•**More unfriendliness, more inflammation.** Researchers at UCLA studied the immune responses of 124 people who were treated poorly by others. In one part of the experiment, the participants delivered an impromptu speech in front of people—who showed no positive reaction whatsoever. In another part, the participants were asked to count backward by 7s and 13s while urged to go faster by "an apparently exasperated experimenter," wrote the researchers in the *Proceedings of the National Academy of Sciences*. Two immune markers of inflammation were measured before and after these difficult encounters, and the markers were much higher afterward. "Acute social stress," wrote the researchers, is linked to "inflammatory responses."

•**Less stress, fewer colds.** Researchers in the Department of Psychology at Carnegie Mellon University in Pittsburgh studied nearly 400 healthy people, infecting them with a cold virus. A much higher percentage of the people with psychological stress in their lives caught colds, compared with people with less stress. "Psychological stress…increased the risk of acute infectious respiratory illness," summed up the researchers in the *New England Journal of Medicine*. In a second study, the psychologists discovered that it was chronic stress—losing a job, or difficulties with family members or friends—that accounted for the higher rate of colds.

•**Suppress your anger, suppress your immune system.** Researchers in the Department of Psychology at the University of Miami studied 61 men, some who usually expressed their anger and some who usually stuffed it. Those who expressed anger had natural killer cells that were more effective at killing antigens.

•**Depression depresses immunity.** In a study from Korean researchers, published in the journal *Medicine*, people who were depressed were more likely to get the herpes virus—a sure sign of lower immunity.

The moral of these studies is clear: You can strengthen or weaken your immune system with your thoughts, feelings, and attitudes.

"Am I in Imminent Danger?"

In terms of an overactive immune system, the key mind-body action is finding a way to calm inflamed emotions—anxiety, worry, and upset of all kinds.

Here's a technique I teach my patients and that they find particularly effective: Whenever you are anxious, upset, or worried, ask yourself this question: "Am I in imminent danger?" Not "Will I be in danger this afternoon, tomorrow, next week, or next month?" Instead, ask yourself: "Am I in danger right now?" Unless you're in the midst of a truly threatening situation—a forest fire in your neighborhood or a burglar in your house—the answer will be "No, I'm not in imminent danger." And this simple realization and assertion will tell the soldiers of your immune system to stand down.

The Write Approach

Many studies show that writing about a past or current trauma—a technique psychologists call expressive writing—can strengthen the immune system.

In one study, researchers from the Department of Psychiatry at Harvard Medical School studied people with AIDS, asking them to take 20 minutes to "describe their thoughts and feelings regarding a stressful life-event." Those who wrote most openly and fully, describing the event in detail, their full range of emotions about it, and how they dealt with the stress, had the highest number of natural killer cells. In other words, said the researchers, expressing and processing your emotions through writing fortifies your immune system. "Higher levels of emotional disclosure and processing of trauma may confer health and immunological benefits," they concluded in the *British Journal of Health Psychology*.

And in a scientific study on expressive writing, published in the *British Journal of Psychology*, researchers from the University of Missouri found that writing just two minutes a day (every day for four weeks) about either a personal trauma or a positive life experience reduced health complaints, compared with people who didn't write regularly.

Here are instructions for expressive writing from James W. Pennebaker, PhD, a social psychologist at the University of Texas at Austin, and author of *Opening Up by Writing It Down...*

"I would like you to write your very deepest thoughts and feelings about the most traumatic experience of your entire life or an extremely important emotional issue that has affected you and your life. In your writing, I'd like you to really let go and explore your deepest emotions and thoughts. You might tie your topic to your relationships with others, including parents, lovers, friends, or relatives; to your past, your present, or your future; or to who you have been, who you would like to be, or who you are now. You may write about the same general issues or experiences on all days of writing or about different topics each day. All of your writing will be completely confidential. Don't worry about spelling, grammar, or sentence structure. The only rule is that once you begin writing, you continue until the time is up."

You can find many other techniques for achieving emotional balance and natural happiness in Happiness Deficiency on page 55.

Smart Treatments for Acute and Chronic Inflammation

The Real Cure Regimens for inflammatory conditions are in many chapters ahead. But in this chapter I'd like to offer a few effective, easy-to-implement, and safe ways to reduce acute and chronic inflammation (and the accompanying pain)—without using deadly anti-inflammatory drugs. As you may have read in Prescription Medications on page 70, the gut-eroding side effects of nonsteroidal anti-inflammatory drugs (NSAIDs) such as aspirin, ibuprofen, and naproxen kill 16,500 people a year and hospitalize hundreds of thousands more.

Sprains, Strains, and Other Minor Injuries

To treat the pain and swelling (i.e., inflammation) of a minor injury, the old standby—rest, ice, compression, elevation (RICE)—works great, as do some other natural remedies.

•**Rest.** This step is pretty obvious. Don't use or put any weight on the body part you've injured, particularly if using or putting weight on it is painful.

•**Ice.** By reducing blood flow to the injury, ice also reduces swelling. There are lots of icing options out there, from ice packs specifically designed for the purpose to a bag of frozen peas. Ice for 20 minutes, four or five times a day. (Ten minutes for areas with little or no fat, such as fingers and toes.) To protect your skin while icing, wrap the cold object in a thin towel. Use ice treatments during the first 24 to 36 hours after an injury, then use heat. (Use a heating pad or any kind of moist heat for 10 to 15 minutes.)

Six Psychological Traits That Boost Immunity

The late psychiatrist George Solomon, MD, a professor of psychology and behavioral sciences at UCLA, was one of the founders of the science he originally called psychoneuroimmunology—the study of the link between your emotions, thoughts, and attitudes and your immune system. As part of his research, Dr. Solomon focused on AIDS patients, people who live or die depending on the strength of their immune systems. He found that those who lived the longest tended to have similar personality traits. For a unique perspective on Dr. Solomon's findings about those traits, we talked with Bernie Siegel, MD, a pioneer in mind-body medicine, author of the bestseller *Love, Medicine & Miracles*, and the creator of the CD *Healing Meditations: Enhance Your Immune System and Find the Key to Good Health*.

The traits of the longest-lived AIDS patients included...

• **Feeling a sense of meaning in work and daily activities.** "If your work feels meaningless—a useless but necessary burden—it's bad for your immune system," said Dr. Siegel.

• **Expressing anger appropriately.** If you suppress your anger, you suppress your immunity, Dr. Siegel told us. "But expressing anger isn't about spewing resentment and hatred. It's about speaking up for yourself when you're not treated with respect."

• **Asking family and friends for help when you need it.** "When your family, friends, and co-workers say, 'Anything I can do for you?' and you keep saying no, you hurt your immune system," Dr. Siegel said.

• **Saying no when you're asked to do something you don't want to do.** "When you say yes to everybody else, you say no to yourself," said Dr. Siegel. "Eventually, your immune system will break down so you don't have to do all those things you don't want to do."

• **Not identifying with a single role.** "If you identify with a role—mother or father, husband or wife, teacher or plumber—what happens when you can't fulfill that role?" asked Dr. Siegel. "You may decide you have nothing to live for—and your immune system may agree with you!"

• **Putting play in your life.** "Play is any activity that is fun and helps you lose track of time," he told us. "That timeless state is uniquely health-giving."

•**Compression.** Applying direct pressure to the injured area also can reduce swelling. Wrap an elastic bandage gently around the swollen area. (If the area starts to throb or tingle, the bandage is too tight. It's also too tight if it simply feels too tight. Rewrap the area so the bandage is looser.) Loosen and rewrap the area every four hours.

•**Elevation.** This also reduces swelling. If you can, place the injured area about one foot above the level of your heart. Twisted ankle? Lie down and prop up your foot on a few pillows.

Use RICE for one or two days. If the area is still inflamed, it's time to see a doctor.

•**Enzymes.** Oddly enough, a supplement intended to improve digestion can also work to reduce inflammation and pain. Digestive enzymes not only digest food, they also "digest" inflammatory immune factors.

I favor using animal-based enzyme products for inflammation and plant-sourced enzymes for indigestion. Take the enzymes between meals so they're used by your body for calming inflammation rather than for digestion. For inflammation, a good option is Mega-Zyme, from Nature's Way. For plant-based enzymes, I recommend CompleteGest from Nature's Way or Similase from Integrative Therapeutics. For acute pain, take them for a few days. For chronic inflammation and pain (discussed more fully below), take two or three tablets, three times a day, between meals, for six to 12 weeks. If they haven't helped after that amount of time, stop taking them. If they have helped, and the pain and inflammation are gone, use them daily as needed.

•**Arnica cream or gel.** The homeopathic remedy arnica is very effective in reducing the inflammation from acute injury. It's an excellent addition to your medicine cabinet. You can find arnica gels and creams it in most stores that feature natural products. Popular brands include Arnicare, from Boiron, and Arnica Pain Relief Cream from MAXRelief.

•**CBD oil.** Hemp oil contains high levels of anti-inflammatory *cannabidiol* (CBD), as well as other inflammation-reducing, pain-relieving cannabinoids. The hemp oil I recommend is Hemp Select, from Terry Naturally, which contains 20 percent CBD.

Local Skin Infection

If you have a boil (carbuncle) or other localized skin infection and inflammation, one of the best ways to treat it is with hot packs, applied for 20 minutes, three or four times a day. This "draws" the infection so that it collects in one area rather than diffusing through the tissues, allowing it to drain on its own or allowing your doctor to drain it more easily. (Don't try to "force" drainage by using the hot pack for more time than I just indicated—let the body go at its own pace!)

To make a hot pack, put a clean washcloth into a pan or ovenproof or microwavable bowl. Next, heat the washcloth on the stove, in the oven, or in a microwave to hot bathwater temperature, about 105° F. (Don't let it get too hot, and you may get burned when you remove it.) Place the pack on the affected area of your body, and cover it with a sheet of plastic wrap—and then cover that with a heating pad or hot water bottle to keep it warm.

Acute Inflammation

Curcumin is a compound known for its anti-inflammatory power and is found in the spice turmeric. The medical database of the National Institutes of Health turns up more than 1,500 studies on curcumin and inflammation (and more than 10,000 on curcumin's many healing powers).

Among the compound's proven anti-inflammatory, immune-strengthening abilities, it…

•**Blocks the production of inflammatory cytokines**

•**Helps white blood cells move faster**

•**Decreases allergic inflammation in laboratory animals**

•**Strengthens cells against bacteria**

But curcumin is poorly absorbed. Problem solved! Curamin and CuraMed, unique curcumin-containing remedies from Terry Naturally, use a form of the compound (called BCM-95) that is absorbed seven times better than 95 percent pure curcumin. (Piperine, an extract of black pepper, also has been used to boost curcumin absorption. But since piperine interacts with certain prescription drugs, I don't recommend these products.)

Curamin is a remarkable pain remedy. Take two or three tabs a day until the pain is gone. It often works very quickly. (Did I mention that this remedy is simply amazing for pain?)

Chronic Inflammation

Of all the natural products on the market to reduce chronic inflammation, one of my favorites is BosMed 500 from Terry Naturally—one twice a day for colitis or asthma. For other inflammation, include CuraMed 750mg, one capsule once or twice daily. This combination supplies two very powerful ingredients: (1) a form of curcumin which increases absorption sevenfold and (2) a special form of the anti-inflammatory herb boswellia (also known as frankincense), standardized to include a high level of AKBA (acetyl-11-keto-beta-boswellic acid), the most potent anti-inflammatory compound in boswellia.

I already discussed curcumin (turmeric) as an excellent anti-inflammatory herb. Let's take a closer look at not only boswellia, but also willow bark, and cherry—three herbs that are effective for calming inflammation.

•**Boswellia.** Boswellia is an herb used for inflammatory conditions in Ayurvedic medicine, the ancient Indian system of natural healing. Many studies and scientific papers confirm boswellia's effectiveness as an anti-inflammatory. For example, a paper from German scientists, in the journal *Phytomedicine*, points out that the "boswellic acids" in the herb…

- •**Increase the production of white blood cells**
- •**Strengthen the ability of the immune system to generate antibodies**
- •**Strengthen the ability of macrophages to devour antigens**
- •**Limit the production of several pro-inflammatory cytokines**
- •**Stabilize mast cells** (which release the histamine that causes allergic reactions)
- •**Reduce the production of leukotrienes,** other inflammatory compounds

"It is not surprising," concluded the researchers, that boswellia has "positive effects" in "some chronic inflammatory diseases, including rheumatoid arthritis, bronchial asthma, osteoarthritis, ulcerative colitis, and Crohn's disease."

•**Willow bark.** Aspirin (salicylic acid) is derived from willow bark. But willow bark is much less toxic and more effective, because it delivers a gentle mixture of anti-inflammatory compounds rather than one ingredient in a concentrated dose.

•**Cherry.** Cherries are a classic remedy for inflammatory diseases such as arthritis and gout. An animal study from the University of Michigan showed that a cherry-enriched diet reduced four inflammatory immune factors (cytokines) by as much as 50 percent. Cherries, concluded the researchers in the *Journal of Medicinal Food*, "reduced both local and systemic inflammation."

PART 2

The Real Cures

Acne, Eczema, Psoriasis, and Other Skin Problems

Real Causes

- **Hormonal Imbalances.** Hormonal imbalances—in puberty or later in life—spark the production of pore-clogging sebum, causing acne to flare (page 84).
- **Nutritional Deficiencies.** Diets too high in sugar and refined carbohydrates—and the accompanying zinc and vitamin A deficiency—imbalance hormones even more (page 3).
- **Chronic Inflammation.** Plugged-up pores become infected and inflamed (page 118).

Everybody knows that acne is the bane of teenagers: 85 percent feel betrayed by their mirrors, either every day or now and then. But what most people don't know is that acne also affects an estimated 40 percent to 55 percent of Americans older than 25—including 12 percent of middle-aged women and three percent of middle-aged men.

The likely reason: a diet rich in refined carbohydrates that spikes blood sugar levels, triggering the hormones that trigger acne.

But before we get into those details of diet and dermatology, let's stop a moment and, well, pick a pimple in print. (That's something you should try not to do on your own face, because if it pops under your skin, it can become inflamed and worsen. So ease up on picking your pimples—even if they're picking on you!)

Your hair follicles are tiny pipes that drain oil-producing glands called sebaceous glands, and they produce sebum. A pimple erupts when a mixture of unshed cells from the walls of the hair follicle and an overload of sebum combine with other local gunk to form a follicle-clogging plug.

The pimple is a blackhead if the plug is open to the air (which oxidizes melanin, the skin pigment that's a portion of the plug). The pimple is a whitehead if the plug is sealed rather than open. At this stage, the pimple is called a comedo. If the plug persists, the immune system is alerted, and the area becomes red and inflamed; then it's called a papule. If the area becomes infected, it's called a pustule.

Acne is mainly a hormonal event. When sex hormones (such as estrogen, testosterone, DHEA) start to skyrocket at puberty, so does the production of pore-clogging sebum, causing acne to flare.

Real Cure Regimen

Here's the proven nutritional reality most dermatologists continue to dismiss or ignore: Diets loaded with sugar and other refined carbohydrates can spike levels of blood sugar (glucose), which in turn stimulates increased levels of those same sex hormones, triggering or worsening acne (which can then bring on the inflammation). Milk products can do the same. So can deficiencies of zinc and vitamin A. This means you can prevent, calm, or even cure acne—with diet.

The scientific literature is definitive about the role of diet in acne. In a paper titled *Does Diet Really Affect Acne?*, a doctor from the Department of Medicine at the George Washington University Medical Center and a registered dietitian from the Physicians Committee for Responsible Medicine reviewed more than 27 studies on the relationship between diet and acne. "There exists convincing data supporting the role of dairy products and high-glycemic-index foods in influencing hormonal and inflammatory factors, which can increase acne prevalence and severity," they concluded in the journal *Skin Therapy Letter*. (The term *high-glycemic-index foods* refers to a scale—the glycemic index—that measures how quickly a food turns into glucose. The faster the rate, the bigger the spike in blood sugar levels, and the greater your risk for acne. White flour is indexed at 100, followed closely by other refined carbohydrates such as soda, ice cream, and corn chips. Sucrose has a GI of 65.)

A team of German researchers dubbed the condition acne alimentaris—acne caused by what you eat, specifically, refined carbohydrates and dairy products—and says "dietary intervention" is the best way to deal with the skin problem.

Here are some of the studies that led to these conclusions…

●**Australian researchers studied 43 teens and young men with acne,** feeding them either a high-protein, low-carbohydrate diet or a diet with no restrictions on carbohydrates (in other words, the typical Western diet). After three months, the group eating the high-protein, low-carb diet had 49 percent fewer acne lesions. "The improvement in acne after a low-glycemic load diet suggests that nutrition-related lifestyle factors may play a role in acne pathogenesis," concluded the researchers in the *American Journal of Clinical Nutrition*.

●**In more research from Australia, doctors studied 12 teenage boys (average age 17).** For one week, seven of the boys ate a high-protein, low-carbohydrate diet (25 percent protein, 45 percent carbohydrate), while five ate a low-protein, high-carbohydrate diet (15 percent protein, 55 percent carbohydrate). Hormonal and metabolic factors that increase sebum production were measured before and after the diet—and all those sebum-increasing factors went up in the boys eating the low-protein, high-carb diet.

●**Researchers from the Department of Nutrition at the Harvard School of Public Health analyzed four years of health and diet data from 4,273 boys** and found that those with the highest intake of skim milk had a 19 percent higher risk of developing acne. The findings were published in the *Journal of the American Academy of Dermatology*.

Based on this, the dietary advice I give my patients for preventing and treating acne…

●**Avoid sugar and high-carbohydrate foods.** As you've just read, such a diet can decrease acne by half after three months.

●**Avoid milk, cheese, and other dairy products.** I recommend a trial run of six weeks of total avoidance. If this regimen helps, permanently reduce the dairy in your diet, or eliminate it entirely.

●**Take the right supplements.** *The three nutrients below have been shown to help clear up acne…*

●Vitamin A: 2,000 IU to 4,000 IU daily. This vitamin can help dry the oily skin of acne. *Caution*: Used long term, more than 4,000 IU a day of vitamin A is bad for bone development;

The Best Face-Washing Regimen for Acne

You'd think that when it came to something as basic as face washing and acne, dermatologists would have figured out exactly what is best. But they haven't.

"Despite the common recommendation [for those with acne] to wash the face twice daily with a mild cleanser, there is little published evidence to support the practice," wrote a team of researchers from Harvard Medical School. To remedy the situation, the researchers conducted a simple study. Guys with mild to moderate acne washed their faces (with a "standard mild cleanser") either once a day, twice a day, or four times a day, for two weeks.

Results? Those washing twice a day had "significant improvements in both open comedones and total non-inflammatory lesions." On the other hand, "worsening of acne condition was observed in the study group washing once a day," with more redness, papules, and total number of inflammatory acne lesions.

The final recommendation: Wash your face twice daily with a mild cleanser. (But excessive face washing isn't as bad for you as was thought, noted the researchers.)

more than 8,000 IU a day can cause birth defects during pregnancy; and more than 25,000 IU a day can cause liver problems. Use these higher doses for limited amounts of time, and only with the supervision and guidance of a qualified health professional, such as a holistic physician or nutritionist. (Higher levels of beta carotene—which is converted to vitamin A in the body—aren't harmful, but they won't help the acne.)

• Zinc: 15 milligrams to 30 milligrams daily. This mineral boosts the action of vitamin A and also speeds skin healing. Zinc is found mostly in foods high in protein—which is one reason why a high-protein, low-carbohydrate diet helps acne.

• Chromium: 200 micrograms to 400 micrograms a day. This mineral can help regulate the blood sugar imbalances that contribute to acne.

• **Increase fiber.** Constipation—less than one bowel movement a day—can create toxins that inflame your skin. I recommend eating a low-sugar, high-fiber whole grain cereal for breakfast, such as Cheerios or Quaker Oatmeal Squares, and eating more vegetables.

• **Slather on these soothers.** *In addition to diet, find relief from breakouts with these skin creams…*

• Topical vitamin A creams such as prescription Retin-A can help dry oily skin.

• Benzoyl peroxide (BPO), an OTC bacteria killer, is also helpful in controlling acne.

• Topical antibiotics, such as *clindamycin* (Cleocin-T) and *metronidazole* (MetroGel), are prescription-only options and a very reasonable approach to controlling acne. Your dermatologist can prescribe a drug that combines a higher-strength BPO (such as 10 percent) and a topical antibiotic, such as BenzaClin (BPO and *clindamycin*).

Oral antibiotics are sometimes needed in the short term to control severe acne, but they're a bad idea for long-term use because they routinely create dysbiosis, a digestive problem discussed in Digestive Difficulties on page 98.

Nutritional Healing for Other Skin Problems

Nutritional deficiencies can play a key role in many other skin problems. Try the nutritional solutions for any of these troublesome conditions.

Eczema

Eczema—a spotty rash of red, itchy, dry, cracked skin—is the number-one reason why Americans see dermatologists, with the problem afflicting more than 20 million adults and 10 million children.

●**Reach for omega-3s.** In a German study of 53 people with eczema, one group took 5.4 grams a day of the anti-inflammatory omega-3 fatty acid docosahexaenoic acid (DHA), and one didn't. After two months, the DHA group had a 23 percent improvement in symptoms, compared with a six percent reduction for the placebo group. The results were in the *British Journal of Dermatology.*

●**Rub in B$_{12}$.** A cream containing vitamin B$_{12}$ improves the itching and redness of eczema by 48 percent more than a placebo cream, reported German researchers in the *British Journal of Dermatology.* And a study in the *Journal of Alternative and Complementary Medicine* found that vitamin B$_{12}$ cream was "significantly more" effective than a placebo in relieving eczema symptoms in 21 children. The cream is theorized to work by decreasing the production of the compound nitric oxide, which feeds the inflammation. B$_{12}$ creams include Vitamin B$_{12}$ Cream from Life-Flo, B$_{12}$ AD Acute Gel from Mavena, and MaxAbsorb B$_{12}$ Vitamin B$_{12}$ cream from Vita Sciences.

Psoriasis

Psoriasis is a skin disease with red, flaky, scaly lesions that can itch, crack, bleed, and hurt.

●**Take in more vitamin E, coenzyme Q10, and selenium.** An antioxidant supplement containing these three nutrients reduced the symptoms of severe psoriasis, reported Russian researchers in the journal *Nutrition.* The daily dosages were 50 milligrams of coQ10, 50 milligrams of vitamin E, and 48 micrograms of selenium.

●**Heal with aloe vera.** Several studies have tested aloe vera as a treatment for psoriasis. In one, from researchers in Thailand, 80 people with mild to moderate psoriasis received either an aloe vera cream or *triamcinolone acetonide* cream (Aristocort, Kenalog, Triderm), which is commonly used for skin problems. After eight weeks, the aloe vera cream was more effective in reducing symptoms. I'm not surprised. In Hawaii, where I live, aloe vera is a respected natural remedy for skin problems. I became a believer in the power of aloe vera when my skin wouldn't heal after tendon surgery and I thought I would need a skin graft. After I drank eight ounces a day of aloe vera juice for two days, the incision healed. I was amazed! And I wasn't drinking any kind of special aloe vera juice—I bought an inexpensive, sugar-free variety, which is available at Walmart and Safeway. If you have psoriasis, consider drinking eight ounces of aloe vera juice daily. You could also try aloe vera cream or gel. Look for a product that contains at least 0.5 percent pure aloe vera. However, if you notice any additional redness or discomfort—always a possibility with super-sensitive skin—stop using aloe.

How to Stop Female Hair Loss

Balding in men is mostly an inevitable process, driven by genetics. But women suffer from hair loss, too—with hair thinning and shedding for no obvious reason, usually starting in your 50s and 60s.

Doctors called this condition Telogen Effluvium. *Here's what's happening…*

Hair follicles have a natural cycle of rest and activity. But in this condition they go into a prolonged resting phase (telogen). And rather than returning to the growth phase, your hair falls out.

In women, the most likely cause is severe stress, showing up as hair loss three to nine months later (when the next growth phase doesn't kick in). Other causes include infections, nutritional deficiencies, thyroid problems, anemia, polycystic ovary syndrome, psoriasis, and autoimmune disease (which is more likely to cause patchy bald spots rather than diffuse thinning).

To address hair loss in women, conventional medicine mainly recommends the drug *minoxidil* (Rogaine) and hair transplant surgery. *Natural medicine offers many effective but little-known cures…*

●**Millet seed oil.** A study in the *Journal of Cosmetic Dermatology* shows this compound is very effective in getting hair out of the telogen phase.

●**Horsetail.** This herb is rich in silica, a mineral that is a must for healthy hair. (It's also good to reverse brittle nails.)

●**Biotin.** This vitamin has been found to support healthy hair.

All of these compounds are combined in the product Hair Renew Formula, from Terry Naturally. Use it for a few months—and see if your hair starts coming back. (Results usually take three to nine months, although hair growth usually starts to markedly improve in two to three months.)

Two other ways to address hair thinning…

●**Optimize overall nutritional support.** A good multivitamin-mineral powder, such as the Energy Revitalization System from Nature's Way, is excellent for this. Plus, you can take a 29 milligram iron tablet for six months to 12 months, until your ferritin is over 100.

Caution: Use supplemental iron only with approval from your doctor. Don't take iron if your ferritin is over 200. And have your doctor check for iron excess (hemochromatosis)—it's a problem that's easy to correct but life-threatening if overlooked.

●**Optimize thyroid function.** See Hypothyroidism on page 254 and follow the recommendations there.

Rosacea

Fourteen million Americans have rosacea, a skin disease with symptoms such as acne, redness, flushing, broken blood vessels, and sensitive skin that can be dry, oily, or both.

●**Consider *metronidazole* cream.** This topical antibiotic reduces inflammation. Use it once or twice daily, or as directed by your doctor.

●**Put zinc to the rescue.** In a study published in the *International Journal of Dermatology*, of 19 people with rosacea, those who took 100 milligrams of zinc three times a day had a significant decrease in symptoms.

●**Check your stomach acid.** I've found that my patients with rosacea often have a deficiency of stomach acid, even if they have acid indigestion. For more on treating this problem, see Heartburn and Indigestion on page 250.

Wrinkles

Those telltale signs of aging—the product of oxidation—aren't completely unavoidable.

●**Go fish to banish wrinkles.** Women ages 40 to 60 who took a fish oil supplement for three months had a 10 percent increase in skin elasticity (a sign of youthful skin), reported German researchers in the *Journal of Dermatological Treatment*. To put more fish oil in your diet, eat three to four servings of salmon or tuna a week. The fish oil supplement I recommend to my patients is Vectomega, from Terry Naturally. One or two tablets of this uniquely concentrated product replaces eight capsules to 16 capsules of a typical fish oil, making it easier to take. Nordic Naturals is another good brand of fish oil. Follow the dosage recommendations on the label.

●**Try antioxidants, too.** Healthy women who took a daily antioxidant supplement for three months that included 4.8 milligrams of beta-carotene had skin that was firmer, moister, and smoother, reported German researchers.

Adrenal Exhaustion

Real Causes

●**Nutritional Deficiencies.** A lack of nutrients—particularly vitamin C and vitamin B_5 (pantothenic acid)—prevents the adrenal glands from recovering (page 3).

●**Happiness Deficiency.** Chronic stress exhausts the adrenal glands (page 55).

●**Hormonal Imbalances.** The nutrient deficiencies trigger imbalances in the hormonal system (page 84).

●**Sleep Problems.** Lack of sleep makes exhausted adrenal glands even more exhausted (page 33).

Let's review some of the ways that your adrenal glands let you know they're worn out. Do any of these descriptions fit you?

●**You're fatigued first thing in the morning and find it hard to get out of bed.**

●**You're tired all the time**—and when you're under stress, you're even more tired.

●**You like the energy you feel when you're dealing with a crisis because it's one of the few times you actually feel energetic.**

•**When you're hungry, you feel intensely irritable.** ("Feed me now, or I'll kill you!" is a thought you might be having. Candy bar advertisers have promoted the term "Hangry." A good term, but candy bars are one of the worst things you can eat when you are Hangry!)

•**You have frequent viral infections such as sore throats and colds,** and they take quite a while to clear up.

•**Sometimes you feel dizzy when you stand up.**

You can find a complete description of this common condition (it afflicts millions of people, the majority of them women) in Hormonal Imbalances on page 84. There you'll discover what your adrenal glands do—how they can become exhausted, the many health problems caused by adrenal exhaustion, and how you can tell if you might have the problem.

But what you won't find in that chapter, and will find in this one, is even better: the Real Cure Regimen to solve the problem of adrenal exhaustion (which I also call adrenal burnout). Like all my Real Cure Regimens, it's easy to implement and (if the experience of thousands of patients is any guide) likely to be very effective.

Ready to start feeling energetic again?

Real Cure Regimen

The regimen consists of three parts that address the real causes of adrenal exhaustion: (1) a diet that normalizes low blood sugar (glucose), a main feature of adrenal exhaustion; (2) nutrients to help your adrenal glands strengthen and recover; and (3) mental and emotional attitudes that reduce adrenal-exhausting stress.

The Adrenal-Strengthening Diet

The first part of this diet is the foods you don't eat—because these foods fatigue your adrenals.

•**Swear off sweets.** Yes, a candy bar and other types of sugar-laden sweets can lift your spirits—for a little while. Sugary sweets first pump up and then deflate your blood sugar levels, and that rapid and repeated rise and fall exhausts your glucose-controlling adrenal glands. *However...*

When blood sugar levels are low—when you feel particularly tired and irritable—try eating just a *little* sugar to help your levels normalize: one-half packet (half a teaspoon) of table sugar. (That's about the amount of sugar in four Tic Tacs.) Place the sugar under your tongue for fast absorption. You'll find just that little bit is enough to increase blood sugar levels and eliminate anxiety and irritability quickly without a ride on the roller coaster of glucose spikes and dips. For sugary sweetness, use natural, nonsugar sweeteners such as stevia (I like NOW foods BetterStevia and Stevia Select) or stevia combined with erythritol (Truvia and Pure Via).

•**Cut the caffeine.** Like sugar, caffeine forces the adrenal glands into action—and eventual exhaustion. Limit yourself to one cup of coffee in the morning, then decaf the rest of the day. Better yet, switch to good-for-you green tea, which has unique components that don't stimulate adrenals—and it contains theanine, a compound that increases both calmness and concentration. One cup contains 25 milligrams of caffeine, so you don't have to worry about overdoing it on the caffeine. (But don't drink more than 10 cups per day—a level of intake you're unlikely to even get close to.)

•**Pig out on protein.** I'm not recommending you overeat, but I am encouraging you to enthusiastically consume protein-rich foods, such as poultry, fish, eggs, cheese, beans, and nuts. They help stabilize blood sugar levels.

Wait a minute: Did I just advise you to eat more eggs, the cholesterol criminal? Here's the breaking news about eggs: Numerous studies show that eating two eggs a day doesn't raise cholesterol levels. Eggs deliver the most balanced protein on Mother Nature's menu. Enjoy them!

And speaking of balance: Include plenty of vegetables (particularly nutrient-dense leafy greens) with your high-protein meals.

•**Eat a little, and eat often.** Three squares aren't the right gastronomic geometry for a person with adrenal exhaustion. Go for five (or even six) smaller, high-protein, low-sugar meals, a style of eating known as grazing. But don't increase your total daily calorie intake.

•**Drink more water, eat more salt.** Here's why. Your adrenal glands are responsible for not only maintaining blood sugar levels, but also regulating blood volume and blood pressure—tasks that require plenty of water and salt. But if you have weakened adrenal glands, your body doesn't adequately retain either water or salt. In fact, two signs of adrenal exhaustion are (1) feeling thirsty and urinating more, and (2) craving salt.

A Meal Plan for Your Adrenal Glands

A day of adrenal-healing foods should look something like this:

•**Breakfast.** Good news for those with weak adrenals: Eggs, meat, and cheese—in a delicious dish such as a ham and cheese omelet—are a great way to start the day. So are moderate amounts of foods such as milk, yogurt, and other dairy products. But avoid high-carbohydrate foods like pancakes, potatoes, and white bread. (One slice of whole grain bread is okay.)

•**Midmorning snack.** A cube of cheese. A handful of mixed nuts. A hard-boiled egg. You get the high-protein picture.

•**Lunch.** Meat is on the menu again—fish, chicken, or a hamburger (skip the bun). Include a vegetable salad, or better yet, have a green salad liberally topped with tuna or chicken.

•**Afternoon snack.** Eat this snack two or three hours after lunch. Use the same types of high-protein foods you munched on midmorning. In fact, make sure to keep them handy!

•**Dinner.** Meat meal number three, with plenty of vegetables on the side. Or have a bean dish. Fresh fruit is a wonderful dessert.

•**Bedtime snack.** A glass of protein-rich warm milk (or almond milk) is soothing and promotes sleep. Add an egg, some cheese, or an ounce or two of nuts. Good night—and good health!

The simple solution: To assist your exhausted adrenals, you need to drink more water and eat more salt. About this time, you might be asking yourself, "Isn't salt like, well, like eggs?" Exactly—it's not bad for you, even though just about everybody says it is. Studies link higher intakes of salt to increased life span. (*The exception:* If you have high blood pressure or heart failure, don't increase your salt intake without your physician's okay.)

Exactly how much water and salt is *more* water and salt? I'm not one for driving yourself crazy by trying to keep perfect track of mealtime measurements such as grams and servings that are so beloved by academics and government officials. If you're thirsty, drink. If you crave salt, add a dash of it to your foods. Let your body tell you what's good for you.

Adrenal-Supporting Supplements

The supplements in the Real Cure Regimen have three purposes: They supply the health-supporting factors your exhausted adrenals can't; they help normalize blood sugar levels; and they help your dog-tired glands start wagging their hormonal tails again.

I think you'll find that taking these supplements boosts your energy levels and once your adrenals are healed, you'll find that you're sick less often. They also smooth out your moods, perhaps saving you thousands of dollars you might have spent on a therapist or divorce attorney!

Here are the supplements I recommend. For simplicity's sake, take Adrenaplex from Terry Naturally. It contains all the nutrients below and is dramatically helpful in countering adrenal exhaustion. However, if you are a woman with a condition that creates high testosterone (polycystic ovary syndrome or diabetes), or you have breast cancer or are a breast cancer survivor, use Adrenal Stress End from Nature's Way instead. It doesn't contain DHEA or pregnenolone, which are contraindicated for those conditions.

•**Adrenal extracts: 200 milligrams to 500 milligrams daily.** An adrenal extract or "glandular" supplement is a nutrient-rich portion of tissue from the adrenal gland of a cow or pig. In my experience with patients, taking an adrenal glandular is one of the fastest ways to supply exhausted glands with the raw material they need to revive and thrive. It's as if your adrenal glands are starving and you feed them—until they're strong enough to start making their own bountiful supply of glucose-balancing, energy-giving hormones.

But not all adrenal extracts are equal in purity or potency. In addition to the ones made by Terry Naturally and Nature's Way, Cortisol Manager from Integrative Therapeutics and Adrenal Complex from Standard Process are other glandular products I suggest to patients.

•**Licorice root: 125 milligrams to 400 milligrams daily.** This herb helps out the adrenals by slowing the body's breakdown of adrenal hormones such as cortisol. As a result, the already-weary adrenals don't need to make as much.

•**Chromium: 200 micrograms daily.** This mineral helps normalize blood sugar, particularly in people under stress—and people with exhausted adrenals always feel under stress.

•**Vitamin C: 200 milligrams to 1,000 milligrams daily.** Your adrenal glands are the spot in the body that contains more vitamin C than any other. (Your brain contains a lot, too.)

The vitamin C is crucial in the manufacture of cortisol and other adrenal hormones—and more vitamin C helps.

•**Pantothenic acid (vitamin B₅): 100 milligrams to 300 milligrams daily.** This B vitamin also helps boost the production of cortisol. In fact, a diet deficient in pantothenic acid can make your adrenals shrink!

•**Tyrosine: 450 milligrams to 1,000 milligrams daily.** Your body uses this amino acid to make noradrenaline.

•**Pregnenolone: 15 mg.** The raw material for all the other adrenal hormones.

Bioidentical Adrenal Hormones

As you can read in the chapter on Hormonal Imbalances (page 84), I'm a great believer in correcting hormonal imbalances with bioidentical hormones—natural and exact replicas of the chemical structure of your own hormones. If the diet and supplements in the Real Cure Regimen for adrenal exhaustion don't solve the problem, then it's time to sit down with a holistic-minded doctor and consider taking bioidentical adrenal hormones. *There are two...*

•**Cortisol.** This adrenal hormone is available by prescription: hydrocortisone from a compounding pharmacy (which creates customized medications on site), or Cortef from a standard pharmacy. When I supplement in my patients, I recommend 5 milligrams to 20 milligrams of hydrocortisone or Cortef. Higher doses can be toxic. I find that these dosages are quite safe for my patients. However, long-term use of higher dosages can be very dangerous: They can suppress the adrenal gland (supplied with too much cortisol, it stops working), causing diabetes, high blood pressure, and/or osteoporosis.

•**DHEA** is a key adrenal hormone linked to energy, youthfulness, and good health. It is available without a prescription. But if you take more than 10 milligrams a day, I recommend you use this hormone with the guidance and supervision of a holistic physician, who can order a test for your blood level of DHEA-S (dehydroepiandrosterone sulfate, a version of DHEA), to help guide dosage.

General guidelines when using this test to determine dosage are...

DHEA 5 mg–50 mg P.O QD (decrease the dose if acne or darkening of facial hair in females occurs)			DHEA-sulfate (mcg/dL) (x 0.02714 = umol/L)		
In Males			In Females		
DHEA-Sulfate		Rx (mg/day)	DHEA-Sulfate		Rx (mg/day)
umol /l	mcg/dl		umol /l	mcg/dl	
0–2.7	0–100	50	0–0.8	0–30	25
2.8–5.4	101–200	40	0.9–2.2	31–80	20
5.5–7.6	201–280	25	2.3–3.0	81–110	20
7.7–8.7	281–320	10	3.1–3	111–114	5

For my patients, I find that an optimal dose is usually 5 milligrams to 10 milligrams for women and 25 milligrams to 50 milligrams for men. As with many supplements, quality is not consistent in the marketplace. I recommend the brand from Nature's Way, which is available in 5 milligram and 25 milligram dosages.

There are several cautions when using DHEA. Too-high doses can cause acne or darkening of facial hair. If you have a hormone-sensitive cancer, such as prostate or breast, don't use this hormone without your doctor's permission.

Alzheimer's Disease and Dementia

Real Causes

- **Chronic Inflammation.** Low-grade, chronic inflammation fuels the buildup of the toxic clumps and tangles of protein (amyloid and tau) that are the hallmarks of the disease (page 118).

- **Nutritional Deficiencies.** Many of the effects of excess amyloid and tau—such as memory loss and disorientation—can be avoided or eased by optimizing nutrition (page 3).

- **Hormonal Imbalances.** Treating hormonal imbalances, particularly low testosterone and thyroid hormone, can help prevent and treat dementia (page 84).

- **Prescription Medications.** For many elderly people, taking multiple medications can muddle the mind; what is diagnosed as Alzheimer's often goes away when the medications are stopped (page 70).

- **Happiness Deficiency.** As cognitive function declines, a person may become depressed, worsening dementia (page 55).

- **Inactivity.** Studies show that regular activity can help prevent Alzheimer's and that inactivity can worsen the condition (page 40).

A lot of Americans have dementia, the gradual loss of memory and other cognitive functions along with a decline into dependence. About 5.8 million have Alzheimer's disease. Nearly one million more have vascular dementia, caused by poor circulation to the brain and strokes. (Many have both.) In the past few decades, the incidence of Alzheimer's has gone up tenfold among people 65 and older, and twenty-four-fold among those under 65.

But here's a surprising fact: Many, if not most, people diagnosed with Alzheimer's do not have the disease. The only definitive "test" for diagnosing Alzheimer's is a postmortem biopsy of the brain to detect the toxic clumps and tangles of protein (amyloid and tau) that are the hallmarks of the disease. But the severe memory loss and chronic confusion that are characteristic of Alzheimer's and are used to diagnose the disease aren't always caused by Alzheimer's.

Cognitive decline also can be caused by a nutritional deficiency, such as low levels of B_{12}. And by a drug side effect. And by depression and other treatable illnesses. In fact, in his book *The Myth of Alzheimer's: What You Aren't Being Told about Today's Most Dreaded Diagnosis*, Peter J. Whitehouse, MD, PhD, says that a diagnosis of Alzheimer's can only be made once other causes are ruled out, including…

- **Hypothyroidism and other metabolic causes**
- **Vascular problems,** such as stroke
- **Vitamin deficiencies,** including B_{12}
- **Hypercalcemia** (high levels of calcium)
- **Normal-pressure hydrocephalus** (an excess of cerebrospinal fluid)
- **Psychiatric difficulties,** such as depression and schizophrenia
- **Head trauma**
- **Structural brain lesions**—brain tumor, injuries, or blood clots
- **Other neurodegenerative conditions,** such as Parkinson's disease
- **Dehydration and other causes of delirium**
- **Brain infections,** such as HIV, encephalitis, meningitis, and syphilis
- **Chronic effects of various substances,** including medications and alcohol

A proper medical evaluation to detect these underlying (and often reversible) causes of dementia takes at least 30 to 60 minutes—an amount of time most doctors don't have, because Medicare pays poorly for visits over five minutes. That's why, when older folks have the symptoms of cognitive decline, they're often automatically diagnosed with Alzheimer's or dementia—and just as automatically get a prescription for *donepezil* (Aricept), an anti-Alzheimer's drug that has very minimal disease-slowing or disease-relieving benefits.

Real Cure Regimen

In my experience with patients, a thorough exam often finds that an older person with cognitive decline doesn't have dementia. Even if they do, natural treatments can often dramatically improve their memory, mental state, and everyday functioning. (And the treatments in this chapter also will improve the memory of most people with age-related memory loss or mild cognitive impairment, the stages of memory loss that can eventually turn into Alzheimer's.) Here are treatments that address the underlying real causes that are worth considering if you or a loved one has been diagnosed with Alzheimer's or vascular dementia.

Receive Vitamin B$_{12}$ Injections

Make sure your doctor checks your blood levels of B$_{12}$. Optimal levels are a must for a healthy brain. That's because B$_{12}$ strengthens the myelin sheath, the protective covering around axons, which are wirelike extensions of brain cells that help relay messages between those cells.

Any reading above 209 picograms per deciliter is designated "normal" by most labs—but it's not necessarily a healthful level. My suggested strategy: If your B$_{12}$ level is under 540, you should receive a series of at least 15 B$_{12}$ shots over three months. (B$_{12}$ shots can take three months to fully kick in and revive memory and cognitive function.) Make sure each injection has 1,000 micrograms to 5,000 micrograms of B$_{12}$. If your B$_{12}$ level is under 340, you should continue to receive B$_{12}$ shots monthly for the rest of your life.

Also, add one tablespoon of apple cider vinegar mixed into some food at each meal (for example, in salad dressing). Low vitamin B$_{12}$ is often linked with low stomach acid, and apple cider vinegar is a simple way to help that problem.

When Dutch scientists studied more than 1,000 older people who didn't have dementia, they found that people with low B$_{12}$ levels (but still well within the "normal" range) had decreased function in their axons (white matter). "B$_{12}$ status in the normal range is associated with severity of white-matter lesions," concluded the researchers in the *Journal of Neurology, Neurosurgery & Psychiatry*. This is one more study indicating that our so-called normal ranges for many blood tests have nothing to do with good health—and that the normal range should be the range that helps your body function optimally.

Five hundred micrograms of B$_{12}$ can often help take care of low levels of vitamin B$_{12}$, even if your doctor won't agree to give you B$_{12}$ injections.

Consume More Fish Oil

The membranes (outer coverings) of brain cells are made of DHA (docosahexaenoic acid), one of the omega-3 essential fatty acids found primarily in fish oil. Without enough DHA, your brain can't function normally.

I recommend eating three to four servings a week of fatty fish, such as salmon, tuna, herring, or sardines. Or take omega-3 supplements. A unique form, called Vectomega, has a chemical structure identical to that found in salmon and dramatically increases absorption. One to two tablets a day are plenty, instead of the typical eight to 16. Another good brand is Nordic Naturals. Follow the dosage recommendation on the label.

In one study, a supplement of 1.7 grams of DHA and 0.6 gram of EPA (eicosapentaenoic acid) improved the appetite of people with mild to moderate Alzheimer's and helped them gain weight, reported Swedish researchers in the *Journal of the American Geriatrics Society*. In another study, published in the journal *Molecular Neurobiology*, Spanish researchers discovered a form of DHA in the brain called neuroprotectin D1 (NPD1) that protects the brain cells against many biochemical stressors, including amyloid-beta.

Try Curcumin and Ginkgo

Studies have shown that Alzheimer's is much less common in India than in the United States, and a dietary factor may be making the difference. It's turmeric, the spice that gives curry its yellow color. The active ingredient in turmeric is curcumin, and studies show that curcumin can dissolve the amyloid plaques that are a hallmark of Alzheimer's. Unfortunately, you have to eat as much curry as they do in India to absorb enough for the protective effect.

An alternative: A unique form of curcumin (BCM-95) boosts absorption of the compound sevenfold. For my patients with memory loss, I recommend one capsule to two capsules a day of a product that contains BCM-95: CuraMed, from Terry Naturally. Also try the herb ginkgo biloba, which can improve circulation to the brain. Use 40 milligrams to 80 milligrams, three times a day, for six weeks, to see if it works for you.

Treat Hormonal Deficiencies

If you have a diagnosis of Alzheimer's or dementia, I would consider treating hormonal deficiencies even if your blood tests for those hormones are "normal." *You'll need to work with a holistic practitioner or a compounding pharmacy for these treatments...*

• **A trial of prescription desiccated thyroid.** For most people with unexplained chronic confusion and memory loss, I recommend a three-month trial of this natural thyroid hormone to see if it helps. If you have risk factors for heart disease—high LDL cholesterol, high blood pressure, and the like—your doctor should start with a low dose and increase it slowly.

In a study by Brazilian researchers, published in the journal *BMC Public Health*, men with subclinical hypothyroidism (low levels of thyroid hormone that are still considered normal) had an eight-times-higher risk of developing Alzheimer's or dementia. And in a study by researchers at Harvard Medical School and Boston University School of Medicine, published in the *Archives of Internal Medicine*, women with low-normal levels of thyroid hormone had a 2.4-times-higher risk of developing Alzheimer's. "The most important thing to take away from this study is the question of whether our currently accepted standard of what normal thyroid levels are is too broad," wrote Zaldy S. Tan, MD, the lead researcher of the study.

• **In men, try testosterone, too.** If the total testosterone is under 400 ng/dl, I recommend using natural testosterone cream to bring the level to 600 ng/dl to 800 ng/dl. (A dose of 25 milligrams to 50 milligrams a day is plenty in older men with decreased mental function. Too much can unmask a hidden case of heart disease, possibly causing a heart attack or stroke.)

• **In women, consider bioidentical estrogen/progesterone.** Synthetic forms of estrogen/progesterone (Premarin and Provera) do not improve brain function and do increase your risk of breast cancer, heart disease, and stroke. However, estrogen affects memory (the brain is packed with estrogen receptors), and I think a six-month trial of bioidentical estrogen/progesterone is worthwhile in women with cognitive decline. Talk to your doctor about whether this treatment is right for you.

Sleep Eight Hours

Sleep protects and restores brain function. (In a 10-year study from the UK of 1,225 men, those with sleep disturbances—particularly daytime sleepiness caused by poor sleep—were 4.4 times more likely to develop vascular dementia.) For those diagnosed with dementia, I recommend a bedtime dose of three milligrams to five milligrams of melatonin, the sleep-inducing hormone. Another excellent sleep-inducing product is the herbal mixture Revitalizing Sleep Formula from Nature's Way (available at Amazon.com).

Also, treat sleep apnea or restless legs syndrome (RLS). These two sleep disorders can also cause insomnia and increase your risk of dementia. In sleep apnea, excess tissue in the throat cuts off breathing during sleep, repeatedly rousing the sleeper to a semi-awake state. Its main symptoms are snoring and daytime fatigue. (You can find treatments for sleep apnea in Insomnia and Other Sleep Disorders on page 268.) In restless legs, you have intensely uncomfortable feelings in your legs that cause you to move them around, seeking relief—particularly when you're trying to fall asleep. Your legs may also jerk around while you sleep. Optimizing blood levels of iron often works to ease or solve RLS. (See Nutritional Deficiencies on page 22 for advice.)

Investigate Your Meds

It is amazing how many people "diagnosed" with Alzheimer's recover normal mental function when they are weaned off unnecessary medications.

Ask your doctor if he's willing to work with you to find out if any (or many) of your medications are contributing to the confusion. The best approach, if it's safe: Your doctor tapers you off your medications, slowly reducing their dosages to see if the lower dose provides relief from any memory loss and other mental difficulties. For a few critical medications (heart medications and

---

A Prescription Option for Dementia

Aricept is a prescription drug used to treat dementia. It works by raising levels of the neurotransmitter acetylcholine, but the effect is minimal. (In fact, I think its main effect is boosting the profits of drug companies.) In an analysis of 13 studies on Aricept and Alzheimer's, researchers found that, on average, the drug raised cognitive function less than three points on a 70-point scale. Also, side effects (most commonly nausea, vomiting, and diarrhea) caused nearly one-third of those taking the drug to stop taking it.

However, if you have been diagnosed with Alzheimer's, and you have insurance that covers prescription medications, I would add Aricept to your Real Cure Regimen. Taking five milligrams (not the standard 10) is optimal, because there's less risk of side effects.

The rest of the treatments in my Real Cure Regimen for Alzheimer's and dementia are probably much more effective than Aricept, but it's worth adding this medication for the small benefit you might derive.

---

the like), your doctor may stop the medication for two to three days to see if your mind clears, or change medications to see if that helps.

Does this sound like a drastic strategy? I don't think it is. I suspect that many of the elderly would be fine without many (if not most) of their medications. For example, a study from the National Institutes of Health showed that, after a few months of use, the arthritis medication *celecoxib* (Celebrex) was no more effective than a placebo. So why continue to take it?

Sadly, it's easier for a physician to *add* a medication (it takes about one minute to write the prescription and discuss its use with the patient) than *stop* a medication (which requires a thorough review of why the medication was started and entails a degree of risk to the physician).

Don't Forget About Other Diseases

Many medical conditions can contribute to cognitive decline: heart disease, diabetes, depression, liver disease, anemia, chronic infections, and others. Make sure your doctor checks to see if another disease is the underlying cause. For this—as with many other health problems—I recommend seeing a holistic physician, who will take the time to conduct a proper evaluation of your condition, rather than blaming something reversible on "old age."

Preventing Alzheimer's With Nutrition

Is there a diet that can lower your risk of Alzheimer's?

Yes, say researchers from the Taub Institute for Research on Alzheimer's Disease and the Aging Brain, at Columbia University, who published their results in the *Archives of Neurology*. They studied 2,148 people over age 65 for four years and found that people with a "dietary pattern" that emphasized vegetables and fruits and limited red meat and dairy products were 48 percent less likely to be diagnosed with Alzheimer's. *The prevention pattern…*

High intake: Dark green, leafy vegetables (such as spinach and kale); cruciferous vegetables (such as broccoli and cabbage); tomatoes; fruits; nuts; fish. Several studies show that nutrients in whole foods like leafy green vegetables can help prevent or treat Alzheimer's disease or dementia.

Low intake: High-fat dairy products; red meat; organ meat; butter.

Niacin (vitamin B$_3$): In a five-year study of more than 3,700 people, researchers at the Centers for Disease Control and Prevention found that the more niacin people consumed, the less likely they were to develop cognitive decline and Alzheimer's, with a daily intake of 45 milligrams offering the most protection. (The RDA is 16 milligrams for men and 14 milligrams for women.)

Folate: Researchers in the Department of Neurology at the University of California, Irvine, analyzed the link between several nutrients and the development of Alzheimer's disease, and found that folate intake at or above the RDA was the most powerfully protective. "The participants who had intakes at or above the 400 microgram RDA of folate had a 55 percent reduction in the risk of developing Alzheimer's," commented the researchers, in *Alzheimer's & Dementia*. "But most people who reached that level did so by taking folic acid supplements, which suggests that many people do not get the recommended amounts of folate in their diets."

Stopping Memory Loss Long Before Alzheimer's

Memory loss proceeds in stages: from age-related memory loss to mild cognitive decline to Alzheimer's and dementia. But specific nutrients have the power to prevent age-related memory loss.

•**Vitamin E.** Researchers at Utah State University conducted a long-term study on people age 65 and older called the Cache County Study on Memory Health and Aging. They found that those with the highest blood levels of vitamin E and vitamin C also had the highest scores on the Modified Mini-Mental State examination. (The researchers also found that those who took antioxidant supplements containing vitamin E had a 36 percent reduced risk of developing Alzheimer's. In a similar study of more than 1,000 older people, Italian researchers found that those with the lowest blood levels of vitamin E were 2.6 times more likely to develop dementia.)

•**Beta-carotene.** Researchers at Harvard Medical School studied nearly 6,000 men older than 65. Those taking 50 milligrams of beta-carotene every other day had "significantly higher" scores on tests of memory and general mental prowess. The results were in the *Archives of Internal Medicine*. And in a study by researchers at the UCLA School of Medicine, high blood levels of beta-carotene were linked to lower risk of memory loss and decline—89 percent lower in those with a genetic predisposition to Alzheimer's and 11 percent lower in those without Alzheimer's genes.

•**Vitamin B$_{12}$.** When researchers at the University of Illinois matched vitamin B$_{12}$ intake and the amount of gray matter in various areas of the brain (gray matter processes information), they found that those with the highest B$_{12}$ intake had the most gray matter. "These effects were driven by vitamin supplementation," they wrote in the journal *Brain Research*. (In other words, it was vitamin supplements and not B$_{12}$ from food that made for bigger, healthier brains.)

In other studies on B$_{12}$ and brainpower…

•Lower blood levels of vitamin B$_{12}$ were linked to poorer performance on memory and mental tests in 84 people age 69 and older who didn't have dementia, reported Welsh researchers in the *American Journal of Clinical Nutrition*.

•Five months of B$_{12}$ injections given to older people with low B$_{12}$ levels improved their scores on memory and mental tests, reported Dutch researchers.

•In a five-year study, researchers at Harvard Medical School found that supplementing the diet with vitamins B$_{12}$, B$_6$, and folate helped preserve memory and mental ability in women over 40 with low dietary intake of B vitamins.

•**Folate.** Commenting in the journal *Lancet* that "low folate and raised homocysteine concentrations in blood are associated with poor cognitive performance" (by which they mean poor memory, less ability to take in and understand information, and slow reflexes), Dutch researchers tested the ability of folate to boost memory and mental performance in 818 people 50 to 75 years old. For three years, half the study participants took 800 micrograms a day of folate and half took a placebo. After three years, the "cognitive functions that decline with age" were "significantly improved" in those who took folate, but not in the placebo group. In fact, on memory tests, the supplement users had scores comparable to those of people 5.5 years younger, and on tests of mental speed, the folate group performed as well as people 1.9 years younger.

•**Zinc.** English researchers studied 387 people ages 55 to 87, giving half zinc supplements (15 milligrams to 30 milligrams daily). After three months, those taking zinc "performed significantly better" on memory tests, reported the researchers in the *British Journal of Nutrition*.

Vitamin K: People with early-stage Alzheimer's had a 55 percent lower intake of vitamin K than people of the same age who didn't have Alzheimer's, reported researchers in the *Journal of the American Dietetic Association.*

Anxiety

Real Causes

- **Nutritional Deficiencies.** Low levels of nutrients—particularly magnesium and the B vitamins—can play a role in anxiety (page 3).
- **Hormonal Imbalances.** An imbalance of adrenal and/or thyroid hormones can cause anxiety (page 84).
- **Happiness Deficiency.** During a period of relative calm (such as while watching TV), buried feelings and worries can rise to the surface and trigger a panic attack (page 55).

You're worried nearly all the time. And because you're constantly worried, you're irritable, impatient, and restless, and have a hard time sleeping. Non-stop worrying is also hard on your health, causing headaches, tight, painful muscles, and digestive upset. And your relationships suffer, too, as family and friends tire of hearing about your constant concerns. That's a description of generalized anxiety disorder, or GAD. Other types of anxiety include post-traumatic stress disorder (PTSD), panic disorder, severe shyness (social anxiety disorder), and obsessive-compulsive disorder (OCD).

Having spent the past 30 years providing effective treatment for those with disabling diseases such as chronic fatigue syndrome, fibromyalgia, and chronic pain (stressful diseases, which can trigger anxiety, are often significant components), I know how devastating an anxiety disorder can be. Unfortunately, all that most doctors have to offer the 10 percent of the population with an anxiety disorder are anti-anxiety medications such as Xanax (*alprazolam*) and antidepressants. Not only are these drugs often ineffective, but they are also rife with side effects and often addictive.

Real Cure Regimen

As a physician and researcher, my job is to find the best combination of natural and prescription therapies that can help patients who haven't been helped by "modern" medicine. That's why I'm very excited to report on several anti-anxiety products with a unique formula of natural compounds. People are amazed at how highly effective these products are in restoring a naturally calm and peaceful state of mind. They also find that it increases their energy and mental clarity.

The Power of Cannabinoids (Hemp)

In December 2018, the federal government finally came to its senses and legalized hemp—a strain of the *cannabis sativa* plant that is used for agricultural purposes such as fiber, rather than to "get high." The legalized hemp plants contain less than 0.3 percent of THC, the "cannabinoid" in cannabis (marijuana) that causes the "high." I think the legalization of hemp is very good news because an enormous body of scientific research—and the clinical experience of untold numbers of clinicians and their patients—suggests that hemp oil can help a wide array of health problems.

Anxiety is one of them.

But don't rush out and buy any hemp oil product. Hemp oil and its active component CBD (cannabidiol) have become very trendy—and many products on the market seem more focused on advertising, network marketing, and pretty labeling than on what is actually in the bottle. So I am very picky about the hemp oils I use with my patients—and you should be picky, too.

Plus, there are at least 10 highly active cannabinoids in hemp oil other than CBD—it's simply that CBD has gotten the most attention. Which is why I recommend you use whole hemp oil, which contains all of those cannabinoids (but, as I said earlier, doesn't contain very much THC).

The product I recommend: Hemp Select, from Terry Naturally. Each capsule has 50 mg of hemp oil and 10 mg of CBD. (Get it without the curcumin, which is more cost-effective.) Another good, full-spectrum brand is CBD Oil from Plus. If you are in a state where medical marijuana is legal, you can also find reliable THC-free or "low-THC" hemp oil products at a marijuana dispensary.

The best dosing? For acute anxiety attacks, take 30 milligrams to 50 milligrams of CBD or 150 to 250 milligrams of whole hemp oil. For preventing anxiety, take the lower end of these doses—30 mg of CBD or 150 mg of whole hemp oil—twice a day. Higher doses are safe. For example, children with epileptic seizures are given over 1,000 milligrams of CBD daily, so it's hard to overdose. But be forewarned: any reliable, effective product will be expensive.

Another Use for Echinacea

Most of us are familiar with using the herb echinacea to prevent and ease viral infections, such as cold and flu. But research has shown that a special extract of echinacea—found in AnxioCalm, from Terry Naturally—was as effective as Valium-type medications (benzodiazepines) for anxiety, after six weeks of use. The recommended dose is one to two tablets, twice a day.

The Best Anti-Anxiety Ingredients

In my clinical experience, one of the best supplements for easing anxiety is a product called Calming Balance, from Roex (available online from various sources). Its ingredients get to the core of some of the real causes of your anxiety, specifically nutrient deficiencies and hormonal imbalances. The product produces an anti-anxiety effect within 30 minutes, but that effect continues to increase over two weeks of continued use—at which point your anxiety should be under control! Once anxiety is normalized, lower the dose (from three capsules, three times daily, to one capsule to three capsules, one time daily). Or take it only as needed.

Now, let's explore the individual ingredients in this wonderful supplement.

•**Thiamin (vitamin B$_1$): 500 milligrams.** Vitamin B$_1$ is critical for proper brain function, mental clarity, and energy production, as well as for preventing the production of excess lactic acid. (A large body of research shows that sensitivity to high levels of lactic acid can cause anxiety attacks in those prone to them.)

At her 93rd birthday party many years ago, the late Dr. Janet Travell told me about a natural treatment for anxiety, a treatment few physicians are aware of. A professor of medicine at the George Washington University Medical School, Dr. Travell was the White House physician for Presidents Kennedy and Johnson, and was the world's leading expert on pain management. At the party, she told me that 500 milligrams of vitamin B$_1$ three times a day was highly effective in treating anxiety. I started using this treatment in my practice and was astounded at its effectiveness. Unlike a drug, which decreases anxiety by numbing you, vitamin B$_1$ decreases anxiety (and improves mental clarity) by helping your body to work more effectively.

•**Niacin: 20 milligrams.** Niacin is a natural tranquilizer. In a study on rats, niacin was similar to Valium in affecting the levels of several neurotransmitters that play a role in anxiety (serotonin, noradrenaline, dopamine, and gamma-aminobutyric acid, or GABA) but without being addictive, like Valium. In fact, some experts call niacin "nature's Valium." Niacin also helps decrease excess lactic acid levels and anxiety-causing episodes of low blood sugar/hypoglycemia from adrenal exhaustion.

•**Vitamin B$_6$ (*pyridoxine*): 10 milligrams.** Vitamin B$_6$ deficiency is common in Americans, and those low levels can contribute to anxiety because the vitamin is critical in the production of two brain chemicals that prevent anxiety (GABA and serotonin).

•**Vitamin B$_{12}$: 600 micrograms.** Low blood levels of vitamin B$_{12}$ have been linked to anxiety, and research shows that many individuals require superhigh levels of B$_{12}$ to get adequate levels into the brain.

•**Pantothenic acid: 40 milligrams.** Pantothenic acid (vitamin B$_5$) is another B vitamin that is critical for the treatment of adrenal exhaustion—and adrenal exhaustion is a very common trigger for hypoglycemia-induced anxiety. If you crave sugar, get irritable when you're hungry, are easily overwhelmed under stress, and/or have low blood pressure with dizziness on standing, you probably have adrenal exhaustion. (For more information on this problem, see Hormonal Imbalances on page 84 and Adrenal Exhaustion on page 138.)

•**Magnesium: 100 milligrams.** This key mineral is lost in food processing, and most Americans are deficient in it. In fact, I consider magnesium deficiency to be the single most important nutritional deficiency in the United States because the nutrient is critical for more than 300 chemical reactions in the body. Among its many functions, magnesium has been called the anti-stress mineral—it relaxes muscles, helps sleep, and relieves tension. Very low magnesium levels can even trigger panic attacks, which can be immediately relieved with magnesium therapy.

Unfortunately, magnesium in the form of magnesium oxide and magnesium hydroxide (the cheapest and therefore the most commonly used magnesium compounds in supplements) is poorly absorbed and consequently less effective. Magnesium citrate, a highly absorbable form, is used in Calming Balance, which you can purchase at EndFatigue.com. (Another highly absorbable form is magnesium glycinate.)

•**Theanine: 100 milligrams daily.** Theanine, a compound in green tea, is another outstanding treatment for anxiety, and it also helps with mental alertness. (In other words, it's calming but nonsedating.) Theanine is most effective in the range of 50 milligrams to 200 milligrams, with the effect being felt within 30 minutes and lasting for eight to 10 hours. Calming Balance includes the natural Suntheanine product, which is derived from green tea and is far more effective than synthetic forms.

Research shows that theanine works by three mechanisms: (1) It stimulates the production of alpha brain waves, creating a state of deep relaxation and mental alertness similar to meditation; (2) it helps in the production of the calming neurotransmitter GABA; and (3) it naturally stimulates the release of serotonin and dopamine.

•**Passionflower extract: 200 milligrams daily.** This is one of the best-known herbs for the treatment of anxiety. Passionflower was first cultivated in the United States by Native Americans, and Spanish conquerors learned of it from the Aztecs of Mexico, who used it as a sedative to treat nervousness and insomnia. The plant was taken back to Europe, where it became widely cultivated and was introduced into European medicine.

•*Magnolia officinalis* **extract: 90 milligrams daily.** Magnolia bark has a long history of use in traditional Chinese formulas that relieve anxiety. Magnolia extract from the bark is rich in two phytochemicals: honokiol, which exerts an antianxiety effect, and magnolol, which acts as an antidepressant. Dozens of animal studies have shown that magnolia extract is a nonaddictive, nonsedating stress buster even at low doses. Take a 30-milligram capsule, three times a day.

Lifestyle Tips for Anxiety Relief

Besides this nutritional supplement, these are other natural, safe, and nonpharmaceutical ways to calm your mental woes.

•**Walk in the sunshine.** This is a great reliever of worries and stress. In a study from Danish researchers, published in *Frontiers in Psychology*, walking in nature improved the feeling of well-being and decreased stress.

•**Use a relaxation technique.** An analysis of 16 studies on relaxation techniques and anxiety showed "the effectiveness of relaxation therapy for people with anxiety."

For those starting with relaxation training, I recommend the classic book *The Relaxation Response*, by Herbert Benson, MD, professor of mind-body medicine at Harvard Medical School and director emeritus of the Benson-Henry Institute for Mind Body Medicine at Massachusetts General Hospital. We talked with Dr. Benson, and he reiterated the simplicity and effectiveness of the book's technique, first introduced to the public in 1975.

1. Pick a focus word, short phrase, or prayer that is firmly rooted in your belief system.
2. Sit quietly in a comfortable position.
3. Close your eyes.
4. Relax your muscles, progressing from your feet to your calves, thighs, abdomen, shoulders, neck, and head.

Panic Attacks and Suppressed Feelings

Panic attacks (panic attack disorder) and hyperventilation are two common medical problems. Although you may have an idea of what a panic attack feels like, hyperventilation can include many other feelings, sensations, and symptoms. These include the feeling that you are unable to take a deep enough breath despite taking a full breath (the hallmark of hyperventilation); lightheadedness; a spacey and disembodied feeling; chest pain; numbness and tingling in the fingers and especially around the mouth; and—when an attack is particularly severe—the feeling of impending death.

I remember the first time I saw a full-blown hyperventilation attack. I was in the hospital carrying the beeper for "code blue" (the term hospitals use when someone's heart is about to stop or has stopped) when the beeper went off and I hurried to the emergency room. The patient there had a pulse of over 200 beats per minute, and she looked like she was about to die. We prepared to do CPR, but the arterial blood gas results—a test for lung function—showed that she was only hyperventilating.

Although both panic attacks and hyperventilation have underlying physical causes (including magnesium and other nutritional deficiencies, and thyroid, adrenal, and other hormonal imbalances), I believe there is also a common psychological component: the burying of feelings.

Most people find that these attacks occur not during a period of stress, but when they finally have a chance to relax, such as when they are driving a car or watching TV. Their feelings finally bubble to the surface, triggering the attacks.

You can short-circuit the biochemical part of the attack by breathing in and out of a bag (raising the carbon dioxide level in your blood) or doing abdominal breathing (the abdomen expands outward during inhalation, allowing you to take a bigger breath). But the most important long-term solution is simply to feel what one is feeling, without resistance. (For more information on this approach, see Happiness Deficiency on page 55.)

5. Breathe slowly and naturally, and as you do, say your focus word, sound, phrase, or prayer silently to yourself as you exhale.

6. Assume a passive attitude. Don't worry about how well you're doing. When other thoughts come to mind, simply say to yourself, "Oh well," and gently return to your repetition.

7. Continue for 10 minutes to 20 minutes.

8. When you stop, do not stand immediately. Sitting quietly for a minute or so, allowing other thoughts to return. Then open your eyes and sit for another minute before rising.

Practice the technique once or twice daily, such as before breakfast and before dinner.

•**Avoid sugar and caffeine.** They imbalance your blood sugar and rattle your nerves, increasing anxiety. Theanine-containing green tea is okay, but no more than 10 cups per day.

•**Express your anger.** Anxiety often is a symptom of repressed anger. These feelings need to be expressed and acknowledged and released (without harming others). You can tell when anger is healthy because it feels good to express it. Also, it's often a healthy way of standing up for yourself. When it starts feeling bad, release it. (See the section on the healing power of feeling your feelings in Happiness Deficiency on page 55.)

• **Treat hormonal imbalances.** Anxiety can be caused by an overactive thyroid, by low progesterone and estrogen in women, by low testosterone in men, and by adrenal exhaustion. Have your hormone levels checked—and, if necessary, corrected—by a holistic physician. (For more information, see Hormonal Imbalances on page 84.)

Arthritis

Real Causes

• **Chronic Inflammation.** Arthritis is a form of chronic inflammation of the joints and the surrounding muscles, tendons, and ligaments, either from years of wear and tear (osteoarthritis) or from an autoimmune disease (rheumatoid arthritis) (page 118).

• **Inactivity.** Studies show that regular physical activity—such as brisk walking—decreases the risk of arthritis (page 40).

• **Nutritional Deficiencies.** Many Americans have low levels of the anti-inflammatory omega-3 fatty acids found in fish oil, contributing to the development of this inflammatory disease (page 28).

Arthritis is the number-one cause of chronic pain and disability in the United States. More than 30 million Americans—about 65 percent of people age 65 and over—suffer with joint pain and stiffness from the wear-and-tear disease of osteoarthritis (OA). Another 1.5 million (most of them women) suffer with the red, hot, swollen, and painful joints of rheumatoid arthritis (RA), a joint-attacking autoimmune disease.

My Real Cure Regimen for arthritis can result in dramatic pain relief and improved everyday functioning for people with either OA or RA—and often with minimal or no use of drugs.

Real Cure Regimen

I prefer using natural rather than prescription therapies for arthritis. That's because the most common class of medications for pain relief in arthritis—nonsteroidal anti-inflammatory drugs (NSAIDs)—are estimated to kill more than 50,000 Americans—every year! They do that by causing somewhere between 4,000 and 17,000 deaths from bleeding ulcers, and by increasing heart attack and stroke risk by 35 percent. These facts are from scientific studies involving more than 500,000 people. Didn't hear about the results in the news media? Wonder why?

Here's a hint: Look at who the biggest advertisers are. *Drug companies.*

To add insult to that incredible injury, NSAIDs don't slow the progression of arthritis—and may actually speed it up! (For more information on the downsides of NSAIDs, see Prescription Medications on page 70.) Fortunately, there's an effective, safe alternative to NSAIDs: the natural program I recommend. It eases pain, decreases inflammation, and helps repair joints. *It has four main components, which we'll look at one by one...*

1. Repair cartilage
2. Reverse inflammation
3. Restore function
4. Rule out and (if necessary) eliminate food allergies, and treat infections

Repair

Cartilage covers and cushions the ends of bones so they don't rub together. In OA, cartilage has thinned or disappeared. Bones rub together and hurt. In RA, cartilage and bones are mistakenly attacked by the body's immune system.

But you can repair cartilage using a combination of two cartilage-building nutrients: glucosamine sulfate (750 milligrams, two times a day, for a minimum of six weeks) and methylsulfonylmethane, or MSM (2,000 milligrams a day). If your arthritis is severe, you can add another cartilage-repairing nutrient, chondroitin (400 milligrams, three times a day). I also recommend daily intake of the nutrients in a good multivitamin-mineral supplement, many of which promote wound healing. Let's look at the ingredients of repair, one by one...

•**Glucosamine sulfate.** This compound is a component of cartilage. Its exact mechanism of action in easing arthritis isn't fully understood. But research shows that when you take it orally, glucosamine is incorporated into the molecules that make up cartilage—reducing pain as effectively as NSAIDs, and stabilizing and healing arthritic joints.

I recommend the sulfate form (not glucosamine hydrochloride) because sulfate also can help with joint healing. A study from the University of Utah School of Medicine showed that glucosamine and NSAIDs work synergistically—taking the two together is more effective than NSAIDs alone. This means glucosamine will help you to either stop taking NSAIDs (if pain reduction is sufficient) or reduce your daily dose of NSAIDs, dramatically improving the drug's safety and reducing its cost. Glucosamine might also spare you from knee replacement surgery.

In a five-year study of 275 people with knee OA, those who took glucosamine sulfate had a 57 percent lower rate of needing surgery to replace the knee joint (because the supplement *repaired* the joint).

Doses of less than 1,000 milligrams a day don't improve symptoms; the standard dose is 750 milligrams, two times a day. You can take it with or without food. It is very safe. After three to six months of use, you can usually stop it, and then use it as needed for pain. (This strategy—stopping the drug after pain relief is achieved, and using it only as needed—is the best strategy for many arthritis remedies.)

By the way: Instead of killing 50,000 Americans yearly, glucosamine probably saves lives—research published in the *American Journal of Clinical Nutrition* links the compound to a 17 percent lower risk of death.

Purple Pectin for Pain Relief

Pectin is a fiber found in fruit—and many people find that taking pectin as a supplement is a safe, cheap way to reduce arthritis pain. If you want to try it, purchase Certo—a pectin-containing thickening agent used to make jams and jellies—in the canning section of your local supermarket. Take one tablespoon to three tablespoons, one or two times daily, in eight ounces of juice.

If pectin is going to help, you'll probably see results in one to two weeks. As pain lessens, you can reduce the dose to one teaspoon, once or twice a day.

Another folk remedy worth considering: Copper bracelets. Although there are studies showing they are ineffective in relieving the pain and stiffness of arthritis, I've seen many patients improve after starting to wear a copper bracelet.

•**Chondroitin sulfate.** This compound also plays a role in creating, maintaining, and repairing cartilage, and it's sometimes added to glucosamine or taken by itself. However, its benefits are modest, because less than 10 percent of it is absorbed (as compared with 90 percent for glucosamine sulfate).

To improve absorption, I recommend using a "low molecular weight" form of chondroitin (look for this phrase on the label), which can help slow down arthritis and is particularly worth adding to your regimen if you're not getting adequate relief with the other treatments. Try 1,200 milligrams in a single dose or 400 milligrams three times daily; they are equally effective.

•**Type II Collagen.** This type of collagen constitutes 90 percent of the collagen in joint cartilage, making it especially important for joint healing. Numerous studies show that it not only helps arthritis pain and function, but also helps produce new cartilage. You can find Type 2 collagen in over-the-counter supplements. The ingredient used in many studies—and found in many supplements—is UC-II.

•**Hyaluronic acid complex.** This compound lubricates joints, skin, and eyes. Numerous studies show supplementation can help ease arthritis pain.

•**Other nutritional support.** The individual compounds just discussed are crucial, but overall nutritional support is also critical for repairing arthritis. And the simplest way to get it is by combining a supplement called Be Mobile, from Terry Naturally, with a good multivitamin-mineral supplement. Give these remedies about six weeks to work.

If you want to add more elements to the "Repair" protocol, here are a few other therapeutic agents that could help...

•**MSM.** Research shows that the sulfur-containing compound MSM (methylsulfonylmethane) helps arthritis. In a study at UCLA, those taking the supplement for six weeks (1,500 milligrams in the morning, 750 milligrams at lunch) had an 80 percent decrease in pain.

Research also shows MSM and glucosamine work together to reduce pain and swelling. In a study from Indian researchers published in *Clinical Drug Investigation*, 118 people with mild to moderate osteoarthritis were treated three times daily with one of four regimens: (1) 500 milligrams of glucosamine; (2) 500 milligrams of MSM; (3) a combination of glucosamine and MSM; or (4) a placebo. After 12 weeks, the combination treatment was the best (and the fastest) for decreasing pain and inflammation. Another study, from Korean researchers, helped explain the mechanism of MSM: It decreases the level of cytokines, inflammatory chemicals that contribute to arthritis pain.

•**Vitamin D.** Low intake and low blood levels of vitamin D have been linked to an increasing risk of worsening OA of the knee. And a study in the journal *Rheumatology International* showed that people with the most severe RA—the most pain and the poorest daily functioning—also had the lowest blood levels of vitamin D.

•**SAMe (S-adenosylmethionine).** This compound plays a fundamental role in dozens of chemical reactions in the body—and it can help reduce OA pain as effectively as NSAIDs. However, SAMe supplements aren't easily absorbed, many products don't deliver the amounts their labels claim, and it's expensive.

A better approach: Take the nutrients your body needs to make SAMe. Research shows that people taking the nutrients in the Energy Revitalization System multinutrient powder (from Nature's Way) had blood levels of SAMe similar to those in people taking 400 to 800 milligrams of SAMe daily.

•**Pine bark (pycnogenol).** Several studies show that this powerful antioxidant and circulation-booster can help with arthritis. In the most recent, pycnogenol reduced pain and stiffness, lowered inflammatory biomarkers, and allowed people to use less pain-relieving medication.

Reverse Inflammation

As I discussed earlier, NSAIDs such as ibuprofen are the standard recommendation for arthritis pain. But there are many natural anti-inflammatory compounds with the same action—and without the deadly side effects.

To treat arthritis inflammation, I recommend a combination of several natural anti-inflammatory compounds: boswellia (also known as frankincense); willow bark (from which aspirin is derived); and cherry extract.

Let's look at each of these natural anti-inflammatory compounds. (You can also read about them in Chronic Inflammation on page 118.)

•**Willow bark.** Willow bark contains salicin, the natural source of aspirin's salicylic acid. But when used as an herbal extract, willow bark is much safer than aspirin—which can cause gastrointestinal bleeding—and effectively decreases inflammation and relieves pain.

In a study published in the *Journal of Rheumatology*, German researchers gave people with OA of the hip or knee a daily dose of willow bark extract, standardized to 240 milligrams salicin. It was significantly superior to a placebo in relieving pain. In another study, willow bark extract was about as effective as an NSAID for pain relief and much safer. A third study found that 240 milligrams of salicin a day was more effective than a placebo in treating OA.

I recommend starting with 240 milligrams a day of salicin until you experience the maximum pain-relieving, anti-inflammatory benefit. At that point, consider lowering the dose to 120 milligrams a day, or take it as needed.

•**Boswellia.** *Boswellia serrata*, also known as frankincense, has been used for centuries in the traditional Ayurvedic medicine of India to treat inflammation and pain. Studies show it's helpful for both OA and RA. In one study, 30 people with knee OA were given 1,000 milligrams of either an extract of boswellia or a placebo for eight weeks; the two groups switched treatments for the next eight weeks. When the patients were on boswellia, they had an improved ability to walk and much less pain. (The pain index fell by a remarkable 90 percent!) In the most recent study, published in *Phytotherapy Research*, a boswellia extract not only reduced pain and stiffness—it also helped stop the destruction of cartilage (the spongy cushion between bones) and prevent bone spurs, a symptom of arthritis.

Research shows that boswellia cools inflammation by blocking the production of several inflammatory immune compounds. A commonly used dose: 150 milligrams to 350 milligrams, three times daily.

•**Tart cherries (*Prunus cerasus*).** NSAIDs work by inhibiting COX enzymes that trigger the production of inflammatory compounds called prostaglandins. Tart cherries, uniquely rich in anthocyanins, a powerful anti-inflammatory, inhibit COX as effectively as NSAIDs. (Tart cherries are available frozen, dried, as juice, and as concentrate—they're not the same as the sweet cherries in the produce department at the supermarket.) A dose of 2,000 milligrams of tart cherry extract contains the active components present in 10 tart cherries or 32 ounces of tart cherry juice. Many people also find that eating 10 to 20 sweet cherries a day also helps ease the arthritis symptoms.

In a study from researchers at the University of Pennsylvania School of Medicine, 58 people with knee osteoarthritis drank either tart cherry juice or a placebo drink. After six weeks, those drinking the juice had less pain and stiffness, and were better able to perform daily functions, such as using the stairs or getting in and out of a car. They also had lower levels of C-reactive protein, a biomarker of inflammation.

•**Fish oil.** Fish oil is another powerful anti-inflammatory, and studies show it's particularly effective with RA. In an analysis of more than 20 studies on fish oil and rheumatoid arthritis, published in the journal *Nutrients*, an international team of scientists found that fish oil decreased RA pain by 21 percent.

As I discuss in other parts of this book, I favor a unique form of omega-3 fatty acid called Vectomega, from Terry Naturally. It has a chemical structure identical to that found in salmon and is combined with natural phospholipids that increase absorption dramatically—50 times as much as other fish oils. One tablet or two tablets a day deliver all the EPA and DHA you need. If you prefer liquid fish oil, good brands include Nordic Naturals. Follow the dosage recommendations on the label.

•**Curcumin.** Another excellent option for pain relief is curcumin, the active ingredient in turmeric. While it takes huge amounts of the spice to achieve therapeutic results, there's

Topical Pain Medication: A Safer Option

As we point out several times in this book (and in this chapter), nonsteroidal anti-inflammatory medications for arthritis kill more than 50,000 Americans a year. But you can use the same medications topically—they're just as effective and a whole lot safer. Researchers in the UK studied nearly 600 people with knee osteoarthritis. Half took oral ibuprofen (Motrin, Advil) and half used topical ibuprofen applied to the painful area. After one year, pain relief was equal in both groups—but three times as many of the oral group had troublesome side effects from the drug.

To optimize topical pain relief, I prescribe a topical Nerve Pain Gel from ITC Pharmacy for most kinds of pain. (It contains *gabapentin*, *ketamine*, *clonidine*, *ketoprofen*, *lidocaine*, *amitriptyline*, and *doxepin*, in various concentrations.) Apply a pea-size amount to the painful area three times a day for two weeks, then as needed. Your physician can simply call in the prescription for "Nerve pain topical 60 gm; apply TID," and it can be mailed to you. The pharmacists at ITC (888-349-5453) are also happy to discuss this option with you and your physician.

Another option: Topical comfrey cream, which has been shown to be as effective as Celebrex after six weeks. However, comfrey has a toxic component in it, so I only use Traumaplant, an OTC product where this component has been removed. I also favor topical aspirin creams, such as Icy Hot, which also includes pain-masking menthol. And don't forget about the newest option: topical hemp oil (CBD), which can be quite soothing when used regularly. I favor Hemp Select, from Terry Naturally.

a form of it—BCM-95, which retains turmeric's natural oils—that boosts absorption seven-fold. You can find BCM-95 in Curamin, a pain relief remedy, from Terry Naturally. Curamin also contains DLPA (DL-phenylalanine, which raises levels of endorphins, your body's natural painkiller), and nattokinase (which breaks down inflammation so healing can occur).

In my anti-inflammation regimen, I recommend patients start with Curamin, which has been shown to be more effective than Celebrex in comparison studies. Give it six weeks to work.

You can then add in Vectomega—especially if you don't have adequate relief after six weeks.

Restore Function

You can restore your ability for everyday functioning with exercise, heat packs, and gentle flexibility exercises.

•**Exercise.** Adding exercise to your lifestyle can help further decrease arthritis pain. Exercise at least 20 minutes a day—swimming, walking, and yoga (or any form of stretching) are good choices. If your arthritis is so painful you can't walk, try walking (and other exercises) in a (preferably) warm pool. The buoyancy and warmth of the water makes it relatively easy to exercise with painful joints. A study by Chinese researchers of 64 people with knee

OA showed that water exercise was more effective than on-land walking in relieving pain (though both worked quite well).

But as you exercise, remember this key point: Pain is your body's way of saying, "Don't do that!" When exercising, don't try to "push through" significant pain.

•**Heating pad or moist heat.** Use for up to 20 minutes at a time. After five to 10 minutes, slowly and gently move the joints, gradually reclaiming your full range of motion.

For hand arthritis, try the herbal-filled "bean bags" you can heat up in a microwave, putting them on your hands for up to 20 minutes a session. After five to 10 minutes, stretch your fingers to help restore their full range of motion and function.

•**Rule out and (if necessary) eliminate food allergies, and treat infections.** Food allergies can aggravate both OA and RA. But most food allergy blood tests are not reliable.

However, a unique approach called NAET (Nambudripad's Allergy Elimination Techniques)—combining a muscle-testing technique called applied kinesiology and acupuncture—is an effective way to test for and eliminate food allergies and sensitivities. (To find more information about this approach, see Food Allergy on page 225.)

If your arthritis doesn't respond well to the Real Cure Regimen, it's time to consider whether or not you have a type of food sensitivity often linked to arthritis: sensitivity to the plants in the nightshade family, which includes tomatoes, potatoes, eggplant, peppers, paprika, cayenne, and tobacco. I recommend eliminating those foods for one month. If you experience significant relief—or if your symptoms come roaring back when you start to reintroduce the foods—do your best to keep them out of your diet.

And speaking of diet: I also think it's prudent for arthritis sufferers to avoid the artificial sweetener aspartame (NutraSweet), which may worsen symptoms. Ditto for the food additive monosodium glutamate (MSG), which can aggravate arthritis pain.

And for those with RA, I recommend an anti-inflammatory, Mediterranean-style diet (more fish, less red meat and dairy products; plenty of vegetables, fruits, whole grains, beans, nuts, and seeds; use of olive oil instead of vegetable oils; minimal processed foods). Studies show the Mediterranean diet reduces inflammation and lowers the risk of cardiovascular disease (CVD) in people with RA (who are at much higher risk for CVD).

I also recommend a trial of the antibiotic minocycline (100 milligrams, twice daily) for extended use in RA. It has been shown to reduce inflammation, swelling, and tenderness, and improve long-term outcomes significantly.

Asthma

Real Causes

•**Nutritional Deficiencies.** Low levels of B vitamins and magnesium can trigger airway spasms (pages 10 and 20).

- **Chronic Inflammation.** This leads to the buildup of airway-clogging mucus (page 118).
- **Hormonal Imbalances.** If adrenal and thymus glands are underperforming, you can be more susceptible to attacks (page 84).

An estimated 25 million American children and adults suffer with asthma—inflammation and spasms of the respiratory "pipes" (bronchi) that carry air in and out of the lungs. Yearly, the disease causes more than 500,000 hospitalizations and 3,500 deaths (from severe, choking asthma attacks). Rates of asthma have been increasing over the past 25 years. The number of people with asthma has quadrupled, and the number of deaths from asthma attacks has doubled. Why? Well, some people get asthma in the genetic lottery: If one parent has asthma, chances are one in three that their children will have it; if both parents have asthma, chances are seven in 10.

But it's important to note that 50 percent of people with asthma have attacks that are triggered by allergens, and there's an ever-increasing level of allergens (such as molds, dust mites, and animal dander) in our homes, offices, and other environments. Add to that the high-sugar, high-fat inflammatory diet that most of us eat; the nutritional deficiencies that make us more prone to any disease, including asthma; an overload of immune-weakening chemicals in the environment (including in our additive-laden food); a tsunami of tension and stress; and more air pollution—and you have the real causes of the ever-increasing worldwide epidemic of asthma.

Asthma attacks can range from mild to life-threatening, with symptoms that include shortness of breath, cough, wheezing, and chest tightness. And there are many different triggers for those attacks (some of which we've already mentioned), including allergens, infections, exercise, abrupt changes in the weather, and exposure to irritants such as tobacco smoke or car exhaust.

Real Cure Regimen

There are many helpful medications to control asthma, and most of them are reasonably prescribed by physicians. But if you have asthma, you'll also benefit from natural therapies that decrease the tendency to inflammation and eliminate allergic sensitivities, along with simple strategies to decrease the level of allergens in your home. These additional treatments will help you feel much better and may decrease your need for medications.

•Load up on nutrients. Many nutrients have been found to help prevent and ease asthma, including magnesium, vitamins B_6 and B_{12}, vitamin C, vitamin D, vitamin E, selenium, molybdenum, beta-carotene, and quercetin. You can find all these nutrients in sufficient antiasthma dosages in the Energy Revitalization System multinutrient powder (a supplement discussed in Nutritional Deficiencies on page 30).

I can't emphasize enough that optimal nutrition is crucial—even lifesaving—in asthma control (see "Breakthroughs in Nutritional Healing: Asthma" on page 164 about the nutrition-asthma link). For example, if asthma patients in the midst of a severe, life-threatening attack were given airway-relaxing intravenous magnesium (up to one gram an hour, six grams to 12 grams daily) and also an ongoing, daily oral dose of nerve-nourishing vitamin B$_6$ (100 milligrams), many deaths from asthma attacks could be prevented and hospital stays avoided or shortened.

Here are some more details about specific nutrients and natural treatments to keep you breathing free and easy…

•**Vitamin D.** Research shows that vitamin D can help ease asthma when it's resistant to treatment with prednisone. D is a powerful immune balancer, also shown to help prevent colds, flu, pneumonia, and autoimmune diseases.

•**Boswellia: 300 milligrams, three times daily.** This anti-inflammatory herb (also called frankincense) wonderfully reduces asthma symptoms after six weeks (and usually within days). It is the number-one treatment I recommend for asthma. I recommend BosMed, from Terry Naturally. (You can read more about boswellia in Chronic Inflammation on page 118.)

•**Adrenal nutrients.** Strengthening the adrenal gland can be very helpful in controlling asthma and can even decrease the amount of prednisone (an anti-inflammatory prescription medication) needed to treat severe asthma. To fortify your adrenal gland, I recommend the product Adrenaplex, from Terry Naturally. It contains therapeutic levels of adrenal-enhancing nutrients and herbs such as vitamin C, B$_6$, pantothenate, and licorice extract, and adrenal cortical extract. Take one capsule first thing in the morning. If needed, you can add a second capsule later in the morning or at lunchtime. (You can find more information on the adrenal gland in Hormonal Imbalances on page 84 and in Adrenal Exhaustion on page 138.)

•**Lycopene: 30 milligrams to 45 milligrams daily.** This powerful antioxidant, found mainly in tomatoes, is very effective in preventing episodes of exercise-induced asthma, according to studies in the journal *Asthma*, and in *Annals of Allergy, Asthma & Immunology*. Several other studies show that lycopene levels are low in people with asthma. Why take supplements and not eat more tomato-laden pasta? Well, it's next to impossible to take in enough antiasthma lycopene by eating tomatoes. To take in the daily dose of 30 milligrams, you'd have to eat about a pound of tomatoes, drink 11 ounces of tomato juice, or somehow consume seven ounces of tomato paste. Domino's doesn't deliver for asthmatics.

•**Omega-3 fatty acids.** The anti-inflammatory omega-3 fatty acids in fish are especially helpful in controlling asthma in children, after environmental triggers have been removed from the home. (More about those triggers in a minute.) Tuna, salmon, sardines, and other fatty fish are good sources of fish oil. (To read more about fish oils, see Nutritional Deficiencies on page 28.) Omega-3 fatty acids are also a good preventive. In one study out of Norway and published in the journal *Nutrients*, one-year-olds who ate fish at least once per week had up to a 34 percent reduction in the risk of asthma at the age of six. Another study, out of Harvard Medical School, showed that pregnant women who ate more fish were less likely to have children with asthma. A study by Egyptian researchers also shows three months of taking fish oil supplements reduces the severity of asthma in adults.

•**Thymus-supporting supplement.** Upper respiratory tract infections such as colds, flu, and pneumonia can trigger asthma attacks. To boost immunity during upper respiratory tract infections, use ProBoost. This supplement energizes the thymus gland, which regulates im-

Breakthroughs in Nutritional Healing: Asthma

Several studies show the power of nutrition to tame asthma.

●**Vitamin C eases exercise-induced asthma.** People with exercise-induced asthma who took 1,500 milligrams of vitamin C for two weeks dramatically reduced the number and severity of their symptoms, reported a team of researchers from the Human Performance and Exercise Biochemistry Laboratory at Indiana University, in the journal *Respiratory Medicine*.

●**More vitamin D, fewer trips to the emergency room.** In a four-year study of more than 1,000 children with mild to moderate asthma, researchers from Harvard Medical School found that those with the lowest blood levels of vitamin D were 50 percent more likely to go to the emergency room or be hospitalized with an asthma attack.

In a study of 100 asthmatic children, those with the lowest blood levels of vitamin D had more allergies (which often worsen asthma) and a higher use of steroid medications (which control the disease but cause many side effects).

When researchers at the University of Colorado studied 54 adults with asthma, they found that those with the highest vitamin D levels had the strongest lungs and airways that were least likely to go into spasm, as well as the smallest production of stress hormones. "Supplementation of vitamin D levels in patients with asthma may improve multiple parameters of asthma severity," concluded the researchers in the *American Journal of Respiratory and Critical Care Medicine*.

●**Magnesium eases asthma symptoms.** Noting that earlier studies linked low blood levels of magnesium with asthma, researchers at Bastyr University in Washington studied 55 adults with mild to moderate asthma. Half received 370 milligrams a day of magnesium and half didn't. After six months, those receiving the mineral had a 20 percent improvement in a measurement of breathing strength and fewer asthma symptoms. There was little change in the placebo group, according to the study, which was reported in the *Journal of Asthma*.

munity via the hormone thymulin. During infections, dissolve the contents of one packet under your tongue, three times a day. During cold and flu season, use one packet a day for prevention.

More Ways to Breathe Easy

There are several other strategies that may help ease asthma symptoms and prevent attacks...

●**Avoid food colorings and additives.** Common asthma triggers include the food dye tartrazine (also known as yellow dye no. 5; benzoates (a common type of food preservative); and sulfites (another type of preservative). Look for them on the label—and stay away!

●**Eliminate food allergies.** Try a "multiple food elimination diet" for seven to 10 days to see if your asthma symptoms improve when you're not eating certain foods. You may find yourself amazed at the connection between foods and asthma. For instructions on implementing this diet, see Food Allergy on page 225.

●**Consider NAET.** A special acupressure technique called NAET (Nambudripad's Allergy Elimination Techniques) can actually help eliminate allergies—an excellent approach for anyone with allergic asthma. For more information on NAET, including how to find a practitioner, see Food Allergy on page 225.

●**Treat leaky gut syndrome.** Asthma treatment with antibiotics and steroids can cause an overgrowth of the yeast candida, damaging the intestinal lining and causing leaky gut syndrome. In this condition, partially digested proteins slip through the injured intestinal wall, enter the bloodstream, and are attacked by the immune system, creating a condition of chronic inflammation that worsens asthma and other conditions and diseases. (For information on treating leaky gut syndrome, see Digestive Difficulties on page 98 and Candida Overgrowth on page 181.)

●**Consider adding an electrostatic air cleaner to your furnace.** This device pulls allergens out of the air. Your heating and cooling service company can guide you in picking and installing a unit. It costs about anywhere from $600 to $2,000, but if you have asthma, it's worth it.

Smart tip: Be sure the air cleaner filters can fit in your dishwasher, and wash them the first of each month. If you can't install an in-furnace air filter, an alternative is a HEPA air filter in your bedroom. It's not as thorough, but it's extremely helpful.

Autoimmune Disease

Real Causes

●**Cellular Toxicity.** The more than 80,000 artificial chemicals in the environment overwhelm and confuse the immune system; no longer able to tell the "good guys" from the "bad guys," it mistakenly attacks the body (page 109).

●**Hormonal Imbalances.** Low levels of adrenal hormones can contribute to the development of autoimmune disease (page 84).

●**Chronic Inflammation.** This is the "collateral damage" from the body attacking itself (page 118).

●**Digestive Difficulties.** Incomplete food digestion combined with "leaky gut" syndrome can trigger a wide array of food allergies—which puts the immune system into overdrive (page 98).

The body's immune system is programmed to detect what is and isn't part of the body—what is "self" and what is "not self"—and then to attack and destroy what is "not self." But modern life has turned that automatic task into a polluted puzzle.

With more than 80,000 synthetic chemicals in the environment—many of them similar to the hormones and other biochemicals produced by our bodies—the immune system has become, well, confused. And when it's confused, it can mistake the body's own organs and tissues for an outside invader and may attack, causing an autoimmune disease.

Americans are in the midst of an epidemic of autoimmune diseases, with tens of millions affected. *A list of some of the most common (and the body part attacked) includes…*

- **Celiac disease** (villi in the lining of the small intestine)
- **Diabetes, type 1** (pancreas)
- **Hashimoto's disease** (thyroid gland)
- **Inflammatory bowel disease** (small and large intestine)
- **Psoriasis** (skin)
- **Sjogren's syndrome** (connective tissue)
- **Systemic lupus erythematosus** (many organs and tissues)
- **Multiple sclerosis** (myelin sheath, the protective covering around the nerves)
- **Rheumatoid arthritis** (joints)

A discussion of all of these autoimmune diseases is beyond the scope of this book. (Excellent books on the topic include *The Autoimmune Epidemic* by Donna Jackson Nakazawa; *The Autoimmune Solution* by Amy Meyers, MD; and *The Wahls Protocol* by Terry Wahls, MD.) But several natural treatments can dramatically improve most autoimmune diseases.

Real Cure Regimen

To address the real cause of cellular toxicity, see what I recommend in Cellular Toxicity on page 109. Chronic inflammation—the primary sign of an overactive disease—is almost always a major component of an autoimmune disease. *Two supplements are standouts in decreasing chronic inflammation…*

- **Omega-3 fatty acids from fish.** Unfortunately, it takes *very* high doses of omega-3s to create the level in the bloodstream and blood cells that can reduce the chronic inflammation of autoimmune disease. I recommend people use a unique fish fatty acid supplement called Vectomega, from Terry Naturally. Its special formulation increases absorption of omega-3s more than fiftyfold compared with other fish oils. One to three tablets deliver the same effect as seven to 21 fish oil capsules (or three to 10 teaspoons of fish oil)—so you spend less time taking supplements and spend less money, too. (For more information on fish oil, see Nutritional Deficiencies on page 28.) If Vectomega isn't your preference, Nordic Naturals also makes excellent fish oils. Or, for the same level of fish oil, eat a serving of fatty fish (salmon, albacore tuna, sardines, anchovies, mackerel, halibut) at least four times weekly.

- **Curcumin and willow bark.** These two herbs are superb at reducing chronic inflammation. I recommend the product Curamin, from Terry Naturally. Take it daily for six weeks, following the dosage recommendation on the label; if you achieve significant symptom relief, lower the dosage. (For more on boswellia and curcumin, see Chronic Inflammation on page 118.)

In addition to those nutrients and herbs, try these other natural remedies…

•**Switch from *prednisone* to Cortef.** Many autoimmune diseases flare up and then quiet down again. If you have a flare-up, your doctor may prescribe somewhere between five milligrams to 40 (or more) milligrams a day of prednisone, a powerful anti-inflammatory corticosteroid (a synthetic version of cortisol, a hormone manufactured by your adrenal glands). When your flare-up ends, your doctor will gradually reduce the dosage, weaning you off the drug. The problem is, prednisone suppresses your body's production of inflammation-calming cortisol, so when prednisone doses are lowered, your inflammatory illness may flare up—and even more severely than before!

The solution: Once the dose is lowered to five milligrams of prednisone a day, ask your doctor to switch you to 15 milligrams to 20 milligrams a day of Cortef. This is a bioidentical form of cortisone, and it can be safely taken at a low dose for extended periods of time (20 milligrams of natural Cortef is like four milligrams of synthetic prednisone). Research and my clinical experience show that long-term use of up to 20 milligrams of Cortef is safe; my own research—summarized in a letter published in the *Journal of the American Medical Association*—also shows it doesn't suppress the adrenal glands. I give Cortef in the morning, before breakfast. (For more information on the safety of this approach, I recommend the book *Safe Uses of Cortisol* by the renowned Cleveland clinic endocrinologist William Jefferies, MD.) I add the supplement Adrenaplex from Terry Naturally to further increase the adrenal benefits.

•**Take DHEA for lupus.** Several studies show that supplementing with 200 milligrams of this adrenal hormone improves symptoms in lupus and slows the development of the disease. Another benefit: If you take DHEA, you may be able to lower your daily dose of prednisone.

Caution: Two hundred milligrams is a high dose of DHEA that can cause acne or darkening of facial hair (in women). Use it only under the guidance of a holistic physician.

Another caution: There are quality problems with many brands of DHEA. I recommend DHEA from Douglas Labs. Or use DHEA from a compounding pharmacy. (See Resources on page 360. For more information on DHEA, see Adrenal Exhaustion on page 138.)

Back Pain

Real Causes

•**Nutritional Deficiencies.** Low levels of muscle-relaxing nutrients such as magnesium can play a role in back spasms (page 20).

•**Chronic Inflammation.** Low-grade, constant inflammation stresses the spine (page 118).

Back pain is one of the most common pain conditions—65 million Americans report a recent episode, and 16 million suffer from chronic back pain. Basically, it's a by-product of evolution.

When our nonhuman ancestors moved from all fours to a standing position, a lot more pressure was put on the bones of the spine. In other words, our backs went ape!

The spine is a column of bones called vertebrae. Separating each vertebra from the next is a disk, a pad of fluid-filled, shock-absorbing cartilage. Inside the column of vertebrae, and protected by it, is a cable of nerves called the spinal cord. These nerves branch out from the front of each vertebra, delivering information from the brain to the body. There are also nerves at the back of each vertebra, carrying information from the body to the brain. The column is held in place by tendons, ligaments, and muscles. It's a complex structure, with a lot of possibilities for pain.

The disks can rupture, leaking fluid that triggers inflammation and swelling, which pinches the nerves and causes pain. Sciatica is a common type of disk-related, nerve-pinching pain (although a tight muscle can also pinch the nerve). There's a compression or irritation of the nerve from the foot as it enters the spine, and pain radiates down the leg.

A self-test for sciatica: Lie on the floor and lift the painful leg straight up without bending it, while keeping the other leg flat on the floor. If the pain worsens, it's likely to be sciatica.

Disk disease is the type of back pain most doctors are trained to identify, which is why they often suggest surgical repair of the ruptured disk. Although damaged disks are the cause that doctors are taught to consider, they aren't the only (or even anywhere near the most common) cause of back pain. Any damage to the spinal nerves—from an injury or from a disease such as cancer—can cause back pain. And any strain or weakness in the muscles and ligaments that support the spine can cause pain. In fact, this is the most likely cause of back pain, even if your x-ray or MRI shows some degeneration of your disks. (Because we're an upright species, with constant pressure on our spines, it's normal to have some wear and tear on disks.)

And just as you can have arthritis in your knees, hips, or hands, you can have spinal arthritis—a common cause of chronic back pain often ignored by physicians and even by some chiropractors, who specialize in back problems. (If you're diagnosed with spinal arthritis, see Arthritis on page 155 for pain-relieving recommendations.)

Real Cure Regimen

Surgery, while often recommended, is expensive, often doesn't work, and may even make you worse. It should be your last resort. "Virtually any non-surgical treatment is worth a try before you resort to surgery," Stephen Hochschuler, MD, co-founder of the Texas Back Institute and author of *Treat Your Back without Surgery*, told us. Back pain is very treatable, most often without surgery. We'll start with nutrition.

Nutritional and Herbal Supplements

Several different supplements are wonderfully effective at relieving chronic back pain. You can take these with pain medications. When you feel better, talk to your doctor about lowering the medication dose (while still making sure you're comfortable).

•**Curcumin, boswellia, willow bark, DLPA, and devil's claw.** This remarkably effective mix can be found in a product called Curamin Low Back Pain, from Terry Naturally.

Boswellia and a special, highly absorbed curcumin (BCM-95) are good for reducing inflammation in lower-back pain. DLPA increases your body's own natural pain relief molecules, called endorphins. And Devil's claw has been shown to dramatically increase the hyaluronic acid needed for the repair of vertebrae. And in one study, published in the journal *Rheumatology*, on back pain, the herb willow bark was just as effective as a powerful NSAID (*rofecoxib*).

You can take this supplement safely with your other pain medications (including aspirin), but it shouldn't be taken by anyone who is aspirin sensitive. Take three capsules daily. You should experience significant pain relief in one to three weeks and optimal pain relief at six weeks. After being pain-free for three months, you can often wean yourself off this product (and other pain medications). (Read more about boswellia and curcumin in Chronic Inflammation on page 130.)

•**Vitamin D: 2,000 IU to 4,000 IU daily.** Scientists are finding that low levels of vitamin D are common in people with chronic back pain. "Our examination of the research, which included 22 clinical investigations of patients with pain, found that those with chronic back pain almost always had inadequate levels of vitamin D," wrote the late Stewart B. Leavitt, PhD, in the publication *Pain Treatment Topics*. "When sufficient vitamin D supplementation was provided, their pain either vanished or was at least helped to a significant extent."

•**Alpha-lipoic acid: 300 milligrams, twice daily.** Alpha-lipoic acid is a powerful antioxidant that helps nerve pain and may also help back pain. In a two-month study by Italian researchers, published in *Clinical Drug Investigation*, 64 people with "acute backache" and "moderate sciatica" were given either 600 milligrams a day of alpha-lipoic acid or another nutrient. Those taking the alpha-lipoic acid had "significant improvements" in sciatic pain and symptoms of back pain, and 71 percent of those taking alpha-lipoic acid were able to take less pain medication. In another study in the *International Journal of Immunopathology and Pharma-*

Don't Let Your Anger Back Up!

Researchers in the Department of Psychology at Rosalind Franklin University of Medicine and Science in Illinois conducted a study on 84 people with chronic back pain. First, they harassed the study participants. Then they had them either verbally express their anger or hold it in. Last, they measured the level of tightness in the muscles along their spines.

Those who held their anger in had higher levels of muscle tension, and that tension took a longer time to dissipate. "Chronic lower back pain patients may be at particular risk for elevated pain severity if circumstances at work or home regularly dictate that they should inhibit anger expression," concluded the researchers in the journal *Psychosomatic Medicine*.

The moral of the study: Be honest with and express your feelings—or be prepared to carry them around as back pain.

You can read more about emotions and chronic pain in Happiness Deficiency on page 55. And an excellent book on the connection between emotions and back pain is *Healing Back Pain: The Mind-Body Connection*, by John Sarno, MD.

Hands-On Help

Research shows that many forms of hands-on professional treatment can help relieve back pain.

●**Chiropractic.** A chiropractor treats back pain by using spinal manipulation or chiropractic adjustment—a gentle or forceful push to spinal joints that have become restricted in their movement. In an 18-month study by researchers at UCLA School of Public Health, people with lower-back pain receiving chiropractic care were 29 percent more likely to achieve pain relief and improved functioning than those receiving conventional medical care.

●**Osteopathy.** A study of osteopathy—which also uses a different type of hands-on spinal manipulation— showed that it reduced pain by 30 percent more than conventional treatments.

●**Massage.** In an analysis of nine studies on massage and back pain, researchers in England found that massage was excellent for a newly aching back (subacute nonspecific lower-back pain).

●**McKenzie Method.** This approach uses a unique system of diagnosis to first find the physical cause of your back pain and then prescribe specific exercises to relieve it. A study by researchers at the University of Oregon showed it was more effective than NSAIDs, strength training, massage, chiropractic, or back exercises at relieving chronic lower-back pain.

●**Physical therapy.** Physical therapists use a range of techniques to improve back pain, including passive motion of your limbs to extend range of motion; exercise regimens; training in how to sit, stand, and walk; and heat and cold therapy. In a study at UCLA on physical therapy, researchers found that it was 69 percent more likely to decrease pain and improve daily functioning than conventional medical care. If you're considering physical therapy (PT), find a professional who is familiar with Dr. Janet Travell's trigger point and spray and stretch methods. (Many PTs don't know about these methods.) It uses a cooling spray (such as Gebauer's Spray and Stretch aerosol spray) along with stretching the muscle, a mainstay in the system of pain relief called trigger point therapy. Elegantly simple, it can often relieve decades of pain in minutes.

●**Acupuncture.** In this modality, tiny, painless needles are inserted along energy pathways called meridians, freeing blocked energy and relieving pain. In an analysis of 11 studies on acupuncture and low back pain, published in the *Clinical Journal of Pain*, acupuncture was more effective than NSAIDs such as ibuprofen for acute back pain.

cology on alpha-lipoic acid and back pain, Italian researchers found that those taking a daily dose of 600 milligrams had less back pain and disability, and also less sciatica.

●**B vitamins.** Brazilian researchers studied 372 people with lower-back pain, treating them with the painkiller *diclofenac* (Voltaren, Cataflam) or *diclofenac* and 50 milligrams of thiamin (and two other B vitamins). After three days, 46 percent of those treated with the drug and B vitamins felt better, compared with only 29 percent of those treated with the drug alone, according to the study in *Current Medical Research and Opinion*.

●**Glucosamine sulfate (1,500 milligrams daily) and chondroitin sulfate (2,500 milligrams daily).** As mentioned earlier, arthritis of the spine is a common but often undiagnosed cause of back pain. That's why it's worthwhile giving these two anti-arthritis nutrients—excellent for relieving arthritis pain—a six- to 12-week trial, to see if they help. You could add 2,500 milligrams to 3,000 milligrams daily of MSM, a nutrient that also can help relieve arthritis pain. (For more information on these nutrients, see Arthritis on page 155.)

Effective, Fast-Acting, Nonaddictive Medications

If needed, medications can also help with chronic back pain. *Here are the ones I favor for my patients...*

●**Lidoderm patches.** You can safely wear these patches—basically Novocain in a skin patch—for up to 16 hours a day over the painful area (though the instructions say to limit their use to 12 hours a day). In some people, the patches help in 30 minutes; in others, relief takes a week or so. The patches are safe and rarely have any side effects. This medication is often sufficient for relieving back pain. But if it's not, you can discuss the following medications with your doctor:

●*Metaxalone* (**Skelaxin**). I find that this is a good, non-sedating prescription muscle relaxant for my patients with back pain.

●**Ultracet.** This prescription drug—a combination of acetaminophen and a unique endorphin-raising medication called *tramadol* (Ultram)—is excellent for pain and is much less likely to be addictive than other narcotic pain relievers.

●*Lamotrigine* (**Lamictal**). This antiseizure medication can also help relieve back pain, particularly in people with severe disk pain who haven't been helped by other treatments. In one study, Lamictal provided a 70 percent decrease in pain in 14 of 21 patients.

Lifestyle Advice

Commonsense precautions and simple therapies can prevent or relieve back pain.

●**Lift right.** Don't bend over from the waist. Instead, squat with your knees apart, with the object between your knees and as close as possible to your body. Using your legs, stand up and lift, bringing the object closer to your body as you stand. Be sure to keep your back straight.

If you can't manage a squat, put one knee on the floor, and then, using your arms, move the object onto the opposite thigh and, with a firm grip on the object, simply stand up.

●**Sleep on a medium-firm mattress.** A team of Spanish researchers studied 313 people with chronic nonspecific back pain (no known cause) who had pain while lying in bed and after getting up in the morning. They assigned the people in the study to one of three types of mattresses: soft, medium-firm, or firm. After three months, those sleeping on the medium-firm mattress had the least pain while sleeping, less pain in the morning, and less daytime disability and back pain. "A mattress of medium firmness improves pain and disability among patients with non-specific low-back pain," concluded the researchers in the journal *Lancet.*

A medium-firm bed can also prevent back pain. Researchers at Oklahoma State University conducted a one-month study of 59 people and found that replacing current bedding with a medium-firm bed decreased back discomfort and stiffness upon waking, while also improving sleep quality and comfort. The findings were in the *Journal of Chiropractic Medicine.* But medium may not work for everybody—try out different mattresses and find the one that feels best for you.

•**Use heat for relief.** In one study, people with chronic lower-back pain using heat wraps around their lower backs had a 60 percent reduction in pain intensity after three days. In another study, the heat wraps worked 25 percent better than *ibuprofen* (Advil, Motrin, Nuprin) or *acetaminophen* (Tylenol) at reducing chronic lower-back pain. "A heat wrap goes beyond the simple pain relief provided by over-the-counter pills," Scott F. Nadler, DO, the study leader, told us. "It increases blood flow to the painful muscles, decreasing pain and improving flexibility and mobility." The product used in the study was ThermaCare Lower Back and Hip HeatWraps.

•**Do yoga.** In a study by researchers at the University of Washington in Seattle, 101 people with chronic lower-back pain were divided into three groups: One group took 12 weeks of yoga classes; one took 12 weeks of exercise classes; and one read a self-help book on back pain. Yoga was more effective than the other approaches at relieving pain and reducing everyday disability.

•**Distract and relax with music.** In one study, researchers found that listening to relaxing music for 30 to 60 minutes daily, for three weeks, decreased back pain by 40 percent. And in a study of people hospitalized for chronic lower-back pain, five days of music therapy—regularly listening to music they found relaxing—reduced disability by 34 percent, anxiety by 75 percent, and depression by 72 percent. "Music therapy can be a useful complementary treatment in chronic pain and associated anxiety-depression," concluded the French researchers.

Breast Cysts

Real Causes

•**Nutritional Deficiencies.** Low levels of iodine are the major cause of breast cysts and tenderness (page 26).

•**Hormonal Imbalances.** Although not the main cause, the swings in estrogen during a woman's menstrual cycle can play a role in this problem—but these hormonal swings are less likely to cause a problem once the iodine deficiency is corrected (page 84).

Breast cysts are so common—occurring in an estimated 48 percent of women—that many doctors now refer to the condition as *fibrocystic breast changes* rather than the older term, *fibrocystic breast disease*. (However, older names are still used, including "benign breast disease" and "mammary dysplasia.") If you're one of the many women with this problem, you know how your breasts feel when the condition is at its worst, usually in the week or two before you menstruate: Your breasts are lumpy; they feel full, swollen, and heavy; and they hurt. (Although they're far less common in postmenopausal women, the symptoms are the same.)

While breast cysts are common in America, they're rare in Japan. What's the difference?

Real Cure Regimen

The Japanese diet is high in iodine (mostly from seaweed and seafood), and the American diet is low. Iodine plays a crucial role in breast health. Iodine reacts with an amino acid on the surface of abnormal breast cells, causing the natural death of the cell. But without iodine, those cells can multiply, leading to breast cysts—and even breast cancer. Yes, there is a link between breast cysts and breast cancer. *The most recent research…*

Doctors at Albert Einstein College of Medicine in New York studied 1,239 women: 615 with breast cysts and 624 without them. Those with breast cysts had a 45 percent greater risk of developing breast cancer. And those with breast cysts that had abnormal cells (atypical hyperplasia—breast cells that are abnormal in size, shape, and appearance) had a 527 percent greater risk of developing breast cancer. The findings were published in the medical journal *Cancer Causes & Control*.

Older research shows iodine can correct the problem. In a study of more than 1,300 women with breast cysts, 74 percent reported improvement when taking daily iodine. Iodine is "beneficial" for breast cysts, concluded the Canadian researchers in the *Canadian Journal of Surgery*. That's why the first (and main) item in my Real Cure Regimen for breast cysts is getting your iodine up. Then I offer a few other nutritional tips to help the pain.

•**Rev up your iodine.** Everyone needs 150 micrograms to 200 micrograms of daily iodine for health. (Using iodized salt to salt your food—which I endorse—will get you to this level. The only people who should restrict salt are those with heart failure.) I recommend a therapeutic dose of 6.25 milligrams (6,250 micrograms) for breast cysts. I recommend using the iodine supplement Tri-Iodine 6.25 mg, from Terry Naturally.

Give iodine treatment three months to work. (It may help sooner.) Very rarely, the iodine aggravates acne or indigestion. Stop the supplement if one of those side effects occurs. And don't exceed the recommended amount unless you are under the care of a holistic health practitioner. Too much iodine can negatively affect the thyroid gland.

I usually recommend the same dosage of iodine for women with breast cancer, or even increase it to 12.5 milligrams, while using thyroid testing to make sure no harm is being caused to the thyroid gland. A recent scientific paper in the *Journal of Cancer*, from a researcher at the Temple University School of Medicine asserts that falling iodine intake is *the main reason* there is an accelerating rate of breast cancer in younger women. (For women with breast cancer, I recommend an excellent book called *Iodine*, by David Brownstein, MD.)

•**Get more vitamin E.** Benign but painful breast cysts or lumps are a common occurrence among menstruating women, and sometimes the condition is at its worst right before menstruation (cyclic mastalgia). In a study in the *Breast Journal*, researchers gave 150 women with cystic mastalgia either vitamin E or a placebo for four months. Vitamin E had a "significant curative result," they concluded. As for vitamin E's effectiveness, the title of an older article in the *Journal of the American Medical Association* puts it succinctly: "Vitamin E relieves most cystic breast disease."

Take 400 IU a day of this nutrient, in the form of "natural mixed tocopherols." (Vitamin E is really a family of nutrients, and employing the entire family—rather than one member, such as alpha-tocopherol—works best.)

●**Avoid or reduce caffeine.** Australian researchers analyzed data from the Nurses' Health Study II—a study of tens of thousands of women—and found that those with the highest intake of caffeine had more than double the risk (2.46 times higher) of developing breast cysts with atypical hyperplasia (AH). The findings were in the journal *Cancer Epidemiology, Biomarkers & Prevention.*

Caffeine isn't just in coffee, of course—you'll also need to avoid or reduce your use of tea, chocolate, and energy drinks. (By the way, the same researchers found that women who took a multivitamin supplement had a 57 percent *lower* incidence of breast cysts with AH.)

●**See your doctor.** If you have a new breast cyst or lump that lasts for more than two menstrual cycles, have your physician check it. Also, see your doctor if one area of your breast has severe or persistent pain that doesn't come and go with your menstrual cycle.

Cancer

Real Causes

Cancer has multifactorial causes, but certain factors can keep the immune system strong so that it routinely eliminates the cancer cells that are a normal result of everyday cell growth and repair.

- ●**Nutritional Deficiencies.** Zinc, selenium, and many other nutrients are critical for immune function (page 3).
- ●**Hormonal Imbalances.** Normal levels of adrenal and thymus hormones are a must for optimal immunity (page 84).
- ●**Chronic Inflammation.** This factor increases the risk that cancer cells will grow and multiply (page 118).
- ●**Poor Sleep.** A good night's rest optimizes the strength of the immune system (page 33).
- ●**Inactivity.** Many studies link low levels of physical activity to an increased risk of developing cancer or a recurrence (page 40).

Most oncologists are well-meaning and caring individuals. But they're also doctors and part of a medical system that emphasizes profits over patients. And cancer treatments such as chemotherapy, radiation, and surgery are extremely profitable.

The typical oncologist attends cancer conferences, finds out what esteemed academicians (who are usually on drug company payrolls) are saying about the newest (and usually most expensive) cancer treatments, and starts using those treatments in his or her practice. And why not? Those treatments have been endorsed by experts, and they're profitable to boot. (A bit more about that. Oncologists make 65 percent of their income based on chemotherapy. So the higher the cost of the chemo they give, the more they get paid.) Meanwhile, it's understood among most oncologists that anyone proposing a natural (and, let us not forget, competing) treatment for cancer must be trying to rip off desperate and vulnerable patients—and therefore the oncologist must protect the gullible public from these charlatans. (Needless to say there are natural treatments for cancer that are nothing but hype and nonsense. But others are helpful.) This pro-medical, antinatural belief system allows the cancer establishment to self-righteously block the public's access to effective alternative and complementary cancer therapies.

Now, I am not saying that you should forgo chemotherapy, radiation therapy, or surgery for cancer. In many cases, these medical treatments reduce suffering and extend or save lives. (For example, the so-called "targeted cancer therapies" that block cancer genes are extending the lives of many people, particularly those with stage IV cancer.) In some cases, however, these treatments offer minimal benefit, along with extreme toxicity and excessive costs. And in a few cases the medical treatment offers no benefit and significant physical and fiscal downsides.

If you find yourself diagnosed with cancer, how do you decide what's best, when your well-meaning oncologist is criticizing natural therapies, and your natural doctor is saying chemo is killing you?

The good news is, there's really little or no conflict between medical and natural cancer treatments—just between the people offering them. I favor what I call *comprehensive* medicine: the use of the best natural and medical therapies for the benefit of the patient, with no prejudice against either. And comprehensive medicine is particularly effective in addressing cancer.

Here's how to find the cancer treatments that will work best for you.

Real Cure Regimen

In spite of what your oncologist believes or may have told you, there are a large number of natural therapies for cancer that scientific research shows can help. And there are folks out there who can make sure you know about them.

Nutritional and Herbal Support

Many nutritional and herbal supplements can help prevent or slow cancer. If you have cancer, discuss your supplement regimen with a holistic physician.

•**Vitamin D.** "More than 17 different types of cancer are likely to be vitamin D-sensitive," reported researchers at the Sunlight, Nutrition and Health Research Center in San Francisco. Among those cancers are breast, colorectal, prostate, pancreatic, bladder, esophageal, gallbladder, gastric, ovarian, rectal, kidney, uterine, and Hodgkin's and non-Hodgkin's lymphoma. According to their study in *Recent Results in Cancer Research*, universal supplementation with 1,000 IU of vitamin D would decrease cancer death rates by up to 20 percent, saving $25 billion yearly in health care costs in America.

When researchers at the Harvard School of Public Health analyzed diet and health data from more than 47,000 men, they found that those with the highest vitamin D levels had a 22 percent lower risk of death from any cancer, compared with men with the lowest levels. The researchers estimate that increasing daily vitamin D intake by 1,500 IU would lower overall cancer death rates in men by 29 percent (85,550 fewer deaths a year).

Some additional data on vitamin D and the four most common cancers…

•Breast cancer (331,000 cases and 42,000 deaths yearly). In a study of more than 2,700 postmenopausal women published in *Carcinogenesis*, those with the highest blood levels of vitamin D had 69 percent less risk of breast cancer than those with the lowest levels.

In a German study of nearly 900 premenopausal women, those with the highest blood levels of vitamin D had 55 percent less risk of breast cancer, reported researchers in the *International Journal of Cancer*.

Researchers at the University of Buffalo found that women who spent an average of two hours or more a day outside had a 20 percent lower risk of breast cancer than women who spent 30 minutes or less outside. (Sunlight generates vitamin D.) The link between time spent outside and breast cancer risk supports the theory that vitamin D may protect against breast cancer, concluded the researchers.

In a study by researchers at the Fred Hutchinson Cancer Research Center in Seattle of 790 breast cancer survivors, 76 percent had very low blood levels of vitamin D—and the lower their vitamin D, the more advanced their disease. "Clinicians might consider monitoring vitamin D status in breast cancer patients," concluded the researchers in the *American Journal of Clinical Nutrition*. I favor a simpler approach. Since tests for blood levels of many nutrients (including vitamin D) are unreliable, take at least 2,000 IU of vitamin D daily.

•Colorectal cancer (145,000 new cases and 51,000 deaths yearly). Italian researchers in the *International Journal of Cancer* analyzed nine studies on vitamin D levels and colorectal cancer involving 2,630 people. For every 10-nanograms-per-milliliter increase in blood vitamin D levels, there was a 15 percent decrease in risk of colorectal cancer. In a European study of more than 1,200 people, those with the highest blood levels of vitamin D had a 40 percent lower risk of colorectal cancer, compared with those with the lowest levels. "Improving vitamin D status could be potentially beneficial against colorectal cancer incidence and mortality," concluded researchers from the Harvard School of Public Health, in a paper summarizing all the research in this area.

•Lung cancer (234,000 new cases and 154,000 deaths yearly). Researchers at Harvard Medical School studied the survival data from 456 patients with early-stage lung cancer. Patients who had high levels of vitamin D and had surgery in sunny months were 2.5 times more likely to be alive five years after surgery, compared with patients with low levels of vitamin D who had surgery in the winter. "The survival advantage at five years is pretty dramatic: 72 percent survival versus 29 percent, when you compare the highest level of vitamin D intake versus the lowest level," noted David Christiani, MD, lead researcher.

•Prostate cancer (174,600 new cases and 31,600 deaths yearly). Researchers at Harvard Medical School analyzed 18 years of diet and health data on nearly 48,000 doctors. They found

To Reduce the Side Effects of Chemotherapy, Try Antioxidants

In a review of 33 rigorous studies evaluating the effects of taking antioxidants with chemotherapy, involving 2,446 people, the supplements were found to reduce the toxic effects of the drugs. Five of the studies found that those taking the antioxidants were able to complete more doses of chemotherapy (which is sometimes stopped because of its toxicity). Antioxidants used in the studies included glutathione, melatonin, vitamin A, N-acetylcysteine, vitamin E, selenium, acetyl-L-carnitine, coenzyme Q10, and ellagic acid.

"This review provides the first systematically reviewed evidence that antioxidant supplementation during chemotherapy holds potential for reducing dose-limiting toxicities," concluded the authors in the *International Journal of Cancer*.

The fact that antioxidants *help* with chemotherapy may be just the opposite of what you've heard from your oncologist: that they harm the power of chemotherapy (and radiation) to kill cancer. That's simply not true. Those taking the nutritional support do better. If I have a cancer patient with an oncologist who voices this concern, I compromise: If the chemotherapy schedule allows it, I stop the supplements for one week before and one week after each round of chemotherapy.

---

that 36 percent were deficient (below 20 nanograms per milliliter) in vitamin D during the winter, and 77 percent had "insufficient" levels (below 32 nanograms per milliliter). Those with the lowest levels had double the risk of developing prostate cancer and 2.5 times the risk of developing deadly, aggressive prostate cancer. "This research underscores the importance of obtaining adequate vitamin D through skin exposure to sunlight or through diet, including food and supplements," concluded the researchers in the *Journal of the National Cancer Institute*.

I recommend that my cancer patients take 2,000 IU to 4,000 IU of vitamin D daily. (If you have high calcium levels from bone metastases, take a vitamin D supplement only under a physician's guidance.)

•**Zinc.** DNA is the genetic material that instructs our cells how to behave, and DNA damage can trigger many diseases, including cancer. Researchers at Oregon State University fed nine healthy men a diet very low in zinc for 40 days—and then found broken strands of DNA in blood cells. But that breakage was quickly repaired when the men started eating enough zinc. "Zinc appears to be a critical factor in maintaining DNA integrity in humans," concluded the researchers in the *American Journal of Clinical Nutrition*.

Researchers from Wayne State University School of Medicine, in the journal *Nutrition and Cancer*, pointed out that zinc can shut down several biochemical factors linked to development and progression of cancer, and that blood and tissue levels of zinc are more predictive of cancer progression than any other nutritional marker (the lower the zinc, the more aggressive the cancer).

•**Iodine and coenzyme Q10.** Iodine is an important nutrient for women with breast cancer. In countries with high iodine intake, such as Japan, women have 70 percent lower rates of the disease. For a woman with breast cancer, I recommend the supplement Tri-Iodine, from

Terry Naturally, which offers a line of products that has from 3,000 micrograms (3 milligrams) to 25,000 micrograms (25 milligrams) per capsule. (Do not take more than 12,500 micrograms of iodine a day, unless you are under the supervision and guidance of a holistic physician.) In one study, women with metastatic breast cancer had significant reduction in the size of their tumors when they took coenzyme Q10. I recommend 200 milligrams to 400 milligrams a day.

●**Flavonoids.** German researchers conducted a study on 87 people who had been operated on for colon cancer or for a precancerous colon adenoma, dividing them into two groups: One took a flavonoid supplement and one didn't. After three to four years, there were no recurrences of colon cancer in the flavonoid group, and one new adenoma. Among those not taking the supplement, 20 had a recurrence of their cancer, and 27 percent had a new adenoma. All in all, there was a seven percent recurrence rate among those taking the supplement and a 47 percent recurrence rate among those not taking it. "Sustained long-term treatment with a flavonoid mixture could reduce the recurrence rate of colon neoplasia [tumors and adenomas]," concluded the researchers in the *World Journal of Gastroenterology*. The supplement taken in the study contained 20 mg/d apigenin and 20 mg/d epigallocatechin-gallate.

●**Curcumin.** Curcumin is an extract of the herb turmeric and is a powerful antioxidant. Because of the breakthroughs in developing highly absorbed curcumin, this is becoming an important supplement for those with cancer. Among curcumin products, I favor CuraMed from Terry Naturally, a form of curcumin with a nearly sevenfold better rate of absorption than other forms of high-potency curcumin. Take one to two of the 750 mg capsules a day for cancer prevention, and two to six capsules a day for supportive treatment.

●**Selenium.** Researchers analyzed the results of three major nutritional studies on diet and colon cancer and found that people with the highest dietary intake of selenium had a 34 percent lower risk of developing colorectal adenoma, a precancerous growth. "Higher selenium status may be related to a decreased risk of colorectal cancer," concluded the researchers in the *Journal of the National Cancer Institute*.

The Promise of Low-Cost, Generic Medications for Cancer

Because cancer cells grow very quickly, they require a lot of energy. This makes them especially vulnerable to being *starved*. How to starve cancer cells is discussed in the book *How to Starve Cancer...Without Starving Yourself* by Jane McLelland. It discusses research on a range of common, safe, and low-cost generic medications that block energy production by specific cancer types.

But although a large body of research supports the efficacy of these medications, the medications themselves are too low-cost to attract the funding needed for large, clinical studies to definitively prove their efficacy. Many groups of physicians and scientists are trying to raise money to fund this research. (One of my favorites among this is the Yu Foundation, which also studies using modified fasting and a ketogenic diet to battle cancer.) But you don't need to wait 20 years until these studies are completed. Buy this book, read it, and talk about it with your oncologist.

In another study, researchers from the Roswell Park Comprehensive Cancer Institute in Buffalo, New York, gave 200 micrograms or 400 micrograms of selenium or a placebo to 424 people for 20 years. The 200-microgram dose (the amount I recommend) decreased "total cancer incidence" by 25 percent; the 400-microgram dose had no effect. The Nutritional Prevention of Cancer study on more than 1,300 people showed that 200 micrograms of selenium specifically decreased the risk of lung, colon, and prostate cancer and the overall risk of developing any type of cancer.

●**Acetyl-L-carnitine.** This nutrient, a combination of two amino acids, improves the body's ability to manufacture energy. In a study of patients with advanced cancer, carnitine (starting at 500 milligrams a day and increasing gradually to 3,000) decreased fatigue, improved sleep, and eased depression.

●**Ginseng.** American ginseng has been shown to be very helpful for cancer fatigue. Newer forms don't have the potency of the wild herb, which now sells for over $700 per pound, and is hard to find. But a new botanical technique has been found that gives cultivated ginseng the same potency as wild forms. It is called HRG80 Red Ginseng Energy. Research is showing that it may also have anticancer properties.

●**CBD (cannabidiol).** A study in the *Journal of Pain and Symptom Management* shows that CBD, derived from the cannabis (marijuana) plant, can relieve chemo-induced nerve pain. Another study in the same journal showed it was effective in relieving cancer pain itself—and didn't lose its effectiveness over time, which is the case with other drugs used to treat cancer pain, such as opioids. And many cancer patients find that cannabis helps ease nausea from chemotherapy, and increase appetite (loss of appetite is a big problem for cancer patients).

●**Grape seed extract.** This compound has been shown to affect more than a dozen pathways that control cancer growth, and animal studies show it can slow breast, colorectal, lung, prostate, and skin cancers. In a recent study from researchers at UCLA and the University of New Mexico, a small group of lung cancer patients received high doses of grape seed extract—and had a 55 percent reduction of a biomarker for the spread of cancer. Writing in the journal *Cancer Prevention Research*, the researchers concluded that grape seed extract should be used to prevent and fight lung cancer.

Most grape seed extracts have a high molecular weight and so are poorly absorbed by the body. That's why I recommend a product with a low molecular weight: Clinical OPC, from Terry Naturally, at a dose of 400 milligrams, three times daily.

●**Andrographolide.** This is an extract of the Asian herb *andrographis*, or green chireta. In a study in *Nutrition and Cancer*, researchers from India reviewed all the research on andrographolide and concluded the extract has "remarkable anticancer activity." It works against cancer mainly by causing *cell-cycle arrest*, a kind of state of suspended cellular animation, in which cancer cells no longer divide and duplicate. It also stimulates the immune system. I recommend Andrographis EP80, from Terry Naturally. Take one capsule, three times daily.

●**Boswellia.** This herb—famously called *frankincense*—fights cancer by stimulating *apoptosis*, the death of cancer cells. In cellular studies—where boswellia is mixed with cancer cells in a petri dish—the herb has been effective against many cancers, including bladder, brain, breast,

Relief from Cancer Pain

It's unacceptable for a cancer patient to be in pain—and there are many ways to stop that pain and other discomforts of the disease (and side effects from its treatments). A few other chapters in this book can help a person with cancer pain.

For bone pain, see the Real Cure Regimen in Osteoporosis on page 302.

For nerve pain, see the regimen in Nerve Pain (Neuropathy) on page 294.

Other pain-relieving tips for cancer pain…

•**Take the medication before the pain.** If you're taking medication for chronic pain, take it before you expect the pain to occur or at the first sign of its return. Don't wait for pain to become severe. If you follow this strategy, you'll need less medication overall and therefore have fewer side effects.

•**Limit side effects from narcotics.** Narcotics may be used to control severe cancer pain, but they have common side effects such as constipation, fatigue, nausea and vomiting, itching, dizziness, dry mouth, and confusion. Ask your doctor about using a lower dose of two different narcotics. This strategy may provide more pain relief with fewer side effects.

Also, if tolerance to one narcotic develops, switching back and forth between narcotics (such as switching from hydrocodone to oxycodone) can restore effectiveness.

Magnesium supplements (such as the level of magnesium in the Energy Revitalization System multinutrient powder) can also help prevent side effects from narcotics.

•**Control uncontrollable nausea.** Ask your physician to talk to a compounding pharmacist about making a multi-ingredient nausea-controlling skin cream, which is applied to an area of soft skin, such as the wrist. The prescription contains *lorazepam* (Ativan), *diphenhydramine* (Benadryl), *haloperidol* (Haldol), and *metoclopramide* (Reglan). Typically, you apply and reapply the cream every six hours, as needed. Nausea often settles within 15 to 30 minutes after applying.

•**If needed, see a pain specialist.** I've treated many patients with cancer pain, and I know their pain can be adequately controlled. The problem is not a lack of effective treatments, but a lack of physician education in pain management. If you have cancer pain and it is not eliminated by your physician, ask for (if necessary, demand!) a consultation with a specialist board certified in pain management. Do not accept being left in pain. It's unhealthy, and during cancer you need to use your energy for maximizing your enjoyment of life, not for trying to cope with pain!

cervical, colorectal, lung, melanoma, ovarian, pancreatic, and prostate, and leukemia. And in a case history reported in *Integrative Cancer Therapies*, a patient with recurrent bladder cancer went into remission after starting boswellia.

Boswellia also works to ease the side effects of cancer treatment. In a paper in the *Journal of the Neurosurgical Sciences*, from Italian researchers, patients with brain cancer who took a boswellia extract had less brain swelling after radiation of the brain. In a similar study, also from Italy, use of a boswellia-based cream reduced skin damage after radiation for breast cancer. I recommend the product BosMed 500, from Terry Naturally. Take one to three capsules, three times daily.

Walk Away from Cancer

Many studies show that regular exercise lowers the risk of developing cancer and helps prevent a recurrence of the disease. For example, in a 17-year study of more than 2,600 men, Finnish researchers found that men who exercised an average of 30 minutes a day had a 37 percent lower risk of developing and dying from any cancer. And when researchers at the Harvard School of Public Health studied 668 men with colon cancer, they found that those who exercised the most had a 53 percent lower risk of dying from the disease, compared with men who exercised the least.

The take-home message is to follow the exercise guidelines, and participate in an exercise you enjoy for at least 150 minutes a week. (Exercise bouts as short as 10 minutes are perfectly okay.)

Work with a Holistic Practitioner

There are many safe, low-cost natural treatments that improve outcomes while decreasing chemotherapy toxicity. A holistic practitioner can guide you on your specific case.

Candida Overgrowth

Real Causes

- **Nutritional Deficiencies.** Excess sugar in the diet feeds the candida fungus, encouraging overgrowth (page 3).
- **Prescription Medications.** Antibiotics kill the good bacteria that help keep the candida fungus in check (page 70).
- **Digestive Difficulties.** Leaky gut syndrome—a weakened intestinal wall—leads to food allergies that can be caused by candida overgrowth (page 107).

Fungi typically grow on other creatures. And that includes the yeast *Candida albicans*, which lives happily and unobtrusively in your gut and mouth. But candida can multiply, overgrowing its normal limits and infesting your gut and sinuses. In your gut, it crowds out "friendly" bacteria that keep you healthy. And wherever it overgrows, it pumps out toxins, sparks inflammation, triggers food sensitivities, weakens the immune system, and generally causes ill health.

Candida overgrowth can occur for many reasons, including nutritional deficiencies, a sugar-loaded diet, insufficient sleep, antibiotics (which kill off friendly bacteria in the gut, allowing yeast to overgrow), steroid medication, diabetes, and digestive problems. (For more about the role of candida infection in causing and complicating digestive problems, see Digestive Difficulties on page 107.)

Standard medicine acknowledges only *visible* candida infections of the skin, nails, hair, or pelvic area (as well as serious blood infections that can kill you). That's because there's no

Should You Stop Eating Yeast?

Many books on yeast overgrowth (such as the classic, *The Yeast Connection*, by the late William Crook, MD, a wonderful physician) advise readers to avoid all yeast in the diet, based on the theory that an allergic reaction to yeast is the cause of the problem. However, the yeast found in most foods (except beer and cheese) is not closely related to candida, the yeast that's usually responsible for the overgrowth. In my experience with patients, many who try to eat a yeast-free diet end up eating a nutritionally inadequate diet that doesn't help them overcome the problem.

Yes, a few people with yeast overgrowth do have a food allergy to yeast, but in my practice they account for less than 10 percent of those with the problem. These people may benefit from a strict yeast-free diet. For most people, a sugar-free diet is enough and much easier.

medical test that can diagnose candida overgrowth of the bowel or sinuses by distinguishing it from the normal presence of candida in the body. As a result, most doctors say yeast overgrowth in the gut or sinuses simply doesn't exist. Tell that to the fulminating fungus—or the millions of Americans who suffer.

You should suspect candida overgrowth—and use the Real Cure Regimen for it—if you have one or more of the following health problems…

•**Chronic sinusitis or nasal congestion** (which is usually caused by yeast)

•**Food allergies** (a result of leaky gut syndrome, in which candida overgrowth affects the lining of the intestinal tract, allowing large, undigested food proteins into the bloodstream, where the immune system attacks them)

•**Chronic fatigue syndrome/fibromyalgia** (If you have either of these health problems, you can assume you also have candida overgrowth.)

•**Sugar addiction** (Sugar is yeast's favorite food, and cravings for sugar and other refined carbohydrates are often a sign of candida overgrowth.)

•**Irritable bowel syndrome** (often caused or complicated by candida overgrowth)

•**Adrenal exhaustion** (For a full list of symptoms, see Adrenal Exhaustion on page 138.)

•**Night sweats** (Many infections can cause night sweats, including C. albicans.)

•**Recurrent, painful canker sores** (inside the mouth, lasting for about 10 days) or inflammation of the corners of your mouth (called angular cheilitis)

•**A history of recurrent or long-term antibiotic use** (especially tetracycline for acne)

When you treat the yeast, these problems usually improve and even vanish.

Real Cure Regimen

This regimen is very effective with my patients, usually eliminating symptoms in six to 10 weeks, although you need to continue the treatment for three to five months. (The yeast organisms are entrenched, so they don't go away overnight.)

•**Avoid sugar.** Yeast eat sugar 24/7. If you feed them, they live and multiply. If you don't, they die off more easily. That means taking sugar off their menu and yours. (Fortunately, carbohydrates other than sugar aren't an issue, so flour and wheat are on the menu.) And that's sugar in all its forms—including fruit juices (a piece or two of fruit a day is okay), corn syrup, jellies, pastry, candy, and soft drinks (there are nine teaspoons of sugar in every 12 ounces!), as well as other sugars such as brown sugar, honey, agave, coconut sugar, and evaporated cane juice.

Use healthful, natural stevia as a sugar substitute. (Despite the misinformation supported by the makers of chemical sweeteners, stevia, an herb, is safe and natural.) The brand of stevia is important, however; some have a bitter aftertaste. Two brands I favor: Now Better Stevia and Stevia Select (which has an awesome line of flavored stevias).

•**Take a probiotic supplement.** These supplements contain the friendly and health-giving bacteria that typically inhabit your gut, such as Lactobacillus acidophilus. Those good-guy bacteria combat the fungi, killing them off. I also suggest you take them whenever you're taking antibiotics (which kill off friendly bacteria) and continue taking them for at least one month (possibly as long as five) after you're finished with your prescription.

All probiotic supplements are not created equal, however. Many don't contain the number of bacteria advertised on the label, or the bacteria in the supplement are dead, or they die in the acid environment of the stomach—all of which means the probiotic isn't doing you much good! In my practice, I use the form of acidophilus called Pearls Elite, from Nature's Way. Take two capsules, once a day, for five months. Follow the rest of this Real Cure Regimen. After five months, your yeast and yeast-caused symptoms should be under control. Then switch to one capsule a day for prevention.

•**Eat acidophilus-rich yogurt.** Another way to ingest friendly gut bacteria is to eat them. Eat a daily cup of unsweetened yogurt with a live culture that is rich in acidophilus. (Some of the sugar-free Greek yogurts are amazingly delicious. I just add some stevia and fresh fruit.)

Take "Yeast Die-Off" into Account

I recommend using the sugar-free diet, the daily cup of acidophilus-rich yogurt, the probiotic supplement, and the natural antifungal supplement for one month before starting to take a prescription antifungal medication. That's because using the medication can cause a massive die-off of yeast, and if you're sensitive to the yeast "body parts," your symptoms may actually worsen. Starting with the natural remedies helps circumvent that die-off and the reaction to it by gradually beginning the process of killing the yeast before you take the medication.

Do You Have Candida? It's Easy to Find Out!

There's no lab test that I find reliable for candida overgrowth. But the simple questionnaire below can give you a pretty good idea as to whether or not you have it. As I noted earlier however, if you have chronic fatigue syndrome, fibromyalgia, chronic sinusitis, or unexplained spastic colon (irritable bowel syndrome), it's reasonable to simply assume you have candida overgrowth—and then to get it addressed.

Yeast Questionnaire

Answer yes or no to each of the questions below. Your total score shows you the probability that yeast overgrowth is a significant factor in your case. To calculate your total score, simply add the point values shown in parenthesis for each of the questions you answer "yes" to.

POINTS

_____ Have you received therapy for acne with tetracycline, erythromycin, or any other antibiotic for one month or longer? (50)

_____ Have you taken antibiotics for any type of infection for more than two consecutive months, or shorter courses over three times in a 12-month period? (50)

_____ Do you have CFS or fibromyalgia? (50)

_____ Do you have sinusitis and/or spastic colon (irritable bowel syndrome)? (50)

_____ Have you ever taken an antibiotic (even for a single course)? (5)

_____ Have you ever had prostatitis or vaginitis? (25)

_____ Have you ever been pregnant? (5)

_____ Have you taken birth control pills? (15)

_____ Have you taken corticosteroids such as Prednisone, Cortef, or Medrol? (15)

_____ Have you ever had a fungal infection—such as jock itch, athlete's foot, or a nail or skin infection—that was difficult to address? (20)

_____ Do you crave sugar or breads? (20)

_____ Do you frequently get painful sores in your mouth (not on your lips)? (10)

_____ **Total**

If your total was 70 or higher, consider implementing the Real Cure regimen in this chapter to rebalance candida.

•**Take** *nystatin* **or an antifungal herbal supplement.** Nystatin is an anti-fungal medication typically used to address candida, but only in the gut. For those of you whose insurance covers medications, it is a reasonable, low-cost alternative to herbal supplements. But if your doctor won't prescribe nystatin for the three to six months it takes to work, or if you prefer natural treatment, some herbals can be very helpful. But there's a caveat.

While many natural antifungals are helpful, when they're used in a dosage high enough to kill the yeast, they can irritate the stomach. To solve this problem, I've found that a buffered caprylic acid called Caprylex (by Douglas Labs) is very helpful and easy on the stomach. Each tablet provides 400 mg of a buffered calcium-magnesium caprylate complex, equivalent to 300 milligrams of caprylic acid. Plus, Caprylex is specially formulated to provide timed, controlled release of caprylic acid throughout the small and large intestine. Take two tablets daily on an empty stomach, at least 30 minutes before a meal. Take it for at least three months. It can be taken at the same time as the probiotic.

Another problem with natural treatments for candida overgrowth: they stay in the intestines, so they can't kill the candida in the sinuses and elsewhere in the body. To do that, I recommend two drugs: Lufenuron and Diflucan. Let's talk about Lufenuron first, which you can combine with natural treatments.

You can order Lufenuron online from Canada, at the website Shop4MyHealth.com. (Otherwise, it's sold only as a treatment for fleas in pets, but it's perfectly safe for humans.) The site sells 800-milligram capsules. The standard, one-day treatment is nine grams, or about 12 capsules (which sell for about $28). I recommend taking the nine grams, repeating the nine grams two weeks later, and then taking it on the first day of each month. (Best to start on the first, take it on the 14th or 15th, and then start the once-per-month on the next first.) You can take it for five months, which should rebalance candida levels in your body. Or continue taking it once-a-month if symptoms recur.

For optimal absorption, it's important to take Lufenuron with a full meal that contains fats. The fat can be any kind, such as cheese, bacon, yogurt, nuts, olive oil, butter, margarine, avocado, salmon, mackerel, or peanut butter. Personally, I take it with a swig of olive oil.

But the first one or two times you take it, *don't* take the full nine grams. Instead, take two capsules per day for six days—which keeps the dead yeast from causing an intensification of your symptoms. (The dosing schedule at Shop4MyHealth.com is different than mine but reasonable, if you want to do it.)

Both Caprylex and Lufenuron can be very helpful—either individually or together. But for more severe cases, talk to your doctor about adding the medication *fluconazole* (Diflucan), at a dosage of 200 milligrams a day, for six to eight weeks. Conventional doctors aren't familiar with treating internal candida, and generally will not prescribe this drug—so it's likely you'll need a holistic doctor to write this prescription for you. (See Resources on page 360 to find a holistic doctor near you.) Get the generic version—and, if it's not covered by insurance, use the free GoodRx phone app, which I also list in Resources. This wonderful, free app can cut costs by over 90 percent for most medications that aren't covered by insurance. You can take Diflucan with the other remedies discussed in this chapter.

Carpal Tunnel Syndrome

Real Causes

- **Nutritional Deficiencies.** Low levels of nutrients—particularly vitamin B_6 (*pyridoxine*)—can cause the tissue swelling that triggers carpal tunnel syndrome (page 3).

- **Hormonal Imbalances.** Low levels of thyroid hormone also can play a role in the swelling (page 84).

- **Chronic Inflammation.** A repetitive stress injury—from a daily activity at work such as typing—can create tissue-swelling inflammation (page 118).

Your hand—maybe one, maybe both—hurts, with burning, tingling sensations and even a kind of itchy, achy numbness. The pain and sensations are mainly in your palm and your thumb, index, and middle fingers. Those symptoms often wake you up at night, and you feel like you have to shake out your hands for the discomfort to go away. What's going on?

You have carpal tunnel syndrome (CTS), an injury to the median nerve, which runs from the forearm to the hand. On its way, the nerve passes through the narrow carpal tunnel, which also is filled with nine tendons. When tendons and other tissues in the nerve are irritated and swell, they can press on the median nerve, causing CTS.

What's behind the irritation? Sometimes it's a repetitive stress injury from performing the same action again and again—working on an assembly line, for example, or typing all day. A nutritional deficiency of nerve-nourishing vitamin B_6 can play a role. Research also shows a link to hypothyroidism. But whatever the cause, a lot of people have the problem: one in 10, according to the American Academy of Neurology. And as many as one in two industrial workers!

The standard medical treatment for the problem: Surgery. It can work. But it's expensive. Plus, sometimes those who have the surgery say they have discomfort from postsurgical scarring or a recurrence of pain two years or more after the surgery.

The good news: If you're willing and able to stop the repetitive action that caused CTS, you can almost always find relief without surgery.

Real Cure Regimen

In almost all my patients with CTS, the problem completely resolves in six weeks with the simple treatments I'll describe. If your physician recommends surgery for CTS, ask if you can try these treatments first, for at least six weeks. It's likely you'll never see the inside of the operating room.

- **Take vitamin B_6.** Vitamin B_6 plays a crucial role in the health of nerves and in decreasing the swelling of the tissues that can compress the median nerve. Studies show that supplementing

A Treatment Worth Trying

Although the regimen described in this chapter is very effective at relieving carpal tunnel syndrome, I'd also like to mention another nonsurgical treatment that a study shows works extremely well.

It's called the CTRAC automatic hand-stretching (or hand traction) device. Somewhat similar to a blood pressure cuff, it wraps around the hand (with a hole for the thumb) and is inflated. It stretches the ligament that surgeons slice up to relieve carpal tunnel, and also stretches the sheath of tissue around the tendons in the tunnel—taking pressure off the median nerve.

In a study by doctors in the former Department of Physical Medicine and Rehabilitation at Saint Vincent Catholic Medical Centers of New York, 19 people with carpal tunnel used the CTRAC device for five minutes, three times a day, for four weeks. They had 92 percent less pain, 93 percent less tingling, 79 percent less numbness, and no pain at night.

"CTRAC is comparable in effectiveness to splints, injections of corticosteroids, and surgery," wrote Humberto Porrata, MD, the study leader, in the *Journal of Hand Therapy*.

You can buy CTRAC at CarpalDoctors.com or call 787-672-7472.

the diet with B_6 can help relieve the symptoms of CTS. "It appears reasonable to recommend vitamin B_6 supplementation to people with CTS," concluded researchers from the Department of Physical Medicine and Rehabilitation at the University of Medicine and Dentistry of New Jersey, in the review of studies on B_6 and CTS in the journal *Nutrition Reviews*.

However, more is not better with B_6: Doses of regular vitamin B_6 over 45 milligrams a day can aggravate nerve problems. So use the safest form of B_6: pyridoxal phosphate.

•**Supplement with a thyroid hormone.** If you have CTS, you will likely benefit from this hormone even if your lab tests for thyroid hormone levels are normal, because thyroid tests interpreted as "normal" are often low, and low levels are a common cause of this problem.

What's the link? Low hormone levels will contribute to the tissue swelling that can pinch the nerve. So taking B_6 and thyroid hormone often decreases the swelling enough to completely relieve the pain and numbness. (For more on the problems with testing for hypothyroidism, see Hormonal Imbalances on page 84 and Hypothyroidism on page 254.)

•**Use a wrist splint.** Most people end up sleeping with their wrists in a flexed rather than straight position, which stretches and strains the median nerve. That's why you wake up in the middle of the night with tingling and numbness. By wearing a "cock-up" wrist splint when you sleep—a splint that keeps your wrist in a neutral position (picture the position of your hand while holding a glass of water)—you take the nighttime stress off the nerve. Wear the splint every night for at least six weeks. You can also wear it during the day, when it's convenient and helpful. Cock-up wrist splints are widely available for under $20 in drugstores and medical supply stores and online.

Cataracts

Real Cause

●**Nutritional Deficiencies.** Too much sugar in the diet can harm the protein in the lenses of the eyes, leading to cataracts. Deficiencies of several nutrients can worsen the problem (page 3).

The lens of the eye—the part that allows us to focus—is filled with clear, liquid-containing proteins. If those proteins start to denature (that is, if they start to lose their structural integrity) they become cloudy, which blurs vision.

Most cataracts are caused by aging: 50 percent of Americans over 65 years old and 70 percent over 75 have them. This process is hastened by diseases such as diabetes and high blood pressure.

Real Cure Regimen

Cataracts aren't dangerous, but they do impair vision. If you're developing one, here are some ways to stop or reverse the process. Start them today—and them for the rest of your life.

●**Maximize the right nutrients.** High-sugar diets speed up denaturing; low-sugar diets protect the lens. But you also want to optimize your intake of eye-protecting zinc, vitamin B_2, and vitamin C, which can help prevent the denaturing of the protein. Research shows, for example, that 80 percent of cataract patients may have a riboflavin (B_2) deficiency (compared to 12 percent of people who don't have cataracts), and that supplementing with 3 milligrams of riboflavin helps prevent cataracts.

In a landmark 10-year study published in the *American Journal of Clinical Nutrition*, researchers analyzed diet and health data from 3,653 people age 49 or older, and found that those with the highest intake of vitamin C from food and supplements were 45 percent less likely to develop cataracts. They also found that a high combined intake of the antioxidants vitamin C and E, beta-carotene, and zinc lowered risk by 49 percent.

Zinc, B_2, vitamin C, and many other nutrients are found in optimal levels in the Energy Revitalization System multinutrient powder (discussed in Nutritional Deficiencies on page 30).

●**N-Acetylcarnosine.** Begin with this treatment—an antioxidant that reduces inflammation, thereby protecting the lens. It's found in eyedrops called Can-C. Use one or two drops in each eye, twice a day. In a placebo-controlled study published in *Rejuvenation Research*, Can-C was quite effective in slowing the growth of cataracts, and reduced glare by 27 percent to 100 percent. (In some people it completely eliminated glare caused by cataracts!)

Try Antioxidant Eye Drops

N-acetylcarnosine is a form of carnosine, an amino acid and antioxidant. In studies by Russian researchers, N-acetylcarnosine eyedrops improved cataracts and eyesight. These eyedrops are available as Can-C Eyedrops. Marc Grossman, OD, LAc, a naturally oriented optometrist, told us that you can help prevent cataracts by applying one to two drops in each eye, one to two times daily. For treatment, he suggests two drops in the affected eye, two times daily. For more on this treatment, read *The Cataract Cure: The Russian Eye-Drop Breakthrough: The Story of N-acetyl-carnosine*, by Marios Kyriazis, MD.

•**Take higher doses of vitamin A, around 25,000 to 50,000 IU daily.** One ophthalmologist jokingly complained that his cataract surgery income dropped by two-thirds when he started adding vitamin A to his patients' regimens. Use vitamin A and *not* beta-carotene.

Caution: This is a high dose, and shouldn't be taken by children, women of childbearing age (it can cause birth defects), or people with liver disease, such as hepatitis C or cirrhosis.

•**Use bilberry, 80 to 160 milligrams, three times daily.** An extract of this antioxidant-rich berry has a long history as an eye-strengthening remedy. In an animal study, Russian researchers found that bilberry extracts "completely prevented" cataracts in animals bred to develop the problem, according to a report in the journal *Advances in Gerontology*. Use a standardized 25 percent extract.

•**Wear sunglasses on bright days.** They help stop sunlight from damaging the lens.

Chronic Fatigue Syndrome and Fibromyalgia

Real Causes

•**Poor Sleep.** Insomnia is a primary symptom of both CFS and FM, and treating it is critical in healing these conditions (page 33).

•**Hormonal Imbalances.** Low levels of adrenal and thyroid hormones, and of testosterone, can contribute to the development of CFS/FM (page 84).

•**Nutritional Deficiencies.** A nutrient-draining addiction to a high-sugar diet can cause CFS/FM (page 3).

- **Inactivity.** The inactivity from the fatigue and/or muscle pain of CFS/FM deconditions the body—and gradually increasing activity is a key part of the cure (page 40).
- **Happiness Deficiency.** Severe stress can aggravate these health problems (page 55).
- **Infections.** Although not one of the Real Causes in Part 1, in this condition several infections often need to be addressed, including *Candida albicans* and Lyme disease.

You go to sleep at night and wake up tired. You nap in the afternoon and wake up tired. You take a two-week vacation and come home tired. You're tired all the time. Really tired.

And that's not all. Your sleep is never deep and refreshing. In fact, it feels like you spend more time awake than asleep, night after night. And you're in pain a lot, mysterious, all-over pain. And you have a hard time thinking—concentrating, remembering, deciding.

If these symptoms sound like your symptoms—severe fatigue that doesn't go away with rest, widespread pain, and brain fog—you probably have chronic fatigue syndrome (CFS) and/or fibromyalgia (FM). (For most people, CFS and FM are two faces of the same illness, which I'll refer to as CFS/FM.)

CFS/FM is an energy crisis: You use more energy than your body can manufacture, usually because of long-term physical or mental stress of one kind or another, and your body blows a fuse. And that fuse is a main fuse: your hypothalamus, a part of the brain that controls sleep, the hormone-producing endocrine system, hunger and thirst, mood, sex drive, blood flow, blood pressure, body temperature and sweating, and bowel function.

If you have CFS-predominant CFS/FM, your main symptoms are severe chronic fatigue and insomnia. If you have FM-predominant CFS/FM, your main symptoms are muscle pain and insomnia. Why muscle pain? Muscles are like a spring: It takes more energy to relax and release than it does to contract. (Think about rigor mortis—muscles that are totally without energy are also totally contracted or stiffened.) The energy crisis, then, has left your muscles shortened, tight, and painful. You might ache all over or in specific areas, with pain that's constant or now and then. And that chronic muscle pain causes the pain itself to generate more pain signals, a problem called central sensitization. You hurt. Probably all over. Probably all the time.

A list of the most common symptoms of CFS/FM includes…

- Exhaustion after even mild activity
- Insomnia
- Achiness
- Forgetfulness
- Brain fog
- Increased thirst
- Bowel disorders
- Recurring infections
- Weight gain (an average of 32 pounds!)
- Low libido

Don't let a doctor tell you these symptoms are "all in your head" or that CFS and FM are not "real diseases." Most physicians aren't trained in recognizing or treating CFS/FM and often even deny their existence. But the National Institutes of Health, the Centers for Disease Control, and the FDA all recognize CFS/FM as real diseases and very common ones. In fact, if statistics include both overt *and* borderline cases, estimates of CFS/FM prevalence have increased markedly, to include more than four percent of the population (about 12 million people).

There are many causes of CFS/FM. As I mentioned earlier, severe physical or emotional stress can cause it. You might have had a sudden infection—what some experts call "the drop-dead flu"—from which you never fully recovered. Nutritional deficiencies are a cause. Or becoming "addicted" to sugar and other refined carbohydrates (which can lead to yeast overgrowth and other chronic infections, exhausting your adrenal glands, which undercuts the hypothalamus and leads to CFS/FM). Or the cause could be any combination of the above factors.

I had CFS/FM in 1975, and it knocked me out of medical school and left me homeless for a year. But I learned how to recover from the illness—and have spent more than four decades helping others do the same.

Real Cure Regimen

The good news is that CFS/FM is very treatable. Just as there is no damage to circuit breakers when they blow in your house, there is also no damage to the hypothalamus. It just goes into "slow" mode until the energy crisis of CFS/FM is properly treated. *I call my treatment for CFS/FM the SHINE protocol, an acronym for...*

- Sleep restoration
- Hormonal support
- Infection treatment
- Nutrition
- Exercise (as able)

In a study published in the *Journal of Chronic Fatigue Syndrome*, my colleagues and I tested the SHINE protocol in 72 people with CFS/FM, dividing them into two groups. One group received the protocol and the other a placebo treatment. After three months, 29 of the 32 people on the SHINE protocol said they felt either "much better" (16) or "better" (13)—they had more energy, deeper sleep, greater mental clarity, less pain, and increased well-being. Among those in the placebo group, only 12 out of 33 people felt either "much better" (3) or "better" (9). And, by the end of the study, those undergoing the SHINE protocol had a 90 percent improvement in their "quality of life."

An editorial about the study in *Practical Pain Management*, the journal of the American Academy of Pain Management, discussed the importance of those results: "The study by Dr. Teitelbaum et al., and years of clinical experience, make this approach an excellent and powerfully effective part of the standard of practice for treatment of people who suffer from fibromyalgia."

Let's look at how you can implement the SHINE protocol.

Sleep Restoration

The hypothalamus controls sleep. In CFS/FM, the hypothalamus is malfunctioning. This means getting seven to eight hours of sleep seems impossible, including the hours of nondreaming deep sleep that are truly restorative and could heal the hurting hypothalamus. Unfortunately, many of the sleep medications on the market only make this problem worse—by actually decreasing the amount of deep sleep (the nondreaming sleep that is most restorative to the body).

If you have CFS/FM, you need to take the right type of sleep medication. That includes *zolpidem* (Ambien), *trazodone* (Desyrel), *gabapentin* (Neurontin), *clonazepam* (Klonopin), and *pregabalin* (Lyrica). You can also take *cyclobenzaprine* (Flexeril) or *amitriptyline* (Elavil) if you don't have restless legs syndrome (those two drugs can worsen the problem).

Over-the-counter medications such as *doxylamine* (Unisom) or *diphenhydramine* (Benadryl) can also be effective in doses of 25 to 50 milligrams at bedtime.

In addition to medications, I also recommend that you try a natural sleep aid, such as the Revitalizing Sleep Formula from Nature's Way, Terrific ZZZZ from Terry Naturally, and five milligrams of a specific form of melatonin called Dual Spectrum, from Nature's Bounty. Both individually and in combination, these natural remedies can be very helpful. (For more on this formula and other natural sleep remedies, see Insomnia and Other Sleep Disorders on page 268.)

Because your sleep center is not working, during the first six months of treatment for CFS/FM, you may need to take as many as six different types of sleep treatments to achieve eight hours of sleep a night, taking a low dose of each rather than a high dose of one. This may seem like a lot of pills and treatments. But think of the treatment for the insomnia caused by your ailing hypothalamus as similar to the treatment for high blood pressure. Your doctor starts with one pressure-controlling medication and adds another and another until control is achieved—and those medications are prescribed for as long as they are needed.

You can probably stop taking sleep medications after six to 18 months of feeling well. But you may need to take one-half to one tablet of sleep medication (or a sleep-enhancing herbal formula) for the rest of your life, particularly during periods of high stress, to make sure you don't relapse. This is similar to a person with high blood pressure or diabetes who stays on medication to control high blood pressure or high blood sugar levels. The doctor doesn't take them off those medications every time pressure or sugar levels normalize! And my experience with more than

Top Natural Supplements for CFS/FM

A patient asked me to list the most useful and effective supplements for people with CFS/FM. On my list, I include the Energy Revitalization System multinutrient powder and ribose, discussed on page 30 and below. *I also recommend…*

- **Revitalizing Sleep Formula,** from Nature's Way
- **Acidophilus Pearls,** from Nature's Way.
- **Adrenaplex,** from Terry Naturally, one to two capsules each morning for adrenal support.
- **Adrenal Stress-End,** from Nature's Way. This product helps revive a weakened adrenal gland, common in CFS/FM. Take one or two capsules each morning (or one or two in the morning and one at noon). If it upsets your stomach, take less or take it with food.

15,000 CFS/FM patients shows that this approach of continuing to regularly use sleep medication is safe. It's also essential if you want to get well and stay well.

Hormonal Balancing

Just as an electric grid control center controls the movement of electricity throughout a city or state, so the hypothalamus controls the dispersion of hormones throughout your body. That's why when your hypothalamus isn't up to par, you have all kinds of different hormonal imbalances and deficiencies—all of which need to be rebalanced and regenerated.

In my experience, it's helpful to treat CFS/FM with bioidentical thyroid, adrenal, ovarian, and/or testicular hormones even if your blood tests for levels of these hormones are normal. (Read page 95 in Hormonal Imbalances to learn more about bioidentical hormones and why many blood tests for hormone levels are inaccurate.)

For example: Bioidentical estrogen and progesterone can help women who have CFS/FM symptoms that are worse around their periods. Bioidentical testosterone can benefit men whose blood tests are in the lowest 30 percent of the normal range (and that's 70 percent of men with CFS). A daily dose of 2.5 milligrams to 20 milligrams of natural hydrocortisone (Cortef) can help reenergize exhausted adrenal glands.

For pain, I combine Curamin and Hemp Select hemp oil by Terry Naturally. These pain-relieving remedies in combination contain herbs and nutrients that help all seven key components of fibromyalgia pain. For more information, see Chronic Pain on page 197.

For anyone with the severe fatigue of CFS or the pain of FM, I also recommend a therapeutic trial of energizing thyroid hormone: specifically, either (1) the prescription desiccated thyroid, or (2) a mix of T4 and T3 thyroid hormones made at a compounding pharmacy (the type of pharmacy that customizes medications on-site).

If your physician won't work with you to find the right mix of bioidentical hormones to treat CFS/FM, I recommend finding a holistic physician who knows how to help you.

Infection Treatment

Most people with CFS/FM have weakened immune systems, resulting in multiple chronic infections. These can include viral infections; parasites and other bowel infections; infections sensitive to long-term treatment with antibiotics such as *ciprofloxacin* (Cipro) and *doxycycline* (Doryx), such as mycoplasma, chlamydia, and Lyme; and, most frequently, fungal/candida infections.

Because most CFS/FM patients have an overgrowth of the fungus Candida albicans, I have found that most benefit from six to 12 weeks of treatment with the antifungal *fluconazole* (Diflucan), as well as the other remedies for candida in Candida Overgrowth on page 181.

Another excellent candida treatment: Sinusitis Nose Spray, a compounded prescription product that your doctor can order from ITC compounding pharmacy. (You can find contact info for ITC in Resources on page 362.) Take it along with Diflucan.

For optimal benefit, add Silver Nose Spray (Argentyn 23). I recommend using one to two squirts of both sprays, in each nostril, two to three times a day, for six to 12 weeks—or until

Are You Dizzy When You Stand Up? If So, Here's the Solution...

Think about it for a moment. We are a big bag of water. Ever wonder why it doesn't all flow down to our legs when we stand up?

It does! Because of this, our autonomic nervous system has to direct the blood vessels in our legs to contract and send the blood back up to our brain and muscles where it is needed.

But when this system is not working properly, your blood pressure can drop significantly when you are upright for an extended period. This can result in low blood pressure (neurally meditated hypertension, or NMH), or a compensatory rise in heart rate, called postural orthostatic tachycardia syndrome (POTS). But whatever name you use, it falls under the umbrella of a problem called orthostatic intolerance. When you stay upright, you get dizzy, exhausted, your heart races, and you have "brain fog," or a feeling of confusion or disorientation, as if your brain isn't working right.

Orthostatic intolerance is a common and very treatable symptom of CFS/FM. And research shows that many people with NMH and POTS actually have CFS/FM. (See page 196 to take a test to see if you have the problem.) *Fortunately, three natural treatments can be very helpful...*

•**Increase salt and water intake.** One of the common hormonal deficiencies of CFS/FM is a low level of vasopressin (antidiuretic hormone), which leaves you dehydrated. You also need to eat large amounts of salt—the sponge that holds water in your body—even licking sea salt from the palms of your hands will help.

•**Use medium pressure (20 mm to 30 mm) compression stockings.** It is remarkable how much improvement many people see by using these. The ideal pair is mid-thigh, but if you can't wear those, knee-high stockings will still help. Wear them during the day when you are active (not when you're lying down for extended periods, such a taking a nap).

•**Improve adrenal function.** Use Adrenaplex, from Terry Naturally, which I discuss in Adrenal Exhaustion on page 138.

•**Talk to your doctor about these medications.** For severe cases, medication may be necessary, including: DDAVP, an antidiuretic hormone (0.1 mg to 0.2 mg orally daily); *midodrine* (ProAmatine), 5 mg to 10 mg twice daily (morning and early afternoon); and medications that increase serotonin and dopamine, such as Zoloft.

---

the problem resolves. (In some cases, people choose to stay on both of these nose sprays long term, which can be very helpful and is safe.) This trio of treatments is wonderful for eliminating chronic sinusitis caused by a fungal infection—a common problem in people with CFS/FM.

If your symptoms persist after several months of following this strategy to treat the candida infection, see a CFS/FM specialist who can test and treat you for other infections.

Nutritional Supplementation

CFS/FM patients need optimal daily nutrition, and they can get it in the Energy Revitalization Formula, the multinutrient powder that I formulated specifically for my CFS/FM patients, but

A New, Ribose-Based Super-Energy Supplement

I have designed a supplement called Smart Energy. It combines the five grams of ribose with the herbal "adaptogens" ashwagandha, rhodiola, licorice and schisandra, all four of which can dramatically increase stamina and energy. And it includes green tea extract (which both energizes and calms). I could write a whole book on the benefits of each ingredient, and their combination—because the benefits of extra energy are, well, amazing.

As a morning routine, I recommend one scoop of the Energy Revitalization System multinutrient powder along with two capsules of Smart Energy—and then a second dose of Smart Energy at lunchtime. You can find both products at my website, EndFatigue.com.

that works to energize and nourish anyone who takes it. (You can read about this supplement and other supplements you may need in Nutritional Deficiencies on page 30.)

I also recommend supplementing the diet with ribose, a compound I consider the ultimate "quick fix" for CFS/FM. Ribose is a healthful sugar that plays a role in the manufacture of RNA and DNA, and is a key building block of cellular energy. In fact, the main energy molecules in your body—ATP, NADH, and FADH—are made of ribose, plus B vitamins and phosphate.

In a study my colleagues and I conducted with the nutrient, published in the *Journal of Alternative and Complementary Medicine*, 36 people with CFS/FM took five grams of ribose, three times a day, for 25 days (after which they lowered the dose to five grams twice a day). Twenty-three of them had more energy, better sleep, more mental alertness, less pain, and greater well-being. On average, the increase in energy was 45 percent.

In a second study (conducted with 257 CFS/FM patients at 53 health practitioners' offices), published in the *Open Pain Journal*, the nutrient increased energy by an average of 61 percent—after only three weeks. That is a very dramatic improvement for a single nutrient.

Ribose is taken in powder form. I recommend five grams of the powder, three times daily, for three weeks, and then two times daily. (Try the SHINE brand, which I formulated—it provides the same quality as any other product on the market, but at half the cost.) You'll usually see a dramatic boost in energy in two to three weeks.

Exercise (moderate)

Exercise is energizing for just about everyone. But if people with CFS/FM exercise beyond a certain point, they feel more fatigued the next day. In fact, they're so fatigued they often have to stay in bed the next day. *Here's a step-by-step approach to exercise with CFS/FM...*

1. Begin with light exercise, such as walking or, if regular walking is too difficult, water walking in a heated pool. Walk only as much as you comfortably can (or start with five minutes). Then increase the time you walk by one minute every one to two days, as is comfortable. When you get to a point that leaves you feeling worse the next day, cut back a bit to the comfortable level and continue that amount of walking each day. Another way to think of the amount to walk each day:

Do You Have Orthostatic Intolerance (POTS or NMH)?

Below is a quick test that has been shown in the *Mayo Clinic Proceedings* to accurately screen for orthostatic intolerance. As I explained earlier: in orthostatic intolerance, when you stay upright you get dizzy, exhausted, your heart races, and you have "brain fog," or a feeling of confusion or disorientation, as if your brain isn't working right. Circle 0-4 below as best applies to you.

A. Frequency of orthostatic symptoms when I stand up
0 I *never or rarely* experience orthostatic symptoms
1 I *sometimes* experience orthostatic symptoms
2 I *often* experience orthostatic symptoms
3 I *usually* experience orthostatic symptoms
4 I *always* experience orthostatic symptoms

B. Severity of orthostatic symptoms when I stand up
0 I *do not* experience orthostatic symptoms
1 I experience *mild* orthostatic symptoms
2 I experience *moderate* orthostatic symptoms and *sometimes* have to sit back down for relief
3 I experience *severe* orthostatic symptoms and *frequently* have to sit back down for relief
4 I experience *severe* orthostatic symptoms and *regularly* faint if I do not sit back down

C. Conditions under which orthostatic symptoms occur
0 I *never or rarely* experience orthostatic symptoms under any circumstances
1 I *sometimes* experience orthostatic symptoms under certain conditions, such as prolonged standing, a meal, exertion (e.g., walking), or when exposed to heat (e.g., hot day, hot shower)
2 I *often* experience orthostatic symptoms under certain conditions, such as prolonged standing, a meal, exertion (e.g., walking), or when exposed to heat (e.g., hot day, hot shower)
3 I *usually* experience orthostatic symptoms under certain conditions, such as prolonged standing, a meal, exertion (e.g., walking), or when exposed to heat (e.g., hot day, hot shower)
4 I *always* experience orthostatic symptoms when I stand up; the specific conditions do not matter

D. Activities of daily living (e.g., work, chores, dressing, bathing)
0 My orthostatic symptoms *do not interfere* with activities of daily living
1 My orthostatic symptoms *mildly interfere* with activities of daily living)
2 My orthostatic symptoms *moderately interfere* with activities of daily living
3 My orthostatic symptoms *severely interfere* with activities of daily living
4 My orthostatic symptoms *severely interfere* with activities of daily living. *I am bed or wheelchair bound because of my symptoms*

E. Standing time on most occasions
0 I can stand as long as necessary without experiencing orthostatic symptoms
1 I can stand *more than 15* minutes before experiencing orthostatic symptoms
2 I can stand *five to 14 minutes* before experiencing orthostatic symptoms
3 I can stand *one to four minutes* before experiencing orthostatic symptoms
4 I can stand *less than one minute* before experiencing orthostatic symptoms

_____ **Total Score**

Scores of 9 or higher (or seven or higher in people with CFS/FM) suggest orthostatic intolerance. You'll find three effective treatments for the problem on page 194: increase salt and water intake; wear compression stockings; prescription medications that can help.

Walk to the degree that you feel "good tired" afterward and better the next day. If you feel worse the next day, stop for a few days and then cut back.

2. After about 10 weeks on the SHINE protocol, your energy production will usually improve dramatically, and you'll be able to continue to increase your walking by one minute, every other day.

3. When you get to one hour a day (or 10,000 steps throughout the day, if using a pedometer to count your steps), you can increase the intensity of the exercise—walking faster, uphill, etc. Again, listen to your body and do only what feels good to you. You'll know the difference between how "good pain" feels versus "bad pain." Bad pain is your body's way of saying, "Don't do that!"

Unless it's cold out and cold flares your pain, I recommend you walk outside so you can get sunshine—your key source of vitamin D, which improves immune function and decreases the risk of hypertension, diabetes, and cancer. (Many people with CFS/FM are vitamin D deficient.) Make a plan to walk daily with a friend, and go somewhere that's enjoyable (on cold days it could be in the mall). That way, you're more likely to have fun and stick with regular exercise.

A Very Promising New Treatment

I have had the honor of knowing fibromyalgia expert Gaetano Morello, ND, for several decades. He serendipitously found that a unique natural (animal serum sourced) treatment was dramatically helping his patients with fibromyalgia—usually in about a week. When they ran out of this unique therapy, symptoms returned and the people taking it were desperate to get more.

We decided to do a study on this promising therapy. You can learn about the results, as well as the treatment we are using, at the website RecoveryFactors.com.

Chronic Pain

Real Causes

- **Nutritional Deficiencies.** Deficiencies in energy-producing B vitamins, magnesium, and ribose can shorten and tighten muscles, causing chronic pain (page 3).
- **Poor Sleep.** Tissue is repaired during sleep—poor sleep equals pain (page 33).
- **Inactivity.** Stretching muscles helps relieve pain (page 40).
- **Prescription Medications.** Cholesterol-lowering statins are common culprits in muscle pain (page 73).

> •**Hormonal Imbalances.** Low levels of thyroid, adrenal, and repro-
> ductive hormones cause muscle pain (page 84).
>
> •**Chronic Inflammation.** An underlying force behind pain (page 118).

About 20 years ago, with 25 percent of Americans suffering from chronic pain, the US government declared a "war on pain"—an all-out effort to solve the problem. Unfortunately, it gave physicians no guidance on how to effectively relieve pain. So, with the encouragement of pharmaceutical companies, physicians increasingly turned to prescribing narcotics for pain relief.

Today, we have just over 20 percent of Americans suffering with chronic pain. Yearly overdose deaths from prescribed narcotics peaked in 2017 to about 17,500 (up from just over 3,400 in 1999), but since then has dropped to about 14,000 a year, according to the National Institute on Drug Abuse. The government has decided to deal with this crisis by seemingly declaring a new war—a "war on people in pain." Prescriptions for narcotic medications are being stopped abruptly—with people given no alternative for pain relief. Sometimes, all they get from their doctor is the attitude, "All pain is tolerable—as long as it isn't mine!"

Meanwhile, the propaganda war against pain is ratcheting up—with the government trying to affix blame rather than solve the problem. Instead of focusing on the deaths from *prescribed* narcotics, the government is lumping in all the deaths from overdose—including deaths from street drugs such as heroin—to inflate the figures and justify their draconian actions.

So, let's take a step back, and get some perspective, by presenting the real numbers...

1. An estimated 50 million Americans suffer from chronic pain, according to a recent study by Brigham and Women's Hospital, more than heart disease, cancer, and diabetes combined.

2. In a survey by the *National Pain Report,* 70 percent of people with chronic pain reported their health care had worsened or they had lost support entirely—and 25 percent had lost access to a primary care physician. Seven percent said they had "reflected" on suicide. People with chronic pain are twice as likely to commit suicide as people who aren't in chronic pain.

3. When yearly deaths from prescription narcotics peaked at 17,500 a year, the biggest culprits were OxyContin and the *fentanyl* patch. But only 5,000 of those deaths were from the narcotics being used as prescribed.

4. There are more than 50,000 yearly deaths from NSAIDs (nonsteroidal anti-inflammatory drugs) such as ibuprofen. Research published in the journal *BMJ* shows an approximate 50 percent increase in the risk of heart attack among regular users of NSAIDs such as *ibuprofen* (Advil) and *naproxen* (Aleve). Another study shows there are more than 16,000 yearly deaths from bleeding ulcers. (I want to add that chronic pain is far more harmful than NSAIDs, but natural options for relief are usually more effective—and much safer—than this overly used pain reliever.)

5. Proton pump inhibitors (PPIs) for heartburn likely cause more than 30,000 deaths a year. Ironically—and tragically—they're often given to prevent an ulcer from NSAIDs! (They're also linked to a 44 percent higher risk of dementia, one of the leading causes of death.)

Translated, these numbers suggests that the current war on prescribed narcotics is causing far more deaths by collateral damage than it prevents—for example, increased use of NSAIDs is *more* deadly than the narcotics. Meanwhile, many people turn to illicit drugs for pain relief, which carry an even higher risk of overdose because they have no idea of what they're taking.

The answer is neither to ignore the threat of overdose nor the suffering of those in chronic pain. There is a third option that has been largely overlooked and that addresses both the pain and the risk of overdose—treat the *root causes* of pain.

For example, research I have conducted and published in numerous journals shows that treating these root causes can dramatically decrease pain and improve daily function—*without* narcotics. Using fibromyalgia as our model, our study showed that a decrease in pain of 50 percent compared to placebo. In fact, by the end of the study a large percentage of the participants experienced so much relief that they no longer qualified for a diagnosis of fibromyalgia!

Bottom line: Using the entire toolkit of treatment—natural remedies; structural therapies, such as physical therapy and chiropractic; and low-cost generic (and safe!) medications—most pain can be effectively controlled and even eliminated...without narcotics. Let's look at the real causes of pain—and its real cure.

Real Cure Regimen

A critical concept in pain management: Pain is not an outside invader. Rather, it is natural part of your body's "monitoring system," telling you that something needs attention—now. Think of it like the oil light on a car's dashboard. And the standard medical approach has been to put a Band-Aid over the oil light or cut it out. Doesn't it make more sense to put oil in the car?

Let's take a look at several types of pain and show how this works...

•**Muscle pain.** This is probably the most common type of pain. And the most underdiagnosed. Because the best test for muscle pain is a good physical exam—which almost no doctors do anymore because they don't know how! And here's another thing most doctors don't know: the essential cause of muscle pain is *decreased energy* in the muscles. *Let me explain...*

Muscles are like a spring—they take more energy to stretch than to contract. But if you get plenty of sleep, balance hormones, regulate the immune system and minimize inflammation, optimize nutrition, and exercise—in other words, if you address the real causes of pain—my research shows you can decrease muscle pain by at least 50 percent (and often completely). And once you've restored energy to muscle, then structural therapies can s-t-r-e-t-c-h the muscle, which offers long-lasting benefits.

•**Arthritis.** Research shows that natural therapies are more effective than NSAIDs for relieving pain. For example, in three comparison studies, the herbal formula Curamin, from Terry Naturally (a combination of a unique, highly absorbed curcumin, boswellia, DL-phenylalanine, and nattokinase), was more effective than Celebrex for both osteoarthritis and rheumatoid arthritis. In another study, from the National Institutes of Health, the natural combo of glucosamine and chondroitin was shown to be as effective as NSAIDs for osteoarthritis. (In fact, many of the study's "data points" showed the natural remedies were more effective.) But the data was manipulated, and the two natural remedies were reported to be *ineffective*...because all but one of the authors of the study were on the payrolls of drug companies!

For those with arthritis, I recommend a combination of Curamin (one to two capsules, three times daily), and Be Mobile (two capsules, twice a day). Give these remedies six weeks to feel their full effect, at which point you may be able to reduce the dose. You can combine these remedies with pain medications.

•**Migraines.** A review of 11 studies, published in the *Journal of Clinical Pharmacy and Therapeutics*, showed that riboflavin (vitamin B_2) is an effective treatment for migraines. In one study, a daily supplement of 300 mg to 400 mg of riboflavin decreased migraine frequency by 69 percent after six weeks. Add magnesium, vitamin B_{12}, and coenzyme Q10 to increase its effectiveness—a combo shown to work in a study published in the *Journal of Headache Pain*. You can find all of these remedies in Neuro Comfort, from Douglas Labs. Take two a day, and give it six weeks to see the full effect.

The herb butterbur (Petadolex) can help relieve the pain of an acute migraine, and can also decrease migraine frequency, according to a study of nearly 300 patients, published in the journal *Phytomedicine*. I favor the product from Nature's Way. To prevent migraines, take 50 milligrams, three times a day for one month and then twice a day. To stop an acute migraine, take 100 mg every three hours, for a maximum of 300 mg in any 24-hour period.

Also, repeated placebo-controlled studies have shown that intravenous magnesium—one gram over 15 minutes—eliminate 85 percent of acute migraines in less than an hour, making it the most effective treatment (short of decapitation). To *prevent* migraines, take 600 milligrams daily, the effective amount used in a study in *Magnesium Research*.

Other natural and conventional non-prescription therapies are also effective for migraine. For example, Excedrin Migraine (which contains *acetaminophen*, aspirin, and caffeine) has been shown to be as effective as prescription triptan medications.

For those who get their headaches predominantly around ovulation and menses, the real cause is hormonal fluctuations. I give bioidentical estrogen and progesterone during these periods to prevent migraines.

•**Central sensitization.** In this problem, the body amplifies the pain signal to make sure that it's not ignored. It does this through the central nervous system, particularly the spine and the microglial cells in the brain. The end result: You're *more* sensitive to pain, with a lower threshold for what causes pain. Although several expensive medications are used to address the problem, they're often ineffectual or inadequate—and they certainly don't reverse the underlying cause.

Several remedies can be very helpful. The most effective is low-dose *naltrexone*—three milligrams to 4.5 milligrams at bedtime. (The drug is typically used in very high doses to reverse the effects of narcotics.) It takes two months to see the effect. See the website LowDoseNaltrexone.org for more information, including compounding pharmacies that can make the medication, which can be prescribed by holistic doctors.

The natural remedy *palmitoylethanolamide* (PEA)—a type of fatty acid manufactured by the body—is also highly effective for migraine. It is available as Mirica, from Young Nutraceuticals, which includes other components that are also helpful. Take two capsules, twice daily, for four weeks, and then twice a day thereafter (or three times a day, if that works better).

An excellent prescription remedy for central sensitization: 3-minocycline or doxycycline (tetracycline family antibiotics), at a dosage of 100 milligrams, twice daily. (It also helps with rheumatoid arthritis.) The pain-relieving effect of this medication is one of the reasons it is so helpful for people with Lyme disease. As with the other remedies, it takes six weeks to show an effect. However, long-term antibiotic use can cause candida overgrowth. So if I prescribe this therapy, I also implement an anti-candida program—see Candida Overgrowth on page 181.

Finally, I'd like to discuss the four natural compounds that I've found are most effective for *any* kind of chronic pain, including a few I've already discussed in this chapter...

•**Curamin by Terry Naturally.** This mix of nutrients is a pain relief miracle for most kinds of pain. Begin with two capsules three times a day. The dose can be lowered after six to 12 weeks.

•**Topical comfrey (Traumaplant Comfrey Cream, from Terry Naturally).** Research shows it's more effective than medications for arthritis, after six weeks. Rub it over the affected joints three times a day.

•**Hemp oil (CBD).** Hemp oil contains CBD and nearly a dozen other cannabinoids that research shows are effective against pain. But I am picky about the brand I use, because many don't contain therapeutic amounts.

My favorite: Hemp Select Hemp Oil, from Terry Naturally. Products from licensed marijuana dispensaries are also usually reliable. The optimal dose for pain is three 50-milligram capsules of hemp oil containing 20 percent CBD. For many, lower doses are just as effective.

•**Kratom.** This herb, a traditional medicine derived from the leaves of an evergreen tree native to southeast Asia, has become controversial because the FDA and the DEA have demonized it, and the media has relentlessly criticized it. *For example:* If any of the herb is found in a person's blood at death, the death is attributed to Kratom—even if the person drank a gallon of tequila and took 60 OxyContin!

Used at a maximum dose of one-half to one teaspoon, three times daily, the herb is a safe treatment for chronic pain. In fact, in a number of patients it has *eliminated* severe, untreatable pain. (For example, I had one patient who was planning on moving to the U.S. from Japan—because her pain went from 10 to zero in one day after taking the herb while in the U.S., but she couldn't get it in Japan.) You can find the herb in vape shops, dispensaries, and online. Use the "Red Bali" or "Red Maeng Da" or "Red Sumatra" forms. You'll know if it is working in 45 minutes.

Remember: In reducing or eliminating chronic pain, it's best to use the *entire* natural tool kit: nutrients, herbs, and medications; structural therapies (chiropractic, osteopathy, myofascial release, physical therapy, etc.); and electromagnetic therapies, such as TENS and magnets. With these tools at your disposal, virtually *all* pain can be treated—usually without narcotics. In the few cases where narcotics are needed, when used in *combination* with these other treatments, they can be a pain-relieving godsend. The problem in relieving chronic pain is *not* lack of effective treatment—it's lack of proper physician education, and access to natural remedies.

Colds and Flu

Real Causes

- **Nutritional Deficiencies.** Many nutrients are critical for the optimal immune function that fights off cold and flu viruses (page 3).

- **Poor Sleep.** Sufficient sleep is a must for a strong immune system (page 33).

- **Hormonal Imbalances.** A weakened adrenal gland and an imbalance of adrenal hormones are risk factors for infections (page 84).

You can find a complete program for optimizing your immune system and preventing infections and other immune problems in Chronic Inflammation on page 118. (Chronic inflammation is a sign of a hyperactive immune system that needs balancing.) This chapter focuses on two of the most common infections: colds and flu, infections of the upper respiratory tract.

Real Cure Regimen

Collectively, Americans cough, sniffle, and sneeze our way through one billion colds a year, spending more than $7.7 billion for doctor's visits and $4 billion on OTC and prescription cough and cold treatments. Fortunately, few people die of a cold. But you can't say that about the flu. On average, the influenza virus hospitalizes nearly one million Americans a year and kills an average of 36,000 a year, many of whom are over age 65 (according to an estimate from the Centers for Disease Control and Prevention for the years 2010 to 2020). And flu shots are no guarantee of protection: the CDC estimates they work only half the time to stop the infection.

If you feel you're coming down with an upper respiratory infection, I recommend the following...

- **Take natural thymic hormone.** The thymus gland—located just below the neck, between the breastbone (sternum) and the lungs—helps power your immune system. Natural thymic hormone—a remedy available in the supplement ProBoost—is a very effective immune stimulant that I think should be in everyone's medicine cabinet. Taken at the first sign of a respiratory infection, it usually stops the infection within 12 to 36 hours. Dissolve the contents of one packet under your tongue three times a day, until the infection clears up.

- **For the flu or flulike symptoms, take Oscillococcinum.** This homeopathic remedy (available at most health food stores, in some pharmacies and supermarkets, and online) can help ease the symptoms of the flu (or the flulike symptoms of a cold), such as chills, fever, achiness, and just plain old feeling bad (malaise). The remedy also speeds healing. For it to work, you need to take it as soon as you have any symptoms, so keep this remedy in your medicine cabinet.

•**Take vitamin C: 1,000 milligrams to 8,000 milligrams daily.** Yes, vitamin C does help the common cold. Finnish researchers analyzed 29 studies on vitamin C and colds, involving more than 11,000 people. They found that taking the vitamin shortened the duration of colds up to 13 percent in adults and up to 22 percent in children. They also found that vitamin C reduced the incidence of colds by 50 percent in endurance and recreational athletes (marathon runners and skiers), and people who spend significant time outside in cold climates. I recommend taking enough vitamin C to cause (harmless) diarrhea (an indication the body has all it needs to fight the infection) and then cutting back to a comfortable level.

•**Suck on zinc lozenges: five to eight daily.** Researchers at Wayne State University in Detroit studied 50 people within 24 hours of their coming down with a cold. Half sucked on zinc lozenges (13.3 milligrams of zinc acetate per lozenge, one lozenge every two to three hours); half sucked on a placebo. The zinc group had shorter colds (an average of four days compared with 7.1 days), and their coughs cleared up more quickly (2.1 days compared with five days). They also had less severe colds, according to the results published in the *Journal of Infectious Diseases*. (In another study by the same team of researchers, published in the *American Journal of Clinical Nutrition*, people 55 and older who took zinc supplements had "significantly fewer infections" of any kind compared with people the same age who didn't take zinc.)

In another, recent study, researchers from Australia and Finland analyzed data from three studies on zinc lozenges and colds—and found that the lozenges decreased: nasal discharge by 34 percent; nasal congestion by 37 percent; sneezing by 22 percent; scratchy throat by 33 percent; sore throat by 18 percent; hoarseness by 38 percent; cough by 46 percent; and the duration of muscle ache by 54 percent. Not surprisingly, they conclude the lozenges are likely to be a "useful treatment" for the common cold.

I recommend lozenges with at least 10 milligrams to 20 milligrams of zinc, taking at least 80 milligrams per day. (These are especially helpful if you have a sore throat.)

•**Take echinacea: 1,000 milligrams a day.** Often recommended for preventing and treating colds, echinacea is the most popular herb in the US (40 percent of people who use natural products using echinacea). But a much-publicized study in the prestigious *New England Journal of Medicine* showed the remedy *didn't* work to stop, shorten, or ease a cold.

Researchers at the School of Pharmacy of the University of Connecticut analyzed results from 14 studies on echinacea and colds, involving nearly 3,000 people. They found that echinacea *did* work, reducing the risk of catching a cold by 58 percent and shortening the duration of a cold by an average of 1.4 days. "The take-home message from our study is that echinacea does indeed have powerful cold prevention and cold treatment benefits," we were told by Craig Coleman, PhD, a professor of pharmacy practice at the School of Pharmacy of the University of Connecticut, who led the study.

Why did the *New England Journal of Medicine* study show that echinacea didn't work? The study had two problems, said Dr. Coleman. It used the least common form of echinacea (*angustifolia*), not the one most people take (*purpurea*). And the dose was three times lower than generally recommended.

To Prevent Colds and Flu

The best defense is a good offense: Keep yourself from getting sick in the first place. *Here's how...*

•**Take vitamin D: 2,000 IU to 4,000 IU daily.** In a study led by James R. Sabetta, MD, an associate clinical professor of medicine at Yale University, researchers took monthly measurements of the blood levels of vitamin D in 195 healthy adults. The measurements started the third week in September and continued for the next four to five months. At the same time, the study participants were asked to report any acute respiratory tract infections.

Those who had blood levels of vitamin D lower than 38 nanograms per milliliter had twice as many upper respiratory tract infections. Among the 18 people in the study who consistently maintained blood levels of D above 38 nanograms per milliliter, 15 were completely free of upper respiratory tract infections—no cases of colds or flu. (Of those 18 folks, 13 were taking vitamin D supplements.) When the above-38 group did succumb to a cold or flu, their illnesses were shorter. Their percentage of days ill with acute respiratory tract infections was 4.9 times lower than in the below-38 group. Of the other 180 participants—all of them with blood vitamin D levels consistently below 38 nanograms per milliliter—81 developed colds and flu.

The study's statistical summary: The 38-plus group had a twofold decrease in the risk of developing a cold or flu. "Maintenance of a 25-hydroxyvitamin D serum concentration of 38 ng/ml or higher should significantly reduce the incidence of acute viral respiratory infections and the burden of illness caused thereby, at least during the fall and winter," concluded the researchers.

How do you know your vitamin D levels? I don't recommend spending money on a test. Instead, take a multivitamin/mineral with 1,000 IU to 2,000 IU of vitamin D3, and get a daily dose of vitamin D—making sunshine by taking a walk outside. (Avoid sunburn, not sunshine!)

•**If you're over 65, to prevent pneumonia, take zinc: 10 milligrams to 20 milligrams daily.** "Low zinc status" is linked to pneumonia in the elderly—more cases, longer bouts, more use of antibiotics, and more deaths, concluded researchers from the Nutritional Immunology Laboratory at Tufts University. Zinc supplementation is a "potential low-cost intervention to reduce" the risk, they concluded in the journal *Nutrition Reviews*. (Low zinc levels are also one reason why the pneumonia vaccine—and perhaps others—are sometimes ineffective.)

•**Take olive leaf extract: 1,000 milligrams, three times daily, for three to seven days.** Although not as effective as natural thymic hormone, olive leaf extract also can rev up the immune system and may help a number of infections. If it causes nausea, cut the dose in half.

•**For sore throat: Gargle with a mouthwash.** I recommend Cepacol or Chloraseptic. You can also gargle with salt water: ¼ teaspoon salt, ¼ teaspoon baking soda (*not* baking powder), and 1 cup lukewarm water.

•**Stop a cough—with dark chocolate.** Yes, believe it or not, dark chocolate is an effective (and tasty!) cough suppressant that works as well as codeine. Eat a square of chocolate from a chocolate bar, two or three times a day when you have a cold. Or drink hot chocolate, made from unsweetened cocoa powder.

●**Drink plenty of water and hot, caffeine-free tea (or hot water with lemon).** Hot liquids loosen mucus, making it easier to cough up. And that mucus you expel contains billions of viruses or bacteria your body no longer has to kill in hand-to-hand combat!

●**Sleep eight hours a night.** Sleep is a must for a strong immune system.

Constipation

Real Causes

●**Nutritional Deficiencies.** Not eating enough stool-bulking fiber or not drinking enough stool-softening water can cause constipation (page 3).

●**Inactivity.** Regular exercise helps with regularity (page 40).

●**Hormonal Imbalances.** Low levels of thyroid hormone slow down the entire system, including the digestive system (page 106).

●**Digestive Difficulties (and Intestinal Infections).** An intestinal over-growth of the candida fungus can lead to constipation (page 107, "Sugar Feeds the Yeast Beast").

Medically, it's considered "normal" to have a bowel movement once every three days—but it's *healthy* to have one every day. Think about it. Would you eat a piece of chewed-up food that had been sitting out on a 98°F sidewalk for three days? No way—it would be rotten and toxic. But if your transit time (the time it takes food to travel from one end of your digestive tract to the other) is three days, that's pretty much the state of the food inside your body (though your immune system and friendly intestinal bacterial help keep the situation somewhat under control).

A healthy transit time? Twelve to 30 hours. That gives your body plenty of time to remove the nutrients from the food and then discard the food residue before it becomes toxic.

Real-Cure Regimen

To test your transit time, eat a can or ear of corn and see how long it takes for the indigestible outer part of the corn kernels to come out the other end. Two days? Three days? You're constipated. If you're constipated, it's time to improve your transit time. *And the most natural ways to do so...*

●**Eat a bowl of high-fiber cereal.** Indigestible fiber provides the "bulk" that helps speed stool through the intestines. An excellent start to your day and your daily fiber intake is a high-fiber, whole-grain cereal such as raisin bran, which supplies eight grams of fiber per serving.

Want more bulk for your buck? Try Grape Nuts, with 11 grams of fiber. If constipation is chronic, try All-Bran, with 19.5 grams of fiber per serving. If none of those cereals appeals to you, choose one you'll enjoy eating regularly that has at least five grams of fiber per serving and a minimum of sugar. And don't skimp on the fruits, vegetables, beans, and whole grains during the rest of the day—they're rich in fiber, too.

•**Stay hydrated.** A cause of stools that are small and hard as rocks, and as difficult to pass: not drinking enough water. Drinking sodas and other sweetened beverages makes the problem worse, because sugar draws water out of the intestines. Tea, however, is a good way to hydrate, and also has a mild laxative effect. (Drink real brewed tea, not the sugar-loaded, soda-like teas that crowd the beverage sections of convenience stores and supermarkets.)

How much water is enough water? You don't have to count glasses. Just keep water on hand, and check in with your mouth and lips every so often. If they're dry, you're dehydrated and it's time to drink up. (You can read more about staying hydrated in Cellular Toxicity on page 111.)

•**Move your feet to move your bowels.** Regular exercise helps keep you regular. So take a walk, play with your kids, or find a physical activity you enjoy with friends.

•**Use natural laxatives.** For symptomatic relief, there are several natural laxatives that are good for you in many other ways...

•Magnesium: 200 milligrams to 400 milligrams daily. This mineral draws water into your bowels, helping to loosen stools. You can take up to 800 mg daily for a few days, every now and then. But if you use that high a dose of magnesium long term, your bowel will become dependent on it, and stop working on its own. (This is called laxative dependency, and it's a common problem with over-the-counter laxatives, which I don't recommend.)

•Vitamin C. In doses over 500 mg, it has a laxative effect. If you take more than 2,000 milligrams a day, use a powdered and buffered form to reduce acidity and increase absorption.

•Pantethine: 500 milligrams, one to three times daily. A chemical cousin to pantothenic acid (vitamin B_5), pantethine directly stimulates bowel function (and also lowers elevated cholesterol).

•**Check for irritable bowel syndrome (spastic colon).** Constipation can be a symptom of irritable bowel syndrome (spastic colon), which is often caused by an unrecognized bowel infection (usually yeast, but sometimes bacterial). For more information on intestinal yeast infections, see Digestive Difficulties on page 98, and Candida Overgrowth on page 181. For more information on irritable bowel syndrome, see Irritable Bowel Syndrome (Spastic Colon) on page 277.

•**Look into your thyroid.** If you have constipation *and* fatigue *and* weight gain *and* cold intolerance, it's likely you have hypothyroidism (low levels of thyroid hormone) and deserve a trial of natural thyroid hormone (prescription Armour Thyroid). This is the case even if your thyroid tests have been "normal." As I discuss throughout this book, those "normal" tests are not an accurate indicator of whether or not you're hypothyroid. (For more on hypothyroidism, see Hormonal Imbalances on page 84 and Hypothyroidism on page 254.)

Depression

Real Causes

- **Nutritional Deficiencies.** Many nutrients play key roles in brain function and in helping depression—particularly the omega-3 fatty acids found abundantly in fatty fish (such as salmon and tuna) and fish oil supplements (page 28).
- **Hormonal Imbalances.** Low levels of thyroid hormones, estrogen, and testosterone can cause or complicate depression (page 84).
- **Happiness Deficiency.** Anger turned inward can trigger depression (page 55).
- **Inactivity.** Studies link regular physical activity to lower levels of depression and show that activity can treat depression as effectively as medications can (page 40).

Every year, doctors in America write prescriptions for antidepressant drugs for an astounding one out of every seven American adults—a rate that has doubled in the last decade. But depression is not a Prozac deficiency. (And, as you can read in "Antidepressants: The Sad Fact about Effectiveness" on page 80, antidepressants aren't particularly effective for mild to moderate depression.) I prefer to address the problem differently, by using natural remedies to support the biochemistry of happiness. Treated this way, most depression can be cured—without the weight gain, fatigue, loss of libido, or increased risk of suicide seen with prescription antidepressants.

Real Cure Regimen

Give this regimen at least six weeks to work. I think you'll be happy with the results.

- **Allow yourself to be angry.** From a psychological perspective, depression is often anger turned inward against oneself. That's why allowing yourself to be angry—even to go into a rage—can be healthy when you're depressed. You can tell when anger is healthy…it feels good!

Remember, however, that you are choosing to be angry, and what you are angry about is nobody else's fault (so don't beat up others with your anger, and don't hurt anyone). When you don't allow guilt over anger to get in the way, notice how your depression decreases and you feel better after a good fit of anger. (For much more on achieving health and happiness by fully feeling your feelings—including anger—see Happiness Deficiency on page 55.)

- **Eat more fatty fish or take fish oil.** An international team of researchers analyzed the results of 31 studies on fish consumption and depression involving more than 250,000 peo-

Antidepressants Don't Work

Major research looking at the effectiveness of the class of antidepressant drugs known as SSRIs (selective serotonin reuptake inhibitors) found that they were no more effective than placebos—the fake, look-alike pills used in scientific studies to test the effectiveness of real drugs.

Medical experts have known for years that SSRIs such as *fluoxetine* (Prozac) were only about 10 percent more effective than placebos in published studies. This study, however, was a meta-analysis by researchers at the University of Connecticut and other institutions that reviewed and analyzed the major research to date on four SSRIs, including the studies with negative results that drug companies usually bury. The antidepressants reviewed were *fluoxetine* (Prozac), *venlafaxine* (Effexor), *nefazodone* (Serzone), and *paroxetine* (Paxil). The researchers' conclusion: The "benefit" of antidepressants "falls below accepted criteria for clinical significance."

In other words, the drugs had no effect on mild depression. None at all.

The researchers noted that the studies showed antidepressants had a "relatively small" effect for the relief of severe depression (as compared with no effect whatsoever for mild to moderate depression, the diagnosis of the majority of people with depression). But, they point out, that was a statistical anomaly produced by the fact that people with severe depression don't respond to placebos—it wasn't a sign of the antidepressant effect of the drugs.

What to do? If you're taking an antidepressant and you feel it's helpful and doesn't cause uncomfortable side effects, you should stay on it. If, however, your antidepressant medication isn't effective—which is common—consider the Real Cure Regimen for depression in this chapter.

ple, publishing the results in the *Journal of Affective Disorders*. They found that those who ate the most fish had a 22 percent lower risk of depression compared to those who ate the least. In a similar study, Chinese researchers analyzed the results of 10 studies on fish oil supplements and depression, and found that the supplements had a "significant anti-depressive effect," reducing depressive symptoms by 69 percent. Other studies show that fish oil can both prevent and relieve: postpartum (after childbirth) depression; bipolar disorder (manic-depression); depression in diabetes (people with diabetes have a 40 percent higher risk of developing depression); and depression in Parkinson's disease (a common problem for people with this disorder).

It's not really a surprise that fish oil can defeat depression when you consider that much of your brain is made of DHA (docosahexaenoic acid), one of the essential fatty acids found in fish oil. If you have depression, try eating three or more servings a week of a fatty fish (salmon, albacore tuna, sardines, anchovies, herring, mackerel, lake trout). Or take a fish oil supplement. (You can read more about fish oil supplements, including the brands I favor, in Nutritional Deficiencies on page 28.)

•**Get the right amounts of nutrients.** More than a dozen nutritional deficiencies can contribute to depression. That's why overall nutritional support is essential for achieving the biochemistry of happiness. You can see the amounts needed in Nutritional Deficiencies on page 3, and I recommend the Energy Revitalization System multinutrient powder (page 30) as an easy way to get all of them.

Also important: Minimize sugary, processed foods, which are linked to depression. In a study in the *Journal of Affective Disorders*, people who drank the most sugar-sweetened beverages were 31 percent more likely to be depressed, compared to people who drank the least.

•**Take curcumin.** Two studies show that a special, highly-absorbed form of curcumin—the active ingredient in the spice turmeric—is more effective for depression than the antidepressant *sertraline* (Zoloft) after six weeks. The formulation studied was CuraMed, and the effective dose is 750 mg, two times daily. And in the newest analysis of seven studies on curcumin and depression, Italian researchers found that curcumin had a "large effect" on symptoms of depression (and anxiety).

•**5HTP (5-hydroxtryptophan).** This compound raises levels of serotonin, the "feel-good" neurotransmitter that controls mood. Take 300 milligrams to 400 milligrams at bedtime, and give it six weeks to work. However, don't combine it with other antidepressants that raise serotonin without checking with your holistic physician. If serotonin is too elevated (a rare problem called "Serotonin Syndrome," which can cause agitation, rapid heartbeat and other symptoms), I lower the 5HTP dose to 200 mg daily.

•**Optimize thyroid function.** Two studies show that treating depression with prescription Armour Thyroid (natural thyroid hormone) is very effective, even when blood tests for thyroid hormone were normal. In fact, taking thyroid hormone helped even when an antidepressant failed. Importantly, only Armour Thyroid (which contains both the T3 and T4 thyroid hormones) worked. Synthroid (a synthetic thyroid hormone that contains only the T4 hormone) did not. (For more information on hypothyroidism and thyroid tests, see Hormonal Imbalances on page 87 and Hypothyroidism on page 254.)

•**Treat other hormone imbalances, too.** Low levels of testosterone (in men) and estrogen (in women) can also contribute to depression. (For more on testing for and treating testosterone and estrogen imbalances, see Hormonal Imbalances on page 92, as well as Male Menopause [Testosterone Deficiency] on page 287 and Menopausal Problems on page 290.)

•**Go for a 45-minute daily walk.** Dozens of scientific studies—in *Mayo Clinic Proceedings*, *Psychiatry Research*, the *American Journal of Psychiatry*, and many other medical journals—show that walking briskly every day is an effective antidepressant.

•**Catch some rays.** Inadequate sunlight is a common cause of depression, particularly the variety called seasonal affective disorder (SAD), depression that worsens in the winter.

Diabetes

Real Causes

- **Nutritional Deficiencies.** A high-sugar, high-fat, low-fiber diet is a risk factor for type 2 (adult) diabetes. Low levels of vitamin D—caused mainly by a lack of sunlight—may be a risk factor in type 1 (juvenile) diabetes, an autoimmune disease (page 15).

- **Hormonal Imbalances.** Low levels of thyroid hormone and low levels of testosterone in men play a role in the development of type 2 diabetes (pages 87 and 92).

- **Inactivity.** A lack of exercise, along with obesity, is a key cause of type 2 diabetes (page 40).

Diabetes is a disease of chronically high blood sugar levels, and there are two main types.

Type 1 diabetes (also called juvenile-onset) is an autoimmune disease. The immune system mistakenly identifies the insulin-generating cells of the pancreas as "foreign" and attacks them. There are more than 15,000 new cases of type 1 diabetes diagnosed in the United States every year.

Type 2 diabetes, on the other hand, is a disease of *habits*, linked to a high-sugar, high-fat diet, overweight, and a sedentary lifestyle. And it's an epidemic, too. More than 30 million Americans have type 2 diabetes: fasting blood sugar levels (measured first thing in the morning, before eating) that are 125 milligrams per deciliter (mg/dl) or higher. Another 88 million have the precursor to type 2 diabetes: prediabetes, with fasting blood sugar levels of 100 to 125 mg/dL.

Why is type 2 diabetes such a huge problem here and around the world? Our bodies make blood sugar (glucose) as a fuel for our cells. For most of human history, we ate a high-fiber diet, which resulted in dietary carbohydrates and sugars (such as sucrose and fructose) being released very slowly and steadily into the bloodstream, over many hours.

Now we eat nearly 140 pounds of sugars a year, or about one out of every five calories. This massive amount of dietary sugar causes huge spikes in blood sugar. This forces our bodies to regulate sugar by churning out larger-than-normal amounts of the hormone insulin, which ushers glucose out of the bloodstream and into cells. Problem is, our cells weren't built to handle all that insulin, and over time they develop "insulin resistance." Glucose tends to stay in the bloodstream—and eventually you develop type 2 diabetes, or chronically high blood sugar. At that point, most physicians will usually offer the person with high blood sugar whatever the newest, most profitable (and, sadly, often toxic) medication the drug companies are marketing.

In summary, there are *several* factors creating a perfect storm for type 2 diabetes. *They include...*

- **Excess sugar and white flour in the diet, combined with low fiber.**

- **The obesity epidemic, which drives insulin resistance.** (Fat clogs insulin receptors.)

- **Sedentary lifestyle.**

•**Toxic chemicals in the environment, which block testosterone in men and increase testosterone in women.** Inadequate testosterone levels in men (anything under 500 ng/dl) have been shown to cause metabolic syndrome, a combination of high blood pressure, high cholesterol and either insulin resistance or type 2 diabetes.

In women, the opposite occurs: An *elevated* testosterone level is linked to an increased risk of type 2 diabetes.

•**Magnesium deficiency is also linked to a significantly increased risk of type 2 diabetes.** Food processing strips whole foods of 50 percent of its magnesium.

To screen for prediabetes, I often check a patient's fasting insulin level—and ignore the so-called "normal" range. (I talk about why "normal" ranges in tests are often misleading in Hormonal Imbalances on page 84.) If the fasting insulin is over 10 uIU/ml, I work with my patient to prevent type 2 diabetes. I will do the same if glycosylated hemoglobin (HgBA1C)—a measure of long-term blood sugar levels—is over 5.7 percent, which is the definition of prediabetes.

If you have diabetes, all that extra blood sugar and insulin can damage your circulation, doubling your risk of heart attack and stroke, and setting you up for long-term circulatory problems. *These complications of diabetes include...*

•**Retinopathy** (damage to the eyes, causing vision loss and blindness)

•**Nephropathy** (damage to the kidneys, causing chronic kidney disease and kidney failure)

•**Neuropathy** (damage to the nerves, causing pain)

•**Ulcers** (hard-to-heal skin ulcers that can lead to amputation of toes, feet, and legs)

The good news: It's not difficult to prevent or control diabetes and its complications. And even *reverse* type 2 diabetes.

Real Cure Regimen

Type 2 diabetes and overweight are so closely related that some experts call the problem "diabesity."

One theory about the connection: The extra fat clogs the insulin receptors on cells. The hormone can't work, and blood sugar levels stay high.

Losing weight (decreasing the fat) and exercising regularly (which tones insulin receptors, too) is one of the best ways to prevent and control the disease.

Eat a Little Less Fat, Walk a Few More Miles

There's good evidence that these two simple lifestyle changes work: the Diabetes Prevention Program study, involving more than 3,200 overweight people with prediabetes, and conducted by researchers at Harvard Medical School and many other institutions.

The researchers divided the study participants into three groups: One group took the glucose-lowering drug *metformin* (Glucophage, Glucophage XR, Fortamet, Riomet); one group took a placebo; and one group followed a Lifestyle Balance Program, eating a diet slightly lower in fat and exercising regularly. After three years, those who followed the lifestyle program had a 58 percent lower rate of developing type 2 diabetes than the placebo group. Those who took metformin had a 31 percent lower rate.

The researchers invited the participants to continue in the lifestyle program or keep taking metformin, and many did. Seven years later, those in the lifestyle group had a 34 percent lower rate of developing type 2 diabetes, compared with the placebo group. Among people 60 and older, the rate was nearly 50 percent lower. Those in the metformin group had an 18 percent lower rate. The lifestyle group gained those benefits by sustaining an average weight loss of five pounds, along with exercising regularly.

"Moderate weight loss through a lower-calorie, low-fat lifestyle and regular exercise—usually walking—seems to be effective in lowering the risk for type 2 diabetes in people at a very high risk of developing the disease," we were told by Jill Crandall, MD, a study author, and director of the Diabetes Clinical Trials Unit at the Albert Einstein College of Medicine in New York City.

The lifestyle elements in the program included…

- **Walking 150 minutes a week** (taking a 30-minute walk at least five days a week)
- **Eating high-fat foods (such as French fries) less often**
- **Eating smaller amounts of high-fat foods**
- **Choosing lower-fat foods over high-fat foods** (such as pretzels over potato chips)
- **Avoiding hidden fat** (such as the five teaspoons of fat in a fried fish sandwich)
- **Trimming fatty meats**

(For more information on exercising regularly, see Inactivity on page 40.)

Avoid Sweets, but Get More Fiber

It's no surprise that a high-sugar diet is a cause of type 2 diabetes, which is also known as "the sugar disease." For example, one study linked drinking two non-diet sodas a day to a 24 percent increased risk of type 2 diabetes.

For a healthy sugar substitute, use stevia, a sweet-tasting herb. (My favored brands are Now Better Stevia and Stevia Select.) You can also use saccharin (Sweet'N Low), which has a long record of safety. I don't recommend aspartame, because some people experience severe reactions to it, including seizures, headaches, nausea, dizziness, depression, and more. (It's surprising to me that it ever received FDA approval for use.) I think the jury is still out on the safety of sucralose (Splenda), although it does cause digestive upset in many people.

One nutrient not to avoid is fiber. By slowing digestion, fiber helps keep blood sugar levels balanced. Easy fiber-increasing strategies include eating a whole grain breakfast cereal and having a slice or two of whole grain toast at breakfast (and don't forget brown rice, millet, quinoa, and other whole grains), including more beans in your diet, and eating more fruits and vegetables.

Nutrients for Preventing and Treating Diabetes

Many nutrients are important in normalizing blood sugar levels and preventing diabetic complications in both type 1 and type 2 diabetes. You can take the individual doses or use the multinutrient powder I created (see Nutritional Deficiencies on page 30). All the optimum doses are in there.

●**Magnesium: 200 milligrams daily.** Magnesium is a key factor in helping prevent metabolic syndrome, a prediabetic condition that is a constellation of several health problems that can include insulin resistance, high blood pressure, extra belly fat, high total cholesterol, and low "good" HDL cholesterol.

Researchers at Tufts University studied more than 500 people over age 60 and found that those with the lowest daily intake of magnesium had a 64 percent higher risk of developing metabolic syndrome. They also linked low magnesium levels to two specific features of metabolic syndrome: a 53 percent higher risk of overweight and a 59 percent higher risk of blood sugar problems. "Older adults should be encouraged to eat foods rich in magnesium, such as green vegetables, legumes and whole-grains," concluded the researchers, in the *European Journal of Nutrition*. That's good advice for everyone, old, young, and in between, but most Americans would do well to take a daily magnesium supplement of at least 200 milligrams.

Magnesium can also prevent type 2 diabetes. In one study, low magnesium levels were 10 times more common in those newly diagnosed with diabetes than in those without the disease. And if you develop diabetes, magnesium can help prevent cardiovascular disease (heart attack and stroke).

●**Chromium: 200 micrograms daily.** In a study in *Diabetes Technology & Therapeutics,* scientists reviewed 15 studies on chromium, involving nearly 1,700 people with different types of diabetes: type 1 (an autoimmune disease); type 2 (the lifestyle disease); gestational (brought on by pregnancy); and steroid-induced (diabetes as a drug side effect). The studies used dosages between 200 micrograms and 1,200 micrograms. In every study, chromium helped stabilize blood levels of glucose and improved the body's use of insulin.

●**Vitamin D: 2,000 IU to 4,000 IU daily.** In one study, researchers found that people with the highest intake of vitamin D were 40 percent less likely to develop type 2 diabetes. "Maintaining optimal vitamin D status may be a strategy to prevent development of type 2 diabetes," they concluded in the *American Journal of Clinical Nutrition*. Vitamin D may also help prevent type 1 diabetes. English researchers found that Finnish children who were given vitamin D–rich cod liver oil during their first year of life were 78 percent less likely to develop type 1 diabetes.

●**Vitamin C: 500 milligrams to 1,000 milligrams daily.** European researchers analyzed 12 years of health and dietary data from more than 20,000 people and found that those with the highest blood levels of vitamin C were 62 percent less likely to develop type 2 diabetes, compared with those with the lowest level. The study was in *JAMA: Internal Medicine*.

●**Vitamin K: 150 micrograms to 500 micrograms daily.** In a three-year study of 355 people ages 60 to 80, researchers at Tufts University found that supplementing with 500 micrograms of vitamin K slowed the progress of insulin resistance.

Hintonia latiflora to the Rescue

There is an amazing herb that can help lower blood sugar: *Hintonia latiflora*. This miracle botanical is an extract from the bark of a shrubby tree that grows in the Sonoran desert (in California, Arizona, and Mexico). For more than 60 years, it's been studied for its ability to reverse high blood sugar—but it only recently became available in the U.S., in a product called Sucontral D, from Terry Naturally. (I'm so enthusiastic about the herb that I also wrote an entire book about it: *Diabetes Is Optional: Hintonia, the Natural Way to Control Type 2 Diabetes*.) How does Hintonia work?

First, it's a rich source of coutareagenin, a special family of flavonoids. This nutrient is found in bark extracts unique to Hintonia—and appears to be responsible for its blood-sugar controlling benefits.

Mexican researchers also found that the plant inhibits the enzyme alpha-glucosidase, which slows the breakdown of carbohydrates, mimicking the effect of a high-fiber diet.

There have been more than a dozen studies on the herb, showing it…

- **Controls and lowers blood sugar**

- **Overcomes insulin resistance**

- **Reduces the need for glucose-controlling drugs**

- **Enhances the effectiveness of diabetes medications**

For example, in a study from German researchers, Hintonia lowered A1c (a measure of long-term blood sugar levels) by 11 percent, lowered fasting glucose levels (blood sugar before a meal) by 23 percent, and lowered postprandial blood sugar (blood sugar after a meal—with higher levels linked to worsening type 2 diabetes and the risk of cardiovascular disease) by 24 percent. In fact, many people in the study went from having type 2 diabetes to no longer having type 2 diabetes—with 39 percent of study participants reducing their medication or stopping it entirely.

If You Have Type 1 Diabetes—Stay Hydrated!

When type 1 diabetes goes out of control, blood sugar levels spiral upward, and the person with diabetes can end up in the intensive care unit with diabetic ketoacidosis—a life-threatening condition in which a total lack of insulin causes the body to start burning fatty acids for fuel, producing toxic "ketone bodies."

One of the most life-threatening complications of diabetic ketoacidosis is massive dehydration. The extra blood sugar that is dumped into the urine pulls water with it like a sponge, causing the dehydration. This is a key part of developing diabetic ketoacidosis. If you have type 1 diabetes and your blood sugar goes too high (frequent urination is a sign that this is happening), see your doctor.

In the meantime, stay well hydrated by drinking a lot of water, and avoid sugar and soda. Those extra glasses of water could save your life—and a hefty hospital bill!

But there's more good news: Hintonia not only lowered blood sugar, it also reduced many of the symptoms of type 2 diabetes, such as fatigue, irritability, lack of mental clarity, thirst, and frequent urination.

The study participants also saw improvements in blood pressure, blood fats, and liver health. Take one capsule, twice daily, at breakfast and dinner. Give it six months to see the full effect.

Another effective herb is berberine, which not only helps lower blood sugar, but also improves other components of metabolic syndrome, including high cholesterol and hypertension. The dose is 500 mg three times a day. If that dose bothers your stomach, decrease to 200 milligrams, three times a day. I combine berberine with Sucontral D for optimal effects.

Use Metformin (Glucophage XR) First

For type 2 diabetes, I prefer this older antidiabetes drug to the newer, more expensive glucose-controlling drugs such as *pioglitazone* (Actos) that have been linked to increased risk of heart disease. In fact, studies show that metformin reduces the risk of cardiovascular disease by 26 percent. (If you take metformin, take a multivitamin containing vitamin B_{12} as well. Studies show that the drug can cause a drop in blood levels of the nutrient.)

Preventing Diabetic Neuropathy

Several nutrients can help prevent diabetic neuropathy (also called peripheral neuropathy, because it usually occurs in the "periphery" of the body: the hands, arms, feet, and/or legs, but not the brain or spine).

•**B vitamins.** The vitamins B_{12}, B_6, and inositol can help prevent diabetic neuropathy. Give these nutrients three to six months to work, since they are helping the nerves heal, as opposed to simply masking the pain.

To help the process occur more quickly, it's very reasonable to add B_{12} shots. In my practice, I give 3,000 micrograms per dose of methylcobalamin, for 15 doses, at whatever rate is best to optimize blood levels (daily to weekly). I continue giving the shots once a month if it's necessary to maintain pain relief or energy levels. In one study, B_{12} shots were four times more effective in relieving diabetic neuropathy than *nortriptyline* (Aventyl), a drug often used for the problem.

•**Alpha-lipoic acid: 300 milligrams, twice daily.** In a Russian study of 28 people with diabetic neuropathy, taking alpha-lipoic acid reduced pain and other symptoms. This is a treatment that requires patience: It can take weeks or even months to work. But the relief is worth the wait.

•**Acetyl-L-carnitine (ALC): 2,000 milligrams daily.** In two studies involving 1,679 people, those who took ALC daily had less pain, improved "conduction" in damaged nerves, and even nerve regeneration. "Data on treatment of diabetic peripheral neuropathy with ALC supports its use," concluded researchers. "It should be recommended to patients early in the disease process to provide maximal benefit." As with lipoic acid, give these supplements at least six weeks to start working. For more on relieving nerve pain, see Nerve Pain (Neuropathy) on page 294.

Dry Mouth and Dry Eyes

Real Causes

- **Nutritional Deficiencies.** Low levels of several nutrients—including magnesium, vitamin B_6, and the omega-3 fatty acids in fish oil—can cause dry mouth and eyes. Dehydration can also contribute to the problem (page 3).
- **Prescription Medications.** More than 400 medications can cause dry mouth and/or dry eyes (page 70).

Dry mouth (xerostomia) affects about 50 percent of people 65 and older, as saliva production sometimes decreases with advancing years. But it's more than an annoyance of aging. Dry mouth can cause or aggravate dental and digestive problems because saliva is critical for washing away gum-damaging, cavity-causing bacteria, and it also provides an enzyme (amylase) that starts the digestion of carbohydrates.

Dry eyes affects about three out of every 10 Americans and is the most common reason people visit ophthalmologists (eye doctors). A disorder of the tear film (the coating that protects and cleans the surfaces of the eyes), it can produce symptoms such as stinging, burning, grittiness, itching, and sensitivity to light.

Common causes of dry eyes include allergies; the skin disorder rosacea; an autoimmune disease (when the immune system mistakes a part of the body as foreign and attacks it), such as Sjogren's syndrome (moisture-producing glands are attacked); perimenopause and postmenopause; and laser or cosmetic eye surgery.

When dry eyes and dry mouth occur together, the condition is called sicca syndrome, and it's often a feature of an autoimmune disease (such as Sjogren's syndrome or lupus) or chronic fatigue syndrome and fibromyalgia.

Real Cure Regimen

There are many ways to ease dry mouth, dry eyes, or both.

- **Check your medications.** More than 400 medications can cause dry mouth and/or dry eyes. If you have one or both of these problems, talk to your doctor about this side effect. A lower dose of the drying drug may be just as effective, without producing the side effect. Or there may be an alternative medication. *The most common pharmaceutical culprits include...*

  - Antihistamines. These include *diphenhydramine* (Benadryl), *loratadine* (Claritin), and *cetirizine* (Zyrtec). Antihistamines also are often found in over-the-counter sleep aids.

The Moisturizing Herb from Scandinavia

Sea buckthorn is a shrub that grows widely in the coastal areas of western Europe, with a particular density in Finland. In several studies, an extract of the sea buckthorn berry has helped relieve mucous membrane dryness—even in Sjogren's syndrome, an autoimmune disease where dryness is extreme. In a study in *The Journal of Nutrition*, Finnish researchers gave 86 people with dry eye syndrome the extract for three months and found that the herb improved the quality of the tear film that wets the eyes, decreasing burning.

The sea buckthorn product I recommend is Omega-7, from Terry Naturally—because many other sea buckthorn oil products do not use the right parts of the plant and are therefore ineffective. The recommended dose is two 500-milligram soft gels, twice daily. It takes two months to see the full effect.

●Antidepressants. *Amitriptyline* (Elavil) is a major trigger of dry mouth and dry eyes, but most antidepressants can cause the problem. So can antianxiety medications such as *alprazolam* (Xanax).

●Birth control pills. Dry eyes are a common side effect. Pregnancy can cause dry eyes too.

●Diuretics. These drugs are mostly used to treat high blood pressure.

●ACE inhibitors (angiotensin-converting enzyme inhibitors). Also mostly used to treat high blood pressure.

●Urinary bladder control medicines. These include *oxybutynin* (Ditropan) and *tolterodine* (Detrol).

●Opiates. This class of drugs includes codeine and morphine, and the much-prescribed synthetic derivatives of codeine, including *hydrocodone* (Vicodin) and *oxycodone* (Oxycontin).

●**Treat nutritional deficiencies.** Low levels of omega-3 fatty acids (found in fish oil) can contribute to both dry mouth and dry eyes. (You can find a complete discussion of omega-3s—including the best dosages and brands—in Nutritional Deficiencies on page 28.)

B vitamins and magnesium can also help with these problems. (You can find the right dosages in the Energy Revitalization System multinutrient powder, which I discuss in Nutritional Deficiencies on page 30.)

●**Relieve dry mouth symptoms.** Always keep a glass or bottle of water with you and drink throughout the day. You can also drink lemon juice, which stimulates the flow of saliva.

Here's a sugar-free recipe: 3½ cups of water; ¼ to ½ cup of fresh lemon juice; and 50 drops of stevia, to taste. And talk to your dentist about saliva substitutes. Over-the-counter spray forms (such as Salivart and Biotene) are effective and best used every 90 to 120 minutes.

●**Give your eyes a break.** Staring at a computer for hours at a time dries your eyes, Robert Latkany, MD, founder and director of the Dry Eye Clinic at the New York Eye & Ear Infirmary and author of *The Dry Eye Remedy*, told us. Worse, staring at a computer that's at eye level or higher keeps your eyes completely open, exposing more of the eye's surface to be dried. The best position for your screen is below eye level (even slightly), which exposes less of the eye's surface. Lower the monitor or raise the chair. If computer work is constant, he also recommends 10-second breaks twice an hour, closing your eyes to allow them to relubricate.

Another excellent option: Cyclosporine (Restasis), FDA-approved eyedrops that actually make your eyes produce more tears. But there are important tips to use it effectively, Dr. Latkany told us. It takes six to eight weeks to start working and doesn't reach peak effectiveness for four to six months—so don't stop using it because you think it isn't working. Also, refrigerate the drops to cut down on the stinging that sometimes occurs when it is applied.

Erectile Dysfunction

Real Causes

- **Happiness Deficiency.** If there is no enthusiasm or excitement for sex, sex is unlikely to happen (page 55).
- **Prescription Medications.** Erectile dysfunction is a side effect of many medications, particularly those for high blood pressure and antidepressants (page 70).
- **Hormonal Imbalances.** Low testosterone in men is a common cause (page 92).

If you watch football, baseball, or most any program that appeals to a predominantly male audience, you know something about erectile dysfunction (ED)—or at least about the drugs used to treat the condition, such as *sildenafil* (Viagra), *vardenafil* (Levitra), and *tadalafil* (Cialis).

ED is the inability of a man to maintain a firm erection long enough to have sex. Although the problem is more common in older men (half of all men 50 and older complain of ED), it can occur at any age (and is increasingly common in men under 40, affecting up to 26 percent of younger men). An occasional inability to maintain an erection is normal, but if the problem persists, it can cause stress, low self-esteem, and relationship problems.

Real Cure Regimen

What causes ED? The condition can have emotional triggers. Fear of not being able to have an erection is self-fulfilling: You can't have one because you're anxious about not having one. Issues with your partner can also affect performance. If you have erections during sleep or when you wake up, the problem is likely emotional and not physical. You and your partner may want to see a counselor to help you with any issues. You can also look at the Happiness Deficiency chapter (page 55) to see if the natural treatments mentioned could bring back some spark.

But there are also many *physical* triggers of ED. Research links ED to both heart disease and diabetes. If you have ED, ask your doctor to give you a thorough workup for these two conditions.

Decreased production of the hormone testosterone can also cause the problem. And you can have ED caused by low testosterone even if your testosterone blood test is so-called "normal." This is especially true if you have metabolic syndrome, a constellation of conditions including high blood pressure and high total cholesterol that is often caused by low testosterone. For more information on accurately and effectively testing and treating low testosterone levels, see Hormonal Imbalances on page 92 and Male Menopause (Testosterone Deficiency) on page 287. Several common medications (antihypertensives and antidepressants) can cause sexual dysfunction, including ED. If you've started one of those medications and developed ED, talk to your doctor about an alternative.

Both natural and medical approaches work well for ED.

•**Take erection-enhancing supplements.** There are many nutritional and herbal supplements that can help increase blood flow to the penis and improve erections. *They include the following…*

   •Arginine, an amino acid: 1,000 milligrams daily

   •Maca root extract, an herb traditionally used for strength and potency: 400 milligrams to 800 milligrams daily

   •*Rhodiola rosea* extract, an energizing herb: 150 milligrams to 300 milligrams daily

   •Epimedium extract, an herb traditionally used for ED: 100 milligrams to 200 milligrams daily

   •Longjack extract, another herb traditionally used for ED: 50 milligrams to 100 milligrams daily

ED Rx

Medications are a very reasonable and effective option in dealing with ED. I think Cialis is particularly good. It starts working more quickly than Viagra and lasts longer—for the same price. It comes in 2.5-milligram and 20-milligram strengths, with prices ranging from $12 to $70 per tablet. To save money, ask your doctor for the 20-milligram tablet and take one-quarter to one-half of a tablet or get the five-milligram pill, and just take it on days that you need it. Dissolve the pill under your tongue for faster action. Don't use ED medications in conjunction with nitrate-containing drugs such as nitroglycerin. The combination can cause very low blood pressure. ED medications may cause problems in patients with heart disease and should be used with caution.

Speaking of medications, several common medications—including statins, blood pressure meds, and antidepressants—can contribute to ED. Turn to Prescription Medications on page 70 to see alternatives, or at least work with your doctor to lower your dose.

- *Panax ginseng*, a strengthening and energizing herb: 100 milligrams to 200 milligrams daily (I'm a big fan of HRG80 Red Ginseng, a wonderful, unique, and new ginseng product from Terry Naturally that contains a high concentration of ginsenosides, the active ingredient).
- Ginkgo biloba extract: 50 milligrams to 240 milligrams daily
- *Diindolylmethane* (DIM): 100 milligrams to 200 milligrams daily
- *Mucuna pruriens* extract (15 percent L-dopa): 50 milligrams to 200 milligrams daily
- *Tribulus terrestris* extract: 100 milligrams to 200 milligrams daily

You can take these nutrients and herbs individually or take a supplement that includes many of them such as Hot Plants–For Him, from Nature's Way.

- **Check testosterone levels, and treat low testosterone with a bioidentical hormone.** By taking a safe level of bioidentical testosterone, you may cause your blood pressure and cholesterol (and high blood sugar) to go down while your erections go up! You can read more about bioidentical testosterone in Hormonal Imbalances on page 92.

- **If you have diabetes, optimize nerve function.** Poor nerve supply from diabetes can cause ED. Optimize nerve function with nutrients such as vitamins B_6 and B_{12}, inositol, and magnesium. Give this treatment two to six months to work.

If you have other symptoms of diabetic neuropathy, such as pain, tingling, burning, and numbness in your feet and/or hands, add alpha-lipoic acid (300 milligrams, twice a day) and acetyl-L-carnitine (500 milligrams, two or three times a day) to help the nerves heal. Give these supplements three to nine months to work. (See also Nerve Pain [Neuropathy] on page 294.)

- **Use the Real Cure Regimen for heart disease.** A common cause of ED is poor circulation to the penis—the same poor circulation that causes heart disease and stroke. (Doctors are now saying that ED in a man in his forties is an early warning sign for heart disease.) You can find the Real Cure Regimen for Heart Disease on page 239.

Fatigue

Real Causes

- **Nutritional Deficiencies.** Many nutrients play key roles in energy production (page 3).
- **Poor Sleep.** The most common cause of daytime fatigue (page 33).
- **Hormonal Imbalances.** Hypothyroidism and other adrenal deficits create an energy drain (page 84).
- **Inactivity.** Exercise energizes the body, mind, and emotions (page 40).
- **Happiness Deficiency.** Engaging in happiness-producing activities is one of the quickest ways to increase energy (page 55).
- **Infections.** Most often an overgrowth of the fungus candida—with telltale signs of candida including nasal congestion, sinusitis, or irritable bowel syndrome (page 181).

If you're feeling fatigued, you're not alone. In one study of 842 parents and their kids, nearly 40 percent of both said they felt fatigued a lot of the time. In another large European study, 31 percent of adults had severe fatigue lasting more than six months.

If you're tired a lot of the time, it's important to have your doctor rule out common fatigue-causing diseases, such as anemia, hypothyroidism, diabetes, and chronic fatigue syndrome or fibromyalgia (CFS/FMS, the two conditions I specialize in treating). Unfortunately, most doctors overlook most cases of hypothyroidism and CFS/FMS.

But most of the time, everyday fatigue isn't caused by those health problems. It's caused by *lifestyle* problems.

Real Cure Regimen

My four key recommendations to overcome lifestyle problems are discussed at length elsewhere in the book. *They are...*

- **Limit sugar and caffeine** (discussed throughout Nutritional Deficiencies on page 3).
- **Get eight hours of sleep a night** (discussed in Poor Sleep on page 33 and Insomnia and Other Sleep Disorders on page 268).
- **Exercise regularly** (discussed in Inactivity on page 40).
- **Get enough nutrients.** Providing yourself with optimal nutrition with a supplement can markedly improve energy.

Along with those lifestyle changes, I'd also like to recommend supplementing your diet with ribose—a unique nutrient that can dramatically help you banish fatigue and restore energy. *Let me tell you more about ribose and why it works so well to banish fatigue and boost energy...*

The Magic of Ribose

Your body produces energy by breaking down the components of food and using them as fuel. But no matter the quality or quantity of the food, you won't produce energy unless your body has enough of three "energy molecules": ATP (adenosine-5-triphosphate); NADH (nicotinamide adenine dinucleotide); and FADH (flavin adenine dinucleotide). If food-derived fuel isn't converted into these three molecules, it's useless.

For many years, I emphasized the importance of B vitamins in forming these three energy molecules, and B vitamins do help a lot. But the energy molecules require two other components for their creation: adenine and ribose. Adenine is plentiful in the body; supplementing the diet with it does not help relieve fatigue. So I turned my attention to ribose, a unique "simple sugar" (carbohydrate) that the body doesn't burn immediately like other sugars (sucrose, glucose, lactose, fructose, etc.). Rather, ribose is preserved for the vital work of making the three energy molecules, and also for making DNA and RNA. Ribose isn't found in significant amounts in food. It's manufactured in your body via a slow and many-stepped process.

We already knew that chronic fatigue and fibromyalgia cause the body to "leak" other key energy-forming nutrients, such as acetyl-L-carnitine. Additional research showed that the body does the same with ribose!

This was a "eureka!" moment for me. Could a lack of ribose be a reason it's hard for people with CFS/FM to start energy production again even after other underlying causes of the condition have been treated—a situation I'd encountered again and again with my patients?

My colleagues and I wondered if supplementing the diets of people with CFS/FM would jump-start their energy production. The answer was a resounding yes! (I'd like to pause and say that I think many treatments that address severe, chronic fatigue may also be effective in relieving everyday fatigue, and, with ribose, that is definitely the case.) In two studies I conducted, on more than 300 patients with CFS/FM, those who took ribose showed an average 61 percent increase in energy after only three weeks, with improvement starting after only 12 days. (By the end of the studies, two-thirds of the participants said their energy levels had improved.)

To put that finding in perspective: A 10 percent energy improvement in a single-nutrient study is considered significant; 61 percent and more was, well, *amazing*. Additionally, "quality of life"—a measurement that takes into account physical health, personal happiness, relationships, and other factors—improved by 37 percent.

Ribose has other benefits as well. Decades of research show that ribose improves heart function. It also relieves pain—probably because chronically stiff, sore muscles can't make enough ribose. And I routinely recommend it to athletes, since ribose assists in muscle recovery after a hard workout or competition.

Recovery with Ribose: A Case History

A case study about ribose was published in the prestigious journal *Pharmacotherapy*. It told the story of a veterinary surgeon diagnosed with fibromyalgia. For months, this dedicated doctor found herself becoming more and more fatigued, with pain becoming so intense she was finally unable to stand during surgery. As a result, she was forced to give up the practice she loved. In fact, she was bedridden.

She heard that a clinical study using ribose for congestive heart failure was under way in the university where she worked. Knowing that fatigue and pain are characteristic of that disease, she asked the study researchers if she could try the remedy to help her overcome the fatigue and pain she was experiencing. After three weeks of ribose therapy, she was back in the operating room, feeling just about normal, with no muscle pain or stiffness—and free of the fatigue that had kept her bedridden for many months.

Being a doctor, however, she was also a skeptic. She couldn't believe a simple sugar could have such a profound effect on her condition. So she stopped taking ribose. And within two weeks, she was out of the operating room and back in bed. She started ribose again, and she was back performing surgery in a few days. But we said "skeptic." She stopped a third time…the symptoms returned…she started ribose again…and the symptoms receded.

Needless to say, she has continued to take ribose.

Energy-Restoring Herbs

Ribose is an energy-restoring sensation. But there are several herbs that also do wonders for relieving fatigue, building stamina, and restoring mental sharpness to a tired brain and foggy mind. *My favorites…*

●**Ashwagandha.** This is the most powerful (and popular) herb in Ayurvedic medicine, the ancient system of natural healing from India. And for good reason. *Extensive cellular, animal, and human research shows it can help…*

- Relieve stress
- Improve memory and cognition
- Strengthen muscles
- Build endurance
- Deepen sleep
- Restore libido and sexual health
- Shed pounds

To get these benefits, however, the brand matters—outright fraud is not uncommon in herbal supplements. I recommend the KSM-66 form, an extract that you can find in many brands. Take 300 milligrams, twice daily.

●**Rhodiola.** This herb was studied by the Russian cosmonaut program, and was found to increase stamina and improve mood, while also boosting the ability to handle stress and exercise harder. It has the unique ability to metabolize the stress hormone cortisol so that cortisol isn't harmful, and to invigorate mitochondria, the tiny energy factories in every cell.

●**Green tea extract.** Chockful of healthy antioxidants, this extract can help normalize blood pressure and blood lipids, and improve memory. In a study from French researchers, it caused an average 2.4 pound weight loss in women—because it speeds metabolism without making you jittery. And it helps skin look younger, according to a study in *Rejuvenation Research*.

I'm so impressed with ribose and these three herbals, that I decided to combine them in a product called "Dr. Teitelbaum's Smart Energy." Each morning, take one dose of the product along with the Energy Revitalization System multinutrient powder. If you'd like even more energy (and who wouldn't?), take a second dose of the Smart Energy at lunchtime.

Within a month, you'll find not only a dramatic increase in healthy energy, stamina, and cognitive function, but most people also find they have a bit of weight loss, their skin, nails, and hair get younger and healthier, and their libido improves! Got fatigue? This simple morning protocol will change your life. In just 30 seconds each day!

●**Ginseng.** Earlier in the chapter, we discussed ashwagandha, the most powerful and popular herb in Indian Ayurvedic Medicine—so let's look at its counterpart in Traditional Chinese Medicine: *Panax ginseng*. Just its name gives you a good idea of how valued it is: *Panax* means "cure for all." Traditionally, it has been valued as a miraculous plant, helping numerous conditions. So it's no surprise that holistic health care practitioners in the know prescribe ginseng if you're feeling exhausted, stressed, brain-fogged, can't sleep, and have the blues. Sound like how *you* feel? You're not alone. Basically, if you have these "symptoms," you're having trouble with the challenges of the modern world.

And Panax ginseng is a great solution, because it banishes fatigue, while improving physical performance and cognitive function. It even helps erectile dysfunction and menopausal symptoms—making it a particular friend of Boomers everywhere.

There's one problem, however. Only *wild* ginseng is potent enough to deliver these benefits. And at more than $700 per pound, it's been overharvested—and now is near-impossible to find. Most of the ginseng left on the market has minimal potency, so I've stopped using it.

But a new development has changed all that. A special form of cultivation and breeding has created a plant extract of ginseng that is 17 times more absorbable and has seven times the rare "noble ginsenosides" (the active ingredient) as standard ginseng. In fact, the product is equivalent in ginsenoside profile to 20-year-old wild ginseng. Without the cost.

This extract is now available in a product called HRG80 Red Ginseng, from Terry Naturally. (This is such a profound development in herbal healing that I was inspired to write a book about it: *The Healing Power of Red Ginseng*.)

Given these amazing tools, optimizing energy has become so much easier!

Looking for Other Causes of Fatigue

There are *many* possible causes of fatigue. If you're tired all the time, I recommend you also read the sections on Nutritional Deficiencies, Hypothyroidism, Adrenal Exhaustion, Male Menopause, Menopausal Problems, and Happiness Deficiency to find common, treatable causes of fatigue.

Food Allergy

Real Causes

- **Digestive Difficulties.** This is the primary cause of food allergies: because of intestinal infections and other digestive problems, proteins are incompletely digested before they're absorbed into the bloodstream, where the immune system reacts to them as if they were foreign invaders (page 98).
- **Hormonal Imbalances.** Imbalanced adrenal hormones weaken the immune system and contribute to food allergies (page 90).

When I say, "food allergy," I'm not talking about a classic food allergy to a food such as peanuts, which produces acute allergic symptoms such as hives and swelling. I'm talking about a type of food allergy also called *food intolerance* or *food sensitivity.*

In this type of allergy, the small intestine absorbs food components (typically proteins) into the bloodstream before they are completely digested. Then the immune system mistakes the remnant of undigested food for a foreign invader—and attacks it. The result is an array of chronic conditions that can include digestive upsets of all kinds, headaches, fatigue, depression, anxiety, joint and muscle pain, and rashes. (And I think this type of food allergy can also cause or complicate many diseases, including arthritis, asthma, ADHD, autism, epilepsy, inflammatory bowel disease, irritable bowel syndrome, psoriasis, and migraines.)

Since food allergies are an underlying cause of so many symptoms and illnesses, if you have one or more of those health problems, it's a good idea to figure out (1) whether you have a food allergy, and if you do, (2) the foods you're allergic to.

But there's a problem. Most blood tests for food allergies are not reliable. They often leave you with the mistaken impression that you're allergic to, well, everything. In fact, my opinion is that food allergy tests are better at driving you crazy than they are at detecting food allergies. And there's a telling scientific study that supports my perspective.

A team of researchers sent the same person's blood to several different laboratories, where it was tested for food allergies. The results? Depends on which laboratory you asked, because no two labs produced the same results! The person tested was found to be allergic to anywhere from 22 to 76 percent of the foods tested. (Are you allergic to eggs? Well, yes and no. And no. And yes.) Then the researchers sent several vials of blood from one person to one lab—and the lab produced *different* results for *each* of the vials.

(There is one laboratory that tests for food allergies—ELISA/ACT Biotechnologies, at ElisaAct.com—that may be more reliable. Duplicate food allergy tests at this laboratory have produced similar results.)

A Simple At-Home Test for Food Allergies

Are you allergic to one or more of the foods you're eating? There's a simple way to tell: Take your pulse and temperature. *Here's what I tell my patients to do…*

1. Find your resting pulse, so you know what it is. Take it first thing in the morning before you get out of bed.

2. Thirty minutes after your next three meals, take your pulse and take your temperature.

3. If your pulse and temperature are elevated—a sign of extra activity, as your immune system begins to respond to the food component it has identified as an allergen—you probably have food allergies.

Testing isn't the only difficulty. Many people aren't just allergic to food(s.) They're also allergic to one or more food *additives*, such as monosodium glutamate (MSG) or aspartame (an artificial sweetener). Figuring out if your allergy is to a food or to an ingredient can be daunting.

Real Cure Regimen

Is there a way out of this labyrinth of allergies? A number of ways, actually. In my experience with patients, I've found that the following approach works well to detect and eliminate food allergies…

Digesting Your Food

As I pointed out a moment ago, incompletely digested food is a common cause of food allergies. You can address this problem by using a supplement of plant-based digestive enzymes (animal-based enzymes don't work for digestion). I recommend CompleteGest, from Nature's Way.

Another effective strategy: Add something acidic to meals, such as the juice of one lemon in water (add Stevia to make lemonade!) or a vinegar-based salad dressing, using a tablespoon of vinegar. (Any vinegar that tastes good to you is okay!)

Healing Leaky Gut

"Leaky gut" is a straightforward term for what's also called "intestinal permeability"—your intestine absorbs food before it's completely digested. The most common causes are: gut infections, such as candida overgrowth (you can find cures in Candida Overgrowth on page 181); overgrowth of bacteria in the small intestine (you can find cures in Irritable Bowel Syndrome on page 277); or the regular use of nonsteroidal anti-inflammatory drugs (NSAIDs), such as ibuprofen (see more in Prescription Medications, page 70, and Arthritis on page 155).

Energize Weary Adrenals

When your adrenal glands are worn out from chronic stress, your immune system is imbalanced—and you're more likely to have food sensitivities. A sure sign of adrenal fatigue is getting irritable when you're hungry. ("Hangry"—a word that's now officially in the *Oxford English Dictionary*—is the term for this increasingly common problem.) You can find cures for adrenal fatigue in Adrenal Exhaustion on page 138.)

In my clinical practice, the symptoms of food sensitivities resolve completely when I treat these three problems. And after doing that, I try to make the sensitivities themselves go away for good using the following method:

Nambudripad's Allergy Elimination Techniques (NAET)

This system of allergy detection and elimination was developed by Devi S. Nambudripad, MD, PhD (she's also a chiropractor and an acupuncturist). NAET is a type of energy medicine, a healing approach that identifies and then balances the subtle energies of the body. This energy is called by different names in different modalities: *chi* in acupuncture and Traditional Chinese Medicine (TCM); *life-force* in homeopathy; *prana* in Ayurveda. NAET combines three types of energy medicine: acupressure, homeopathy, and a muscle-testing technique called applied kinesiology.

Here's how it works: The NAET practitioner asks you to hold a vial with a homeopathic amount (basically, the energy signature, or essential quality) of a specific food or food ingredient. If you are allergic to the contents of the vial, the energy flowing in acupuncture meridians (invisible channels of energy) weakens—and so do the muscles of the arm holding the vial. The weakness is detected by a testing system called "applied kinesiology."

I recommend you ask the NAET practitioner to first test you for the most common food allergens: milk, wheat, eggs, soy, citrus, monosodium glutamate (MSG), aspartame, cane sugar, alcohol, chocolate, and coffee.

After NAET determines what you're allergic to, the NAET practitioner can desensitize you to that food or food ingredient by stimulating specific pressure points while you again hold the vial. Each NAET treatment can eliminate one allergy. Since, like most people, you probably have multiple allergies and sensitivities, it will probably take eight to 15 desensitization visits for you to start seeing benefits, and 25 to 50 treatments to free yourself completely from allergies. The fewer allergens that are detected, the fewer desensitization treatments you'll need.

Does NAET sound a little weird to you? Well, I thought it was weird, too—a couple of decades ago. That was when I was living in Annapolis, Maryland, and had a horrible, lifelong case of hay fever. A friend and NAET practitioner kept telling me she could help. And I kept telling her, "There is no way that voodoo is going to help me." One day, however, when I was sniffling and sneezing and suffering, she said, "Stop being a nitwit and let me treat you." I figured I had nothing to lose, so I let her do it.

Twenty minutes later—after a single treatment—I felt as though someone had finally turned off the faucet in my nose. My severe, lifelong hay fever was gone. That was in the 1990s—and it's still gone. I was so impressed with the results that I flew to Los Angeles to meet Dr. Nambudri-

The Many Names of MSG

Many people are sensitive to MSG (the food additive, monosodium glutamate). But eliminating MSG isn't as simple as not eating in Chinese restaurants. MSG is a very common ingredient—and it's often not called MSG on the label! *Beware of the following ingredients…*

The ingredients below usually contain MSG…

- sodium caseinate
- yeast extract
- maltodextrins
- autolyzed yeast

- textured protein
- calcium caseinate
- yeast food
- hydrolyzed oat flour

The ingredients below often contain MSG…

- malt extract
- malt flavoring
- bouillon
- broth
- stock
- flavorings

- natural flavoring(s)
- natural beef flavoring
- natural chicken flavoring
- natural pork flavoring
- food seasoning

pad. (I also married the woman who treated me, and not because I was grateful she had cured my hay fever.)

To give you an even better sense of the power of NAET, my colleagues and I conducted a scientific study using NAET to treat autism, published in the medical journal *Integrative Medicine*. After one year of 50 treatments, 23 of 30 autistic children were able to return to regular school—compared with none of the autistic children in another group of 30 who weren't treated with NAET.

I highly recommend NAET to my patients and to you. Find out more about the technique—and locate one of the more than 20,000 worldwide practitioners near you—at NAET.com.

Multiple Food Elimination Diet

The advantages of this approach are that, like NAET, it's accurate and effective in helping you find and eliminate food allergies, and it's inexpensive.

The disadvantage: A multiple food elimination diet is a bit difficult and time-consuming to implement. But my patients who have done it say it was worth the time and effort. *Here's how it works…*

First, you stop eating (eliminate) the most common problem foods and food ingredients for one to two weeks. They are milk, wheat, eggs, soy, citrus, MSG, aspartame, sugar in any form, alcohol, chocolate, and coffee. You'll probably go through a "withdrawal period" after you cut out your allergens, so expect three to 10 days of feeling worse. But once you've gotten over the hump, you'll probably feel a whole lot better.

After the elimination phase is over, you begin to reintroduce the eliminated food groups, adding one group (and only one) every three to four days. For example, you start drinking milk on days one, two, three, and four, and you start eating wheat-containing products on days five, six, seven, and eight, etc. If your symptoms start to return during a particular reintroduction period, you know that you are sensitive to that food group or ingredient.

Does that mean you have to stop consuming it for the rest of your life? Not necessarily. After several months of not eating the food or ingredient, try eating it again. You'll probably find you can eat it without your symptoms returning, as long as you eat it in only modest amounts and only once every three to seven days. Eating it more often can reignite the allergy. NAET, however, can often eliminate the allergy.

Glaucoma

Real Cause

•**Hormonal Imbalances.** Both high and low levels of thyroid hormone can increase the risk of developing glaucoma. Poor adrenal function increases the intraocular pressure of glaucoma (page 84).

Inside your eye there's a pool of fluid called the vitreous humor. It's not a stagnant pool, though—the fluid constantly flows into and out of the eye, refreshing and nourishing cells.

But if that flow slows down, pressure (intraocular pressure, or IOC) can build up inside the eye, damaging the optic nerve, the cable-like bundle of nerve fibers that sends sight-creating electrical signals into the brain.

This problem is called glaucoma, and it leads to a gradual narrowing of the visual field that can end in blindness. (Glaucoma causes one out of every 10 cases of blindness in the United States.) In fact, glaucoma has been called the "sneak thief of sight," because the damage can be so gradual that it's not even noticeable until it's quite advanced.

An optometrist or ophthalmologist can quickly, easily (and painlessly) check your IOC with a machine that blows a puff of air on the eye—a good reason to have an eye exam at least once every two years. That exam is particularly important for people at higher risk for glaucoma: African Americans over age 40; everyone over age 60 (with elderly Latinos particularly prone); and people with a family history of the disease.

Real Cure Regimen

IOC-lowering drugs or surgery can correct the problem and are often necessary to save sight, so follow your doctor's advice if you have glaucoma. But there are also natural ways that may bring

---

Acute Glaucoma: A Medical Emergency

Acute glaucoma is a sudden buildup of pressure inside the eye—and it's a medical emergency. Symptoms can include severe, throbbing pain in one eye; blurred vision; the pupil not becoming smaller when you shine a light on it; and nausea and vomiting. Immediate surgery (within 12 hours of the start of symptoms) is required to prevent blindness. Acute glaucoma is uncommon, but if you have the symptoms just described, call 911 or have someone immediately drive you to the emergency room.

---

down difficult-to-control elevations in IOC and allow you to stop taking glaucoma medication (with your doctor's okay).

• **Take vitamin C.** It's a particularly important nutrient in the control of glaucoma; several studies have shown that vitamin C can decrease eye pressure. If you have glaucoma, take 500 milligrams to 2,000 milligrams of vitamin C daily. Use a buffered vitamin C powder, such as Perque or Ester-C.

• **Take other supportive nutrients and food extracts.** Research and my clinical experience show that several other nutrients can strengthen the eye and help control IOC. *They include…*

  • Mixed bioflavonoids (500 milligrams to 1,000 milligrams daily)
  • Magnesium (200 milligrams daily)
  • Chromium (100 milligrams to 250 micrograms daily)
  • Bilberry, 25 percent extract (80 milligrams, three times daily)
  • Fish oil (1,000 milligrams daily, or eat three to four servings a week of fatty fish such as salmon, tuna, mackerel, or sardines)

• **Support your adrenal glands.** Nourishing and regenerating weary adrenal glands can help control IOC. Paradoxically, high doses of synthetic adrenal steroids such as prednisone can cause the disease. (For more information on adrenal support, see Hormonal Imbalances on page 90 and Adrenal Exhaustion on page 138.)

• **Check for thyroid problems.** Thyroid problems are another unrecognized hormonal cause of glaucoma. In a study of more than 12,000 people, researchers found that those with thyroid problems (high or low levels of thyroid hormone) had a 50 percent increased risk of the eye disease. "The results of this study lend support to the hypothesis that thyroid disorders may increase the risk of glaucoma," concluded the study authors in the *British Journal of Ophthalmology*.

In hyperthyroidism (Graves' disease), expansion of tissue within the eye can cause the problem, the researchers speculated. In hypothyroidism, the system that drains the eye may become clogged. (For more information on thyroid problems, see Hormonal Imbalances on page 87 and Hypothyroidism on page 254.)

Reverse Glaucoma Damage with Ginkgo Biloba

Ginkgo biloba is an herb that's often touted as good for the brain. Well, the optic nerve that is damaged in glaucoma is a direct extension of the brain, and ginkgo may help protect it, too.

In a scientific paper titled "Complementary Therapy for the Treatment of Glaucoma: A Perspective," Robert Ritch, MD, the founder of the Glaucoma Center at the New York Eye and Ear Infirmary of Mt. Sinai Hospital in New York, says ginkgo biloba extract (GBE) has the "greatest potential value" of all natural agents in treating the disease, because it increases blood flow to the eye, is a powerful antioxidant, and protects nerves. Several studies show that it works.

•**Slowing progression.** In a study published in the *Journal of Glaucoma*, researchers conducted a 12-year study on 42 people with glaucoma who took GBE—and found the herb slowed the progress of the disease by about 50 percent, compared to people who didn't take GBE.

•**Better blood flow.** Doctors at the Glaucoma Research and Diagnostic Center at Indiana University gave 11 people with glaucoma either 40 milligrams of GBE or a placebo, three times a day, for two days. Those taking GBE had a 23 percent increase in blood flow to the eye. (Blood flow to the eye is lower in glaucoma patients, and worsens the disease.)

•**Improving vision.** In a one-month study from Italy, 27 people with glaucoma took either 40 milligrams of GBE three times a day or a placebo. While the participants in the supplement group were taking GBE, their visual field (the total range of peripheral and central vision) improved by 23 percent—compared with no change for the placebo group.

And when Brazilian researchers tested the herb on people with glaucoma, they found that 40 milligrams of GBE improved two measurements of visual field by 29 percent and 23 percent. "Ginkgo biloba extract administration appears to improve preexisting visual field damage in some patients" with glaucoma, concluded the researchers in the journal *Ophthalmology*. If you have glaucoma, talk to a holistic practitioner about whether GBE might help you.

Hay Fever and Other Airborne Allergies

Real Causes

•**Chronic Inflammation.** Lowering chronic inflammation by strengthening the immune system can ease allergies (page 118).

•**Nutritional Deficiencies.** Low levels of many different nutrients weaken the immune system, worsening allergies (page 3).

Every spring, summer, or fall, do you start to sneeze…have red, itchy eyes…and a stuffed, runny nose…and feel really tired and out of sorts? If so, you probably have hay fever (called seasonal allergic rhinitis by doctors). Medical scientists don't know why humans have allergies. Your immune system has mistaken pollen from grass, trees, or weeds for a foreign invader and revved up its defenses, triggering those symptoms. (Mold, animal dander, the floating feces—yuck!—of microscopic dust mites, and dust itself can also cause airborne allergies.)

Allergies love company. Hay fever affects an estimated one in 10 Americans. So-called "nonsedating" over-the-counter medications such as *loratadine* (Claritin) and *cetirizine* (Zyrtec) can keep mild and occasional hay fever symptoms under control during the day, though they can also make you feel tired. So-called "sedating" *diphenhydramine* (Benadryl) can do the same at night. And those drugs are typically well tolerated if they're not used on a daily basis.

Real Cure Regimen

Even though the cause isn't known, there are effective ways to control symptoms. If your airborne allergies are persistent—and persistently troublesome—I recommend natural remedies for short- and long-term relief. There are many different natural approaches to allergy relief.

Take these nutritional supplements. *Scientific studies provide support for the allergy-easing effectiveness of several nutritional supplements...*

•**MSM (methylsulfonylmethane): 3,000 milligrams to 6,000 milligrams daily.** I've found that this supplement (which calms inflammation, improves circulation, relaxes muscles, and eases pain) can help decrease allergy symptoms after about four weeks of regular use. And there are several studies that support my clinical experience.

In one study, led by a researcher from Central Michigan University, people with hay fever were divided into two groups, with one group taking MSM daily for two weeks. Daily use of the nutrient decreased symptoms by 54 percent—nasal obstruction; runny nose; watery, itchy eyes and nose; and sneezing.

In another experiment, researchers at the Genesis Center for Integrative Medicine in Graham, Virginia, studied 50 people with hay fever, dividing them into two groups. One group took 2,600 milligrams of MSM daily, for 30 days; the other didn't. At the beginning of the study, and every week until it ended, the participants answered a questionnaire about their symptoms and energy level. After one week, those taking MSM had a significant reduction in respiratory symptoms—a nose that wasn't so stuffed and runny, and fewer sneezes. Those symptoms stayed under control during the one-month duration of the study. There was no improvement in the placebo group. "MSM supplementation may be efficacious in the reduction of symptoms associated with seasonal allergic rhinitis," wrote the researchers in the *Journal of Alternative and Complementary Medicine*. And, they noted, MSM has "few side effects."

•**Vitamin C: 500 milligrams to 1,000 milligrams daily.** Vitamin C strengthens the immune system, and several studies show that it can help weaken the symptoms of hay fever. In one, vitamin C reduced hay fever symptoms in 74 percent of those who took it. In another, involving 16 people with hay fever, a dose of 2,000 milligrams of vitamin C reduced the effect of histamine, the biochemical that causes allergic symptoms.

•**Magnesium: 200 milligrams daily.** Noting that the mineral magnesium has "antihistamine-like action," a team of Italian researchers studied 38 people with hay fever, giving half of them a daily magnesium supplement. After one month, those taking the mineral had noses that were less stuffy and runny, fewer sneezes, and eyes that were less teary, and they used fewer tissues. Magnesium has "clinical efficacy…in the control of seasonal allergic rhinitis symptoms," concluded the researchers in the journal *Magnesium Research*.

•**B vitamins.** Treatment with an injectable multinutrient formula (including 100 milligrams of most of the B vitamins, 250 milligrams of pantothenic acid, and 1,000 micrograms of B_{12}, as well as magnesium and vitamin C) was effective in reducing the symptoms of hay fever, reported Alan Gaby, MD, in the journal *Alternative Medicine Review*.

•**Eliminate allergies with Nambudripad Allergy Elimination Technique (NAET)** (For more information, see page 227). This technique combines elements of Chinese medicine, pain management, chiropractic, and homeopathy to help your immune system get back in harmony with the environment and stop reacting to things that are harmless.

To detect the allergies, the practitioner uses a method called muscle-testing (also called applied kinesiology): You hold a particular substance (in this case, an allergen) in your upraised hand while the practitioner evaluates the strength of the arm holding the substance. If an arm muscle is weaker than normal—a sign of disturbances in the body's energy flows—you're allergic to the substance. (This type of testing is very much an art. Some do it well and some don't.)

After allergens are determined, you hold each allergen for about 20 minutes while the practitioner presses on specific acupressure points. Remarkably, this procedure often eliminates the allergic sensitivity.

You can find out more information about NAET at NAET.com, including how to find a practitioner in your area from among the more than 20,000 practitioners worldwide.

Headaches

Real Causes

•**Nutritional Deficiencies.** Low levels of magnesium and vitamin B_6 play a role in headaches. Detecting and eliminating food allergies can often clear up chronic migraines (page 3).

•**Hormonal Imbalances.** Imbalances in thyroid and adrenal hormones, and in estrogen (in women), can cause and worsen headaches (page 84).

•**Chronic Inflammation.** Sinusitis—and subsequent sinus headaches—are often caused by overgrowth of the yeast *Candida albicans*, which sparks inflammation (page 118).

●**Poor Sleep.** Muscular tension is a common cause of tension headaches—and getting a good night's sleep is a must for relieving muscular tension (page 33).

The two most common types of headaches are migraines and tension headaches: More than 35 million Americans have one or the other on a regular basis. Fortunately, both are very treatable (and preventable) with natural remedies. But the different types need to be treated a bit differently to find relief.

Real Cure Regimen
For Tension Headaches

Tension headaches account for about 75 percent of all headaches. They start and fade away gradually, with moderate pain on both sides of the head and across the forehead. The immediate cause is, well, tension—in the muscles of the neck, specifically the sternocleidomastoid muscles (for you anatomy buffs out there), which turn your head from side to side. In fact, you can often find a tender knot or "trigger point" right in the middle of that neck muscle. This point "refers" pain and tenderness to the sides of your forehead (the temples) and across it.

Some people get tension headaches at the base of the skull, on the top of the head, and/or behind the eyes. With these headaches, the immediate cause of the pain is often a different set of tight neck muscles: the suboccipital muscles, at the top of the neck and the base of the skull. If you push on these muscles during a non-headache period, and they are tender and the push reproduces the headache pain, the tension in these muscles is the cause of your headache.

However, a number of remedies can provide immediate relief from the pain of tension headache…

●**Use a hot compress on your neck.** Putting a hot compress on your temples and forehead can provide relief. But remember: The pain in your forehead is referred pain; its source is your neck muscles. So putting the compress over the tender knots on both sides of your neck will work better. And if, as we just discussed, the muscles that are causing your headache are at the top of your neck and the base of your skull, put the compress there.

●**Take a pain-relieving herbal formula.** I favor the supplement Curamin by Terry Naturally. (To read more about this, see the chapters Arthritis on page 155 and Chronic Pain on page 197.) Also try topical comfrey (called Traumaplant), using it over the neck muscles below the earlobe, and at the base of the skull. You can also try CBD (cannabidiol) ointment, rubbing it liberally in the area just described.

●**Use menthol-containing cream.** Rubbed on your forehead and temples, a menthol-containing cream or oil, such as Vicks VapoRub or Tiger Balm, can relieve the pain of a headache. (Make sure to keep the cream/oil out of your eyes.)

Stop Tension Before the Headache Starts

What causes chronic muscle tension? It could be that you're deficient in a muscle-relaxing nutrient, such as magnesium. (Most Americans are magnesium deficient.) It could be poor sleep. (Tens of millions of Americans have insomnia.) It could be lack of exercise. (Only about 20 percent of us are regular exercisers.) For solutions to all of these problems, check out Nutritional Deficiencies (page 3), Poor Sleep (page 33), and Inactivity (page 40).

For more on permanent relief from tight muscles, see the SHINE protocol in Chronic Fatigue Syndrome and Fibromyalgia on page 189.

●**Take** *acetaminophen* **(Tylenol), and only use** *ibuprofen* **(Advil, Motrin) or aspirin if the acetaminophen doesn't help.** Occasionally taking one or two Tylenol to relieve the pain of a tension headache is a safe and effective strategy. On the other hand, *ibuprofen* (Advil, Motrin), aspirin, and other nonsteroidal anti-inflammatory drugs can cause a number of health problems. Better to use these drugs to relieve headache pain only if the other options don't work for you. And never exceed 3,200 milligrams per day of ibuprofen.

See a massage therapist or physical therapist who knows myofascial release. This technique can release the muscle tightness that causes most headaches. To find a therapist, Google (in quotes) "myofascial release therapist near me."

Real Cause Regimen
For Migraine Headaches

Migraines cause intense pain on one side of the head. The onset of a migraine is often signaled by an "aura" of visual disturbances, such as flashing lights. When the migraine arrives, it can be accompanied by nausea, sweating, dizziness, slurred speech, and sensitivity to light and sound. And the migraine itself is often an "episode" lasting for a couple of (miserable) days. If you go to sleep with a tension headache, it's usually gone when you wake up. That's not always so with migraines.

There's a lot of debate about what causes migraines. For decades, many researchers thought they were caused by blood vessels in the brain that tightened and widened too much. Others theorized the cause was low levels of serotonin, a brain chemical (neurotransmitter) that controls sleep and mood, and also plays a role in the widening and tightening of blood vessels. I think migraines are probably a single endpoint of many underlying problems, including nutritional deficiencies, food allergies, and hormonal imbalances.

Natural treatments are more effective at helping prevent migraines. Those remedies typically take about six weeks to start working, so you can continue to take your over-the-counter or prescription medications while you're waiting for the natural remedies to fully kick in.

•**Take the herb butterbur.** In a study by doctors in the Department of Neurology at Albert Einstein College of Medicine in New York, 202 people with migraines took either 50 milligrams or 75 milligrams of butterbur or a placebo. Those taking the 75-milligram dose of the herb had a 58 percent decrease in the number of migraines; those taking 50 milligrams had a 42 percent decrease; and those taking the placebo had a 26 percent decrease. "This level of therapeutic effect is comparable to that achieved by prescription medications," said Richard B. Lipton, MD, the study leader. "Butterbur is an effective preventive therapy for migraine."

I recommend taking 50 milligrams, three times daily, for one month, and then 50 milligrams twice a day. Use only high-quality brands of butterbur (such as Petadolex from Nature's Way or Integrative Therapeutics). Tests show that many other brands of butterbur contain impurities or don't contain the amount of the herb listed on the label. (In other words, they don't work and might even hurt you.)

For an acute attack, butterbur can work to treat a migraine attack, but at a higher dosage than is used preventively: 100 milligrams every three hours, for up to 12 hours.

•**Take magnesium.** Studies show supplementing the diet with magnesium can be as effective in preventing migraines as taking the drug *amitriptyline* (Elavil). In one 12-week study, migraine patients took either 600 milligrams of magnesium daily or a placebo, and there was a significant drop in migraine frequency among those taking the mineral. Another study showed magnesium can prevent menstrual migraines. If you have migraines, I recommend taking 150 milligrams to 200 milligrams of magnesium, twice a day, in the morning and again at dinner or bedtime. (Take less if the supplement causes diarrhea.)

•**Take vitamins B_2 and B_{12}.** In a three-month study from Belgium, migraine patients given 400 milligrams of riboflavin (B_2) daily had a 67 percent decrease in migraine frequency, and the migraines they got were less severe. In another study, 100 milligrams daily had a similar effect. And in a review of 11 studies on riboflavin and migraines, published in the *Journal of Clinical Pharmacy and Therapeutics*, researchers concluded the nutrient had "demonstrated efficacy in the reduction of adult patients migraine headache frequency." I recommend staying on the 400 milligrams for three months and then switching to the 100-milligram dose. In another three-month study from the Netherlands, migraine sufferers who received 1,000 micrograms of B_{12} a day via a nasal spray had an average decrease of 43 percent in migraine frequency.

Neuro Comfort, from Douglas Labs, contains high-dose riboflavin, B_{12}, and magnesium. Take two a day, giving the remedy six weeks to work. And work it does: It usually markedly decreases migraine frequency.

•**Get enough fish oil.** Two studies show that people with migraines who didn't respond to medication found relief by taking fish oil, a natural anti-inflammatory. I recommend one tablespoon to two tablespoons a day for six weeks, or one tablet to two tablets of Vectomega, from Terry Naturally, a highly concentrated and absorbable form of fish oil that is now my "fish oil of choice." If the treatment is effective, cut back to the lowest dose that keeps you migraine-free (or switch to eating three to four servings of fatty fish a week, such as wild-caught salmon, albacore tuna, mackerel, herring, sardines, or anchovies).

Medications for Migraine

Sumatriptan (Imitrex) and other "triptans" are the first choice of doctors for stopping a migraine attack. Advancements in migraine research have led to newer medications, such as gepants, which target and reduce CGRP (calcitonin gene-related peptide, a protein that causes brain inflammation), according to the American Migraine Foundation.

However, the old combination of aspirin, acetaminophen, and caffeine—i.e., Excedrin Migraine or Excedrin Extra Strength, with a cost of 20 cents per dose versus $10 to $25 per dose for sumatriptan—can be effective. You can take up to eight a day of Excedrin medications (every three hours), as long as the caffeine doesn't make you hyper. (The dose recommendations on the bottle are low.)

A fascinating study can guide you as to when to use a triptan to knock out a migraine. During a migraine attack, 75 percent of migraine sufferers have painful sensitivity to normal touch around the eyes, such as wearing eyeglasses. The study showed that if you use a triptan before that sensitivity develops, the drug stops a migraine 93 percent of the time. If you use a triptan after the eye pain/sensitivity sets in, the drug stops the headache only 13 percent of the time (though it still eliminates the throbbing).

Put another way: If you're one of the lucky 25 percent of migraine sufferers who don't get pain around the eyes, a triptan will work no matter when you take it. But if you're one of the 75 percent who do get pain around the eyes, it's a race against time to take the drug before eye pain kicks in.

Bottom line: For those who get pain around the eyes, take a triptan as early as possible in the attack—usually in the first five to 20 minutes. Once the sensitivity has set in, use the Excedrin Migraine instead.

If all other remedies fail to reduce the incidence and severity of your migraine headaches, preventive use of prescription medications can reduce the number of migraine headaches you suffer by 50 percent. Also discuss with your doctor recently FDA-approved remedies, such as anti-CGRP treatments that are injected, oral gepants (mentioned above), dihydroergotamine mesylate nasal spray, and neuromodulation devices that involve nerve stimulation. *Others include...*

- **Gabapentin** (Neurontin)
- **Beta-blockers,** a class of medications used mostly for hypertension and heart disease, such as *propranolol* (Inderal); avoid them if you have asthma or chronic fatigue
- **Calcium channel blockers,** a class of medications used mostly for heart disease and high blood pressure, such as *nifedipine* (Procardia, Adalat)
- **Topiramate** (Topamax), an antiseizure medication
- **Amitriptyline** (Elavil), an antidepressant
- **Doxepin** (Adapin), an antidepressant

•**Try my complete prevention regimen.** Different supplements and regimens work for different people; experiment to see what works for you. *However, the regimen that works best for most of my patients is…*

1. The Energy Revitalization System multinutrient powder in the morning, which contains several of the nutrients recommended above, such as riboflavin, B$_{12}$, and magnesium. For many, the powder alone will markedly decrease or eliminate migraines in six to 12 weeks. (You can read more about this supplement in Nutritional Deficiencies on page 30.)

2. Neuro Comfort from Douglas Labs contains high-dose riboflavin, B$_{12}$, and magnesium. Take two a day. After six weeks, the effect can often be maintained by simply using the Energy Revitalization System vitamin powder.

3. Butterbur (Petadolex), 50 milligrams, three times daily.

I have seen this approach completely eliminate frequent and severe migraine problems. But remember that it takes six to 12 weeks to work. When you're better, begin to lower or stop the treatments one by one, to see which of them you need in order to keep migraines at bay. Continue taking the multinutrient powder, however; it's a superb support for migraine prevention and general health.

Target Other Potential Triggers

If herbal and nutritional supplements don't solve the problem, consider adding the following…

•**Eliminate food allergies.** Several studies show that an estimated 30 to 40 percent of people with migraines find marked improvement by avoiding the foods that trigger their headaches. In fact, one study showed 85 percent of people became headache free when they discovered and eliminated their triggers. However, most migraine sufferers don't know their food triggers.

In one study, the most common triggers of migraines were…

1. Wheat (78 percent)
2. Oranges (65 percent)
3. Eggs (45 percent)
4. Tea and coffee (40 percent)
5. Milk (37 percent)
6. Chocolate (37 percent)
7. Beef (35 percent)
8. Corn (33 percent)
9. Cane sugar (33 percent)
10. Yeast (33 percent)

Some experts say the artificial sweetener aspartame (NutraSweet) can trigger migraines, though this is controversial. Others claim that monosodium glutamate—in all its common forms—is a frequent migraine trigger. "I would say that 80 percent to 90 percent of my migraine patients can avoid headaches completely if they eliminate all sources of MSG from their diets," Gerard L. Guillory, MD, an internist in Colorado, told us.

MSG-containing ingredients include hydrolyzed protein, sodium caseinate, yeast extract, yeast nutrient, maltodextrins, autolyzed yeast, textured protein, calcium caseinate, yeast food, and hydrolyzed oat flour.

To determine if foods are playing a role in your migraines, consider going on an elimination diet, described in Food Allergy on page 227. However, instead of spending the rest of your life avoiding foods and ingredients that trigger your migraines, consider the powerful allergy detection and elimination technique called NAET, which is described in Food Allergy on page 227.

•**Consider acupuncture treatments.** Acupuncture is an excellent option for both migraine and tension headaches. It can reduce pain, reduce the frequency of headaches, improve day-to-day functioning, and increase energy. In one study, published in *BMJ*, people with chronic headaches receiving acupuncture had 22 fewer headaches per year, 15 percent fewer sick days, and 25 percent fewer doctor visits.

•**Women, treat estrogen imbalance.** If most of your migraines are around your period, you may be able to prevent them by controlling fluctuating estrogen levels. One way to do this is to use an estrogen patch (Climara, 0.025-milligram patch) for one week, along with the bioidentical prescription progesterone called Prometrium 100 mg to 200 mg, beginning a few days before your period.

Heart Disease

Real Causes

•**Nutritional Deficiencies.** A lack of many different nutrients can harm the heart, particularly magnesium and the B vitamins. A high-fat, high-sugar, low-fiber diet is also a risk factor (page 3).

•**Inactivity.** Many studies link low levels of physical activity to a higher risk of heart disease (page 40).

•**Hormonal Imbalances.** Low levels of thyroid hormone in women and low levels of testosterone in men are linked to heart disease (page 84).

•**Poor sleep.** Research shows that sleeping less than seven to eight hours a night can double the risk of heart attack and stroke (page 33).

•**Chronic Inflammation.** This is the process that underlies the development of heart disease (page 118).

•**Prescription Medications.** NSAIDs increases heart attack risk at least 35 percent (page 70).

Heart disease is the leading cause of death in America—every year, it kills 659,000 of us. Add another 150,000 deaths from stroke, and you've got the full picture of the devastation that is cardiovascular disease, or CVD. But CVD doesn't have to be your destiny, or that of your loved ones. As you'll read in this chapter, CVD *is preventable*.

More good news: Even if you've been diagnosed with heart disease…even if you've had a heart attack and have heart damage…even if your doctor has given you a "death sentence," telling you there's nothing more to do to improve the functioning of your heart—heart function can be dramatically improved. (For a complete description of the process of CVD, read "Your Overheated Heart" in Chronic Inflammation on page 121.)

Real Cure Regimen

The recommendations in this chapter are excellent both for preventing cardiovascular disease and for controlling and even reversing it. Why aren't more doctors familiar with the methods presented here? The reason is simple. These methods are natural and low cost—and most doctors are only familiar with high-tech, high-cost treatments.

High Blood Pressure

Doctors call it hypertension, and since it's a leading risk factor for CVD, thinking about it might make you a little hyper and tense!

To picture the problem, imagine water flowing out of a garden hose. Now imagine a narrower garden hose. Narrowing that hose increases the pressure inside it, and the water flows out more forcefully. Similarly, when your arteries are narrowed, pressure increases and blood flows through them more forcefully. That higher pressure damages arterial walls and strains your heart, raising your risk of heart attack, stroke, peripheral artery disease (clogged arteries in your legs), and congestive heart failure (a weakened heart muscle that can't pump blood as forcefully).

Many factors can narrow arteries, increasing your risk for high blood pressure. They include smoking, overweight, inactivity, prediabetes and diabetes, and chronic stress. Addressing one or more of these problems—with the Real Cure Regimens for Diabetes on page 210, and with the activity-boosting and happiness-boosting techniques in Inactivity on page 40 and Happiness Deficiency on page 55—can help lower high blood pressure.

Because normal blood pressure is so vital to good health, and because hypertension is easy to detect, doctors measure blood pressure whenever patients visit. And 116 million Americans have hypertension—nearly half of all adults! That's a reading consistently above 130/80. (The top, or systolic, number in that reading indicates the pressure when the heart beats; the bottom, or diastolic, number indicates the pressure when the heart relaxes between beats.)

If blood pressure is high, I'm in favor of controlling it using medications. Unlike medications for high cholesterol (which I'll talk about later in the chapter), medications for high blood pressure save a lot of lives.

Once blood pressure is normalized, however, natural therapies can help keep your blood pressure at a healthy level, as your doctor gradually weans you off the drugs. And that drug-decreasing process can often begin as soon as three months after you've begun the hypertensive medications. (Most doctors think that if you're diagnosed with high blood pressure, you have to be on hypertensive medications for the rest of your life. Most doctors are wrong about that.)

Here's what I recommend for my patients with hypertension to help them control their high blood pressure…

•**Lose weight.** In a study published in the *Journal of Public Health*, researchers analyzed 10 studies on high blood pressure and weight loss, involving more than 170,000 people. They found that being *overweight* (up to 30 pounds above normal weight) raised the risk of high blood pressure by 32 percent, and being *obese* (30 or more pounds overweight) by 47 percent.

In a six-month study by Italian researchers, 50 percent of overweight people with high blood pressure who lost weight normalized their blood pressure. "The first step in blood pressure treatment should be to help the overweight person lose weight," said the study leader, who suggested that medications be used only after a six-month weight-loss program failed. (Although he also said that anyone with a pressure reading of 160/100 or higher should immediately go on medications.)

The simplest, most effective (and scientifically proven) way to shed pounds without counting calories is to eat a diet that emphasizes filling, low-calorie foods, such as vegetables (leafy greens are the low-calorie champs), fruits, beans, whole grains, fish, and chicken. Nutritional scientists call these foods *low-calorie-density foods*. They satisfy your appetite without adding pounds.

Low-calorie soups are particularly filling. In a study of people on a low-calorie diet for one year, those who ate two servings of low-calorie soup a day lost 40 percent more weight than those who didn't eat soup.

You also should minimize high-calorie-density foods—foods you can eat a lot of and hardly notice or feel full afterward. I'm talking about cookies, doughnuts, chips, and the like—in other words, junk food. (Nuts are the exception—they're good for your heart.)

A diet that emphasizes low-calorie-density foods is very similar to the Dietary Approaches to Stop Hypertension (DASH) diet, which recommends eight to 10 servings a day of fruits and vegetables. One study, from the Duke University Medical Center, showed that the DASH diet, combined with weight loss, lowered blood pressure by an average of 16/10—a big drop.

•**Exercise regularly.** Pick the activity or activities you like (or love), and you're more likely to do them regularly, whether it's swimming, jumping rope, or dancing the cha-cha. But most people who are successful at exercising regularly are walkers—and research shows that just a 10-minute walk lowers systolic pressure by three points.

Nonexercisers should start with as little as one minute a day and increase by one minute per day. That might not sound like much, but you'll be walking 30 minutes a day in just one month! And if you walk 30 minutes a day, five days a week, you'll meet the official recommendations for the amount of physical activity you need to prevent high blood pressure and other health problems. (Walking outdoors is best, as sunshine triggers the production of vitamin D, a nutrient that can help reduce blood pressure.) You can also find a day-by-day walking program in the 28-Day Life-Change Cure (page 329).

•**Limit caffeine and alcohol.** Both these beverages can boost blood pressure. Try cutting them out of your diet for two weeks to see if your pressure is lower. If it is, cut back to an average of no more than one cup of coffee (or, better, tea) and one serving of alcohol daily.

•**Get the right nutrients.** As you know if you've read a couple of other chapters in this book, the multivitamin/mineral supplement I recommend is the Energy Revitalization System multinutrient powder. It supplies just the right amounts of many pressure-lowering nutrients, such as magnesium (34 studies support a pressure-lowering effect) and vitamin C (29 studies). You can also see the amounts needed for each individual nutrient in Nutritional Deficiencies on page 3. *For my patients with high blood pressure, I also like to add the following nutritional supplements and foods...*

•Calcium: 400 milligrams to 500 milligrams. Have one cup of fat-free or low-fat milk or yogurt daily. I don't recommend taking calcium supplements, as they have been shown to increase heart attack risk by 21 percent. This is also a concern with people doing chewable antacids, which are basically calcium. This can be avoided by using an antacid that also includes vitamin D and magnesium.

•Coenzyme Q10: 200 milligrams daily. I have seen this heart-protecting nutrient lower systolic pressure as much as 30 to 40 points. It's especially worth trying if you have medication-resistant hypertension or if you're on cholesterol-lowering medications (which block the production of coenzyme Q10). You need to take it with a meal that has fat for it to be absorbed.

•Potassium. The amount found in one banana or one cup of coconut water (or tomato or V8 juice) can normalize blood pressure. Studies show that a high intake of tomatoes also can lower total cholesterol and LDL cholesterol. *An important point*: Getting plenty of potassium is *far more important* for controlling blood pressure than salt restriction. In fact, the most severe salt restriction only lowers blood pressure an average of one to three mm, so I don't generally recommend that people restrict salt for their high blood pressure.

•Dark chocolate. Studies show that less than an ounce a day can lower systolic blood pressure by three to four points. That intake is also linked to a 45 percent lower risk of heart attack death.

•**Blow off some steam.** Some of us are "pressure cookers" with steam release valves that have been shut down. In other words, you feel angry, but you don't blow off steam, and as your emotional pressure rises, so does your blood pressure. The solution? Give yourself permission to have a good hissy fit once in a while. (But don't hurt anyone.) And feel free to do it in private: Roll up your car windows and scream at the world; pound on the bed with a tennis racket; or punch out your pillows. If it feels really good, you definitely need to do it!

Controlling Cholesterol

Lowering cholesterol gets the most attention as *the* way to prevent CVD. But I think moderately high cholesterol is not necessarily the most important—or even an especially significant—risk factor for CVD.

For one thing, scientific research shows that many other factors are far more important in decreasing the risk of heart attack. They include exercising regularly, controlling high blood pressure, treating diabetes, eating healthfully, stopping smoking, receiving nutritional support from supplements, and optimizing thyroid function.

{}

Magnesium and Stroke

The mineral magnesium plays a role in more than 300 biochemical reactions in the body, including those that maintain the health of the heart and the circulatory system. So it's not surprising that a study in the *American Journal of Epidemiology* shows that people with low blood levels of magnesium have a 25 percent higher risk of stroke. And in a study published in the *JAMA: Internal Medicine,* of more than 26,000 smokers—smoking is the number-one risk factor for cardiovascular disease—those with the highest magnesium intake had a 15 percent lower risk of stroke.

The researchers who conducted the first study noted that the mineral may protect against stroke by lowering blood pressure and normalizing blood sugar (high levels of blood sugar damage arteries and veins).

I think magnesium deficiency is probably the most damaging nutritional deficiency in the United States, with more than half of American adults having intakes below the recommended dietary allowance of 310 milligrams to 420 milligrams per day.

To protect your heart and brain, maximize magnesium intake by eating more magnesium-rich vegetables (standouts include spinach and other leafy greens, avocados, and potatoes), whole grains, beans, and nuts and seeds, and by taking a magnesium supplement.

And don't forget zinc—research in the journal *Nutrients* shows that people with the lowest blood levels of zinc are twice as likely to develop heart disease, compared to people with the highest levels. And zinc may be particularly if you've already had a stroke. Italian researchers studied people who had recently suffered a stroke, giving half of them 20 milligrams of zinc a day. After one month, those taking the zinc had a 30 percent greater recovery in brain function than those not taking the mineral, reported the researchers in the journal *Nutritional Neuroscience*.

For another, levels of cholesterol that are too low may be unhealthy, because cholesterol serves a critical function in your body. It's essential for the manufacture of key hormones, such as cortisol, DHEA, estrogen, progesterone, and testosterone.

The bottom line: Cholesterol-lowering medications are lifesaving in people who have already had a heart attack or stroke, or have angina. There is no question in my mind that these folks should be taking statin medications for what is called "secondary prevention."

But taken by those who have never had a heart attack and are simply being treating for high cholesterol (an approach called "primary prevention"), these medications have a negligible impact, decreasing the risk of death from heart disease by about two to 10 percent.

Let's put that statistic in perspective. A meta-analysis of 11 studies on chocolate, published in the journal *BMJ Heart*, and involving more than 150,000 people, found that regularly eating the sweet lowers the risk of heart disease by 29 percent and the risk of stroke by 21 percent. And a 20-year study, presented at the annual scientific meeting of the American Stroke Association, showed that people who never owned cats were 40 percent more likely to die of a heart attack than cat owners, and 30 percent more likely to die of any cardiovascular disease,

Risk Factors for Hypertension Most Doctors Ignore

If you have high blood pressure, ask your doctor to check for and treat these often-ignored risk factors.

●**Testosterone deficiency.** Middle-aged men with metabolic syndrome—a constellation of symptoms that can include high blood pressure, prediabetes, overweight, and low HDL ("good") cholesterol—often have testosterone deficiency. Treatment with bioidentical testosterone (in gel form) can reverse all those problems, including high blood pressure. For more information on testing for and treating testosterone deficiency, read Hormonal Imbalances on page 92 and Male Menopause (Testosterone Deficiency) on page 287.

●**Sleep apnea.** In this condition, extra fat in the throat plugs airways during sleep, stopping breathing for repeated, brief periods throughout the night. But how do you know if you have sleep apnea? Well, if you snore, you're overweight, your spouse says you stop breathing during the night, and you're tired during the day—chances are nearly 100 percent that you have sleep apnea.

Remedies for sleep apnea include: Losing weight; not sleeping on your back or stomach; using a mouth guard-like oral appliance made by a dentist (it pushes the lower jaw and tongue forward, opening your airway); using a continuous positive airway pressure (CPAP) machine during sleep (it blows air into the throat, preventing the airway from narrowing, and is the most effective treatment—though less than half the people who start the therapy stick with it); or undergoing a simple outpatient surgery (see page 277 for more information).

●**Allergies.** Food allergies can trigger high blood pressure. If your pulse or temperature regularly goes up after you eat, consider going on an elimination diet or detecting and eliminating your food allergies using the NAET technique, discussed in Food Allergy on page 227.

including stroke and heart failure. In other words, chocolate and cats can be more effective than cholesterol-lowering drugs!

So why the big push to prescribe cholesterol-lowering medications? Two reasons. There's a test to measure cholesterol levels—and wherever there's a test, there's a treatment. And drug companies earn more than $19 billion yearly from selling the medications. As I discussed in Prescription Medications on page 73, the statin medications that lower cholesterol are not without risk.

For example, statins work by blocking the action of HMG-CoA reductase, an enzyme that helps create cholesterol. But at the same time, they also block the production of coenzyme Q10, which supports the function of mitochondria, tiny energy factories in every cell. The compromised mitochondria contribute to the muscle pain (weakened muscle cells), the memory loss (weakened brain cells), and a host of other side effects that often accompany statins. In fact, people on statins often develop heart failure—the inability of the heart to adequately pump blood to the rest of the body—which is then blamed on the high cholesterol. But I suspect that much of this heart failure is actually caused by coenzyme Q10 deficiency from the statins. (These side effects are largely preventable by giving 200 milligrams daily of coenzyme Q10 with the medications, a therapeutic option that doctors usually ignore.)

For my patients without known heart disease, if total cholesterol is under 250, I skip the cholesterol-lowering medication. However, if you want to lower cholesterol, there are safe, natural ways to do so without medication. *They include…*

•**Eat oatmeal for breakfast.** An oat-based cereal—whether it's cooked oatmeal or a dry cereal such as Life, Cheerios, or Quaker Oatmeal Squares—is a tasty way to lower cholesterol. Add some antioxidant-rich berries to protect your heart even more.

•**Season with garlic.** Eating one to three cloves of fresh garlic a day is a good way to control cholesterol. Crushed into olive oil, garlic is a yummy treat that can drop your cholesterol by 10 to 12 points. (In fact, simply eating garlic and oatmeal can lower cholesterol almost as much as medications do.)

•**Snack on a handful of "tree nuts" daily.** In a review of 61 studies on tree nuts (walnuts, pistachios, macadamia nuts, pecans, cashews, almonds, hazelnuts, and Brazil nuts), researchers from Tufts University found eating the nuts regularly lowered LDL cholesterol and other heart-hurting floods fats such as triglycerides. The type of nuts didn't matter much; eating enough—one ounce a day, or about a palmful—made all the difference.

•**Don't worry about eggs.** Studies show that eating even six eggs every day has no effect on blood cholesterol levels. In fact, a study showed that regular egg consumption lowered total cholesterol and increased "good" HDL cholesterol. "In the majority of healthy adults, an addition of one egg per day to a normal fat diet could raise HDL-cholesterol levels and decrease the ratio of total cholesterol to HDL [a good development]," wrote the researchers. "Therefore, egg consumption might benefit blood cholesterol." A recent review of all the research on eggs and the heart, from researchers at the University of Connecticut, summed up the scientific situation: "…large-scale studies have found only tenuous [weak or non-existent] associations between the intake of eggs and cardiovascular disease risk." Yet the myth persists that eggs are bad for your heart. Don't believe it.

•**Take red rice yeast.** This natural supplement contains monacolins, which were later synthesized into a statin drug. It lowers cholesterol very effectively and is linked to a significantly decreased risk of heart attack.

For this supplement, brand is very important: I recommend the one made by Sylvan, which has been proven effective in clinical studies. Try a a dose of 1,200 to 2,400 milligrams daily, taken before bedtime. That's because the cholesterol-lowering compounds in red yeast rice has a short duration of action, and work best when the body is producing the most cholesterol, which is during sleep. Also take coenzyme Q10 with the supplement, for maximum protection.

•**Take berberine.** This herb not only lowers cholesterol, but also helps diabetes and high blood pressure. The best dose is 200 milligrams to 500 milligrams, three times a day. (If it bothers your stomach, use the lower dose.)

High or Low Cholesterol—You Need Vitamin D

Optimizing vitamin D levels may be more than a hundred times more protective against a heart attack than taking cholesterol-lowering medication.

In a 10-year study, researchers from the Harvard School of Public Health looked at more than 18,000 men without diagnosed heart disease. They found that those with vitamin D deficiency were more than twice as likely (209 percent) to have a heart attack compared with men with adequate blood levels of the nutrient. And the researchers noted that even men with "intermediate levels" of D—levels between deficiency and normal—were 60 percent more likely to have a heart attack.

That increased risk of a heart attack was independent of any other risk factor, including high LDL cholesterol level, low HDL cholesterol level, high triglycerides, a family history of heart disease, overweight, high alcohol intake, low physical activity, diabetes, high blood pressure, and low intake of fish oil.

I recommend 1,000 IU to 2,000 IU of vitamin D daily.

Men: If testosterone is low or low-normal, consider using bioidentical testosterone. In middle-aged men, many of the risk factors for CVD can be caused by low levels of testosterone, including high cholesterol, overweight, high blood pressure, and prediabetes or diabetes. In my male patients, I prescribe testosterone if the patient has a total testosterone level that is under 500 nanograms per deciliter and has one or more of the symptoms of low testosterone, such as high blood pressure, high cholesterol, depression, or erectile dysfunction. I use bioidentical testosterone gel (AndroGel or Testim, or a testosterone gel from a compounding pharmacy that customizes medications). I aim for a testosterone level of over 700. Talk to your doctor about this treatment option. (You can read more about testing for and treating low testosterone in Hormonal Imbalances on page 92 and in Male Menopause [Testosterone Deficiency] on page 287.)

Women: If thyroid levels are low, or you have fatigue, weight gain, or cold intolerance, consider a trial of prescription natural thyroid hormone. High cholesterol in women is often caused by low thyroid levels, which stop the body from efficiently using and burning blood fats. If you have high cholesterol, a trial of thyroid hormone may be worthwhile even if your lab tests for thyroid levels are normal—because those tests are unreliable.

Caution: In women with low thyroid, consider an exercise stress test before beginning exercise or thyroid treatments, because you may have heart disease and severe arterial blockages and not know it. (Just like exercise, thyroid hormone is beneficial for the heart but could trigger a heart attack if you're on the edge of having one.)

(For more on testing and treating low levels of thyroid hormone, read "Hypothyroidism: Millions of Missed Diagnoses" in Hormonal Imbalances on page 87 and read Hypothyroidism on page 254.)

Heart Disease

High blood pressure and high cholesterol are *risk factors* for heart disease. But an ailing heart is heart disease. *There are four main types of heart problems that fall under the category of heart disease...*

1. Angina (chest pain) and heart attack (a blockage of one or more of the coronary arteries that supply blood to the heart muscle)

2. Congestive heart failure (CHF)—weakness of the heart muscle, with shortness of breath and swollen ankles

3. Heart valve problems (a malfunction in one of the four valves that control blood flow to the four chambers of the heart)

4. Abnormal heart rhythms (arrhythmia, a risk factor for heart attack and stroke)

Research and my experience with my patients show that several natural treatments can strengthen the heart muscle, improving its efficiency and lessening symptoms (particularly in CHF, but also with other heart conditions). By using the following remedies, under the supervision of a holistic health practitioner, you should start feeling much better in about six weeks.

•**Ribose.** I discuss this supplement in Chronic Fatigue Syndrome and Fibromyalgia on page 189. Essentially, ribose is a special (and healthful) sugar that plays a key role in the body's production of energy. The heart is the hardest-working muscle in the body, and people with heart disease (particularly CHF) need more energy. Ribose supplies it.

Here's how one scientific paper reviewing ribose and heart disease summed up the findings to date: "D-ribose, a naturally occurring carbohydrate, has demonstrated significant enhancing abilities in replenishing deficient cellular energy levels following myocardial ischemia [heart attack]. Subsequent clinical trials have further substantiated these benefits of D-ribose in patients afflicted with ischemic cardiovascular disease and those carrying the diagnosis of congestive heart failure."

As a supplement, ribose comes in powdered form. I recommend five grams (one scoop of the SHINE brand), three times daily for six weeks, then twice daily. In my experience with patients, this is *the* most important nutrient for optimizing heart function. I predict you will be amazed at the results—the increase of energy and easing of symptoms—after taking it for six weeks or so.

•**Coenzyme Q10.** Like ribose, this nutrient boosts the heart's production of energy, and it's particularly effective in CHF. In fact, a study shows that blood levels of coenzyme Q10 are linked both to the severity of CHF and to who will and won't die from CHF. Those with high blood levels of coenzyme Q10 have less severe disease and usually survive; those with low levels have more severe disease and usually don't. In one of the most recent developments, cardiologists from the Duke Heart Center at the Duke University School of Medicine affirm that the nutrient can strengthen the heart of those with heart failure, helping prevent heart attacks and other "cardiovascular events"—and that coQ10 should be seriously considered as a safe and effective therapy.

I recommend my patients take 400 milligrams for six weeks and then switch to a maintenance dose of 200 milligrams daily. As discussed earlier, this nutrient is especially critical for anyone taking cholesterol-lowering medications, which deplete it. For optimal absorption, take coenzyme Q10 with a meal that contains fat.

●**Magnesium orotate.** In a one-year study in the *International Journal of Cardiology*, 79 people with CHF who took a magnesium orotate supplement had a 76 percent survival rate, compared with 52 percent of CHF patients who took a placebo. Those on the supplement also had a 39 percent improvement in their symptoms, while those on the placebo had a 56 percent worsening. I think the benefit is from both the magnesium and the orotate—a compound that is manufactured in the body by good bacteria and was once considered a B vitamin (B_{13}). I recommend 6,000 milligrams daily for one month, followed by 3,000 milligrams daily for 11 months.

Caution: In the rare patient with kidney failure, magnesium can build up to excessive levels. If you have kidney disease, use the nutrient only under a physician's supervision. It can also cause loose stools. If that happens, use only ½ scoop of the multinutrient powder and take 200 milligrams of the sustained-release magnesium by Jigsaw Health, which does not cause loose stools.

●**Omega-3 fatty acids from fish.** Looking at all the available research, the American Heart Association (AHA) endorses the use of omega-3 fatty acids for secondary prevention of heart disease—prevention of angina, heart attacks, strokes, or other "cardiovascular events" in people with diagnosed cardiovascular disease. It also recommends omega-3s for people with heart failure to reduce hospitalizations and death rates. And those are smart recommendations.

The AHA recommends an average of one gram per day of a mixture of docosahexaenoic acid (DHA) and eicosapentaenoic acid (EPA) found in fish oil. There are several ways to get that dosage (the fatty acids are stored in your cells, so it's not necessary to consume them every day).

●One tablespoon of fish oil, four times a week.

●One serving of a fatty fish such as salmon or tuna, four times a week. (Canned white albacore tuna has three times the amount of fish oil than in chunk light tuna.)

●A daily fish oil supplement that supplies one gram of DHA/EPA. I recommend a highly absorbable supplement from salmon called Vectomega. One tablet daily can supply very high levels of omega-3s because the body absorbs it about 50 times better than omega-3s from regular fish oil supplements. I would increase your fish intake along with the supplement. But not with a fast-food fried fish sandwich—research shows they worsen omega-3 deficiency.

●**Omega-3s also decrease the risk of abnormal heart rhythms and sudden cardiac death** (a heart attack without diagnosed heart disease—which is more than 50 percent of all heart attacks, and 64 percent of heart attacks in women). And a study published in the *European Journal of Clinical Nutrition* shows that people with the highest blood levels of brain-nourishing, heart-soothing omega-3 fatty acids are less likely to be hostile—and hostility (an attitude of cynicism and mistrust) is a risk factor for heart disease. In fact, a study by researchers at the University of Pittsburgh showed that the higher the blood levels of DHA and EPA, the more agreeable the person!

•**B vitamins.** Many studies show that people with congestive heart failure (CHF) are deficient in B vitamins and that supplementing the diet with B vitamins improves the condition. For example, a study in the *Journal of the American Dietetic Association* showed that 27 percent of patients with CHF had riboflavin (B_2) deficiency and 38 percent had B_6 deficiency—compared with two percent and 19 percent of people without CHF. In a scientific paper in the journal *Nutrition in Clinical Practice*, a doctor observed that treatments in CHF deplete the body of thiamin (vitamin B_1) and that supplementation with the vitamin should be "routine practice" in patients with CHF.

B vitamins may also help slow heart disease in its early stages by protecting you from homocysteine. Homocysteine is an amino acid derived from the normal breakdown of methionine, a component of protein. The B vitamin folate (along with B_6 and B_{12}) triggers the body to either excrete homocysteine or turn it back into methionine. When folate intake is low, homocysteine levels are high. Some (but not all) experts think that extra homocysteine damages the cells that line artery walls, stimulating overgrowth, and that it also releases a substance that destroys the flexibility of the artery. The end result: thickened, tough, inelastic artery walls lined with plaque.

Researchers in the Atherosclerosis Research Unit of the Department of Preventive Medicine at the University of Southern California studied people who had very high homocysteine levels (above 9.1 micromoles per liter). They found that taking a daily supplement containing five milligrams of folate, 0.4 milligram of B_{12}, and 50 milligrams of B_6 for three years caused a "statistically significant lower rate" of plaque buildup, compared with people who didn't take the supplement. "High-dose vitamin B supplementation significantly reduces progression of early-stage subclinical [not normally detected] atherosclerosis," concluded the researchers.

Though the role of homocysteine in cardiovascular disease is still controversial, I recommend all my patients supplement their diets with folate and other B vitamins.

•**Acetyl-L-carnitine.** This nutrient helps the mitochondria (the tiny energy factories in every cell, including the cells of the heart muscle) make energy—and it's routinely deficient in people with heart failure. For people with heart failure, I recommend 500 milligrams, three times daily, for six weeks, then 500 milligrams daily. (I don't recommend it as a general, long-term supplement for healthy people, because one study raised concerns that it might increase heart disease risk. But I think it's a very worthwhile supplement for people with heart failure.)

•**Zinc and other antioxidants.** Research shows that a low blood level of the antioxidant zinc (along with high levels of the oxidant nutrients iron and copper) increases risk of heart attacks. In a recent study, in the journal *Nutrients*, Australian researchers found that women with the lowest dietary intake of zinc had *double* the risk of developing cardiovascular disease. Foods rich in zinc include red meat, shellfish, legumes (beans, lentils, peas), nuts, and seeds.

"Zinc may have protective effect in atherosclerosis," concluded researchers from Wayne State University in the *American Journal of Clinical Nutrition*. Additionally, a study by Mexican researchers found that zinc supplements reduced cardiovascular risk factors in people with diabetes, a disease that doubles the risk of heart attack or stroke. The Energy Revitalization System multinutrient powder (page 30) has an optimal level of antioxidants: a "just-right" level of zinc (too much can decrease HDL cholesterol), very little copper, and no iron.

•**Hawthorn.** An analysis of 14 rigorous studies, involving more than 1,000 people, showed that an extract of the herb hawthorn was helpful in treating congestive heart failure, decreasing symptoms and improving the ability to exercise. The herbal extract worked by improving the strength of the heart muscle and improving blood flow to the heart. "Hawthorne has significant benefits for patients with chronic heart failure," concluded the researchers in *Cochrane Reviews*. And in a recent analysis in the *American Journal of Cardiovascular Drugs,* researchers at the Boston Medical Center write that hawthorn is "safe and beneficial," and can "close the therapeutic gap" where drugs for heart failure don't work. I recommend Hawthorn Berries 510 mg from Nature's Way, taking three capsules daily.

Heartburn and Indigestion

Real Causes

•**Nutritional Deficiencies.** The lack of digestive enzymes in processed and packaged foods is a major cause of heartburn and indigestion (page 3).

•**Digestive Difficulties.** Insufficient stomach acid is a cause of indigestion (page 98).

•**Prescription Medications.** Acid-blocking drugs for heartburn can worsen indigestion. They can also have a rebound effect that causes hyperacidity, possibly addicting a person to the medication (page 77). Arthritis medicines also cause 17,000 U.S. deaths a year from bleeding ulcers.

The esophagus is the food tube that extends from the mouth to the stomach. At the bottom is a miniature door of muscle—the esophageal sphincter—that opens to let the most recently chewed-up mouthful into the stomach.

In heartburn, the food-dissolving hydrochloric acid of the stomach "refluxes" up through the esophageal sphincter, burning the vulnerable lining of the esophagus and throat. An estimated 60 million Americans have regular bouts of heartburn, which is also called acid reflux and gastroesophageal reflux disease (GERD). No wonder we spend nearly $13 billion a year on heartburn drugs to prevent and stop the pain.

There is an in-depth discussion of heartburn in two other sections of this book:

1. A section on the dangers of regular, long-term use of the class of antacids called proton-pump inhibitors (PPIs); you'll find that discussion in Prescription Medications on page 77.

2. In Digestive Difficulties on page 98, which presents my perspective on the real causes of and real cures for heartburn and indigestion.

In this chapter, I present the Real Cure Regimen that I've found works best for my patients with heartburn and indigestion.

Real Cure Regimen

The surprising feature of this regimen is that it works to *increase* stomach acid, not *decrease* it. Your body produces stomach acid for a reason: to start the process of digesting your food. (In fact, Mother Nature has gone to a lot of trouble to produce stomach acid in a way that doesn't digest the stomach itself!)

Yes, turning off that stomach acid with PPIs can decrease the pain of heartburn. But it doesn't treat the indigestion that is the cause of the heartburn. In other words, your real problem is not excess stomach acid; your real problem is poor digestion. And that's the problem solved by this Real Cure Regimen.

Here's what I recommend for most of my patients with heartburn and other forms of indigestion, such as stomachache, ulcers, and gastritis, a pre-ulcer inflammation of the stomach lining. (You can continue to take antacids while following this regimen, which will enable you to stop taking antacids after a month or two.)

•**Take digestive enzymes.** One of the primary causes of indigestion in the United States is the lack of enzymes in food, which have been removed during processing. Those enzymes are critical for optimal digestion. And that's why taking a nutritional supplement containing plant-based digestive enzymes is a very effective way to counter indigestion. (Enzymes from animal sources don't hold up well in the acid environment of the stomach.) Long-term use of digestive enzymes also can dramatically improve your health and well-being. I recommend

---

Acid Indigestion? Try an Old-Time Remedy First

For acid indigestion, most Americans rely on proton-pump inhibitors (PPIs), superstrong medications that squelch all acid production and have a lot of side effects from long-term use. But there's no need to fire a cannon when a BB gun works just as well.

Acid indigestion is often easy to clear up. Half a teaspoon of alkaline bicarbonate of soda mixed in 4 ounces of water can quickly neutralize stomach acid and relieve pain. This is especially helpful at bedtime for acid reflux. Do not use bicarbonate in children without your physician's guidance, as children can easily overdose.

For acid reflux that occurs while you are in bed, use gravity to keep acid down in your stomach. Simply raise the head of your bed around 3 or 4 inches. While most pillows won't work to raise your head this far, there is one that works well, the Sleep Improving Pillow Wedge from Hammacher. com. It's worth its weight in antacids!

---

the product CompleteGest from Nature's Way. Take two capsules with each meal to help digest food properly.

Some people find that digestive enzymes irritate the stomach. If it causes irritation, don't use it. Instead, use the DGL licorice and mastic gum remedies (discussed in a moment) until your stomach feels better (usually in a month or two), and then start taking the CompleteGest digestive enzymes.

•**While eating, sip warm liquid rather than cold.** Cold drinks slow and stop digestion. Drink warm liquids during meals to aid digestion. Tea is delightful, as is warm water with a squirt of lemon. Save those iced drinks for between meals.

•**Avoid coffee, colas, alcohol, and non-steroidal anti-inflammatory drugs such as ibuprofen and aspirin.** All of them can hurt your stomach. Once your stomach has healed and indigestion and heartburn are a dim memory, you can use them again, in limited amounts. (You'll know you're using too much if indigestion and heartburn return.)

•**Take deglycyrrhizinated (DGL) licorice.** This herb is often powerfully effective in resolving the symptoms of heartburn and the underlying indigestion. In fact, research shows it's as effective as *cimetidine* (Tagamet), but unlike Tagamet, it's good for you. I recommend taking Stomach & Intestinal Relief from Terry Naturally. Use one capsule, twice daily, with lunch and dinner.

Caution: You must use the DGL form of licorice; other forms can cause high blood pressure.

•**Take mastic gum.** This is the gum (resin) from an evergreen tree, and it's a wonderful remedy for heartburn and indigestion. Take mastic gum in supplement form, one or two 500-milligram capsules, twice a day, for two months.

•**Check for too little stomach acid.** As I said earlier, it's likely that too little stomach acid is a common cause of indigestion. Without enough acid, food doesn't digest well, sloshing around in the stomach—and then refluxing into your esophagus, causing heartburn. To see if this is an issue for you, add two to three teaspoons of vinegar to a meal (as part of a salad dressing) and see if this helps your heartburn and indigestion. If it does, it means you're probably producing too little acid, and you should make two tablespoons of a vinegar-containing salad dressing a regular feature of your lunch and dinner. Use any type of vinegar you like—apple cider, balsamic, rice, wine, you name it. (*Bonus:* studies show vinegar also helps control blood sugar levels.)

•**Treat for *H. pylori*.** *Helicobacter pylori* is a bacteria that can infect the stomach, a common cause of stomach upset and ulcers. Most doctors treat the infection with antacids like omeprazole (Prilosec) combined with two or three antibiotics—a lot of drugs!

Another, more natural approach if you're diagnosed with an H. pylori infection: Use both DGL licorice and mastic gum until your indigestion has settled down, and then add the remedy limonene (an antibacterial essential oil derived from citrus). Limonene is a primary ingredient in the product Heartburn Rescue by Terry Naturally. Use one gel cap once or twice a day. As they kill the bacteria, these remedies may temporarily aggravate your heartburn symptoms. But by killing the infection, they should also slay your heartburn permanently!

If you decide to use the drug-based regimen, I recommend adding 500 milligrams to 1,000 milligrams a day of vitamin C. Research shows it can increase the germ-killing power of the antibiotics.

Melatonin for Indigestion

You probably think of this hormone—available in supplement form—as a remedy for insomnia. But research shows it can also put indigestion to sleep.

Polish researchers studied people who were diagnosed with indigestion (functional dyspepsia—a stomachache with no known cause, as opposed to one with a known cause, such as *H. pylori* infection), dividing them into two groups. One group took five milligrams of melatonin daily at bedtime. The other took a placebo.

After three months, indigestion was "completely" gone in 56 percent of the people in the melatonin group, reported the researchers in the *Journal of Clinical Gastroenterology*. The other people in the melatonin group saw a "partial improvement" in their symptoms, especially at night. Only seven percent of the placebo group had any improvement.

• **After one or two months, stop prescription PPIs.** These drugs include *rabeprazole* (AcipHex), *dexlansoprazole* (Dexilant), *esomeprazole* (Nexium), *lansoprazole* (Prevacid), *omeprazole* (Prilosec, Zegerid), and *pantoprazole* (Protonix)—and using them long term is dangerous, as I discuss at length in Prescription Medications on page 70.

But after you follow the Real Cure Regimen for heartburn and indigestion for one to two months, your heartburn and indigestion should be under control, with no further need for the long-term use of PPIs.

At that point, ask your doctor if you can stop your prescription PPIs and switch to Tagamet (a safer drug, because it decreases stomach acid rather than totally turning it off) and/or stay on DGL licorice and mastic gum.

Once the PPIs have been stopped and you're on only Tagamet and/or the DGL/mastic gum combination, gradually decrease the dose of those remedies, until you're able to stop using them without your heartburn and indigestion returning. (Most people can stop the DGL/mastic gum after two months of use. However, you can use them as long as you want without risk.)

And if your symptoms recur, just use the DGL licorice again for a few days. If you need to, you can even repeat the DGL licorice/mastic gum regimen for a month. You can also add Heartburn Rescue if the *H. pylori* infection recurs.

Bottom line: You'll have broken your addiction to antacids and allowed your stomach to produce the acid you need for proper digestion.

• **Don't chew on plain calcium.** Research shows that taking calcium supplements for osteoporosis (if the supplements do not also include vitamin D or magnesium) increases heart attack risk by 31 percent. Unfortunately, this is also the case with most calcium chewable antacids. The solution? Use a chewable antacid that contains plant-based digestive enzymes (such as Acid Soothe by Enzymedica) for quick and healthy relief.

Hypothyroidism

Real Causes

- **Nutritional Deficiencies.** A lack of many nutrients can affect the thyroid, but the primary nutritional cause is a low level of the mineral iodine (page 26).

- **Cellular Toxicity.** Many of the thousands of chemicals in the environment can disrupt thyroid function (page 109).

- **Hormonal Imbalances.** Hypothyroidism is often an autoimmune disease (Hashimoto's disease) that attacks the thyroid gland, interfering with its ability to produce thyroid hormones (page 87).

Located in the neck, the thyroid gland is the body's gas pedal: It controls how fast or slow just about every part of you goes.

There are two key hormones produced by the thyroid gland…

- **Thyroxine (T4).** This is the stored form of thyroid hormone. *When T4 is ready for use, the body turns it into…*

- **Triiodothyronine (T3).** This is the active form of thyroid hormone.

When your thyroid doesn't produce enough thyroid hormone, you have hypothyroidism, and you're likely to be slow all over. Your metabolism could be sluggish, making weight gain easy and weight loss difficult. Your digestion could be pokey, and you're probably constipated. Your body temperature may be set too low, and you may be cold all the time. Your brain could be plodding, and you probably can't think clearly.

But before you read any more about hypothyroidism here, I'd like you to read another part of the book, if you haven't already: "Hypothyroidism: Millions of Missed Diagnoses" in Hormonal Imbalances on page 87. There I discuss a number of topics that will help you understand the Real Cure Regimen for hypothyroidism that is presented in this chapter. *Those topics include…*

- **A list of the many possible symptoms and conditions that can be caused by hypothyroidism.**

- **Why the problem is so common, affecting an estimated 20 million Americans.**

- **Why the standard test for hypothyroidism is unreliable, resulting in tens of millions of missed diagnoses.** ("The prevalence of undiagnosed thyroid disease in the United States is shockingly high," said Hossein Gharib, MD, past president of the American Association of Clinical Endocrinologists and a consulting physician at the Mayo Clinic.)

- **A simple way to test yourself for possible hypothyroidism.**

•**Why, if you have one or two of the possible symptoms of hypothyroidism** (unexplained fatigue, persistent depression, achy muscles and joints, miscarriages, infertility, heavy periods, constipation, easy weight gain, cold intolerance, dry skin, thin hair, or a body temperature on the low side of normal), you should be treated for the condition—even if your thyroid tests are "normal."

Once you've read that section of the book, come right back to this one and read about how to solve this widespread problem.

Real Cure Regimen

The treatment for hypothyroidism is straightforward: Replace the missing thyroid hormone. The medication doctors typically prescribe is a synthetic form of stored T4 hormone, called Synthroid or Levothroid. If the dose is optimally adjusted, this treatment works fine for many people. Problem is, many others with hypothyroidism can't convert stored T4 into active T3, so they need a medication that also contains the active T3 hormone.

I usually prescribe several different forms of thyroid hormone for my patients, to see which works best for every individual: either desiccated thyroid (a natural form that contains both T3 and T4) or a compounded (customized) thyroid medication that combines T3 and T4. If they don't work, I try Synthroid.

Let me walk you through these options, one by one.

•**Desiccated thyroid.** This natural form of the hormone contains both T3 and T4. I start with ¼ grain (15 milligrams) a day, increasing the dose to ½ grain (30 milligrams) a day by the end of the first week of treatment. Then I increase the dose by ½ grain every one to six weeks. I stop when the patient finds the dose that feels best, where they feel good and the symptoms of hypothyroidism are dramatically reduced or gone. If at any point the patient is shaky, feels hyper, or has a racing heart (a persistent resting pulse over 90 beats per minute), I lower the dose.

Hashimoto's Thyroiditis: When Your Immune System Attacks Your Thyroid Gland

In Hashimoto's thyroiditis, the immune system mistakes the thyroid gland for a foreign invader and attacks it. The "anti-TPO antibody" blood test can easily diagnose Hashimoto's thyroiditis. If you take the test and your anti-TPO antibody is elevated, you probably have the disease and will feel much better on thyroid hormones. (Also see Autoimmune Disease on page 165 for natural ways to calm the immune system.)

A Few Words of Caution

Thyroid medication and exercise are both healthful. And both can trigger a heart attack in a person on the edge of having one.

So if you have significant risk factors for heart disease (smoking, high blood pressure, a total cholesterol level above 260, a family history of heart attack, or stroke under the age of 65), consider seeing your cardiologist for an exercise treadmill test before you start thyroid therapy. The test will detect arterial blockages—which, in a few rare cases, can trigger a heart attack when a person begins taking thyroid medication.

Also, if you have heart palpitations or chest pain after starting thyroid medication, stop taking the drug and see your doctor.

One month after the patient and I have found a dose that works best or we've reached the two-grain (120-milligram) level of dosing, I order a Free T4 blood test to make sure the thyroid levels are in the normal range (too high is unsafe).

In some cases, it's necessary to adjust the dosage slowly upward or downward for the patient to remain in the normal range.

When treating hypothyroidism, most doctors use the TSH (thyroid stimulating hormone, or thyrotropin) test to determine dosage.

This is a mistake: The test is not reliable. Once the TSH is below 2, I would use only the person's symptoms and Free T4 test.

●**Compounded thyroid hormone.** A compounded drug is a customized medicine prepared by a compounding pharmacy. In some patients, I start with a compounded medication containing T3 and T4, using the same dosage and testing regimen I just described for desiccated thyroid.

●**Synthroid.** Often, one hormone treatment works when another does not. If the treatment with desiccated thyroid (Armour Thyroid) or a compounded drug doesn't work, I try Synthroid. One hundred micrograms (0.1 milligram) of Synthroid "equals" one grain of Armour Thyroid. I gradually adjust the dosing upward in the same way I described for desiccated thyroid. It takes one to six weeks to know if a level of dosing is working or not.

Other tips for maximizing the effectiveness of thyroid medication include…

●**Take it first thing in the morning.** It works best when taken on an empty stomach with a full glass of water.

●**Or take divided doses.** Take the first half of your dose first thing in the morning and the second half in the afternoon or at bedtime.

●**Don't take it with a supplement containing calcium and/or iron.** The calcium or iron in nutritional supplements or in iron-rich or calcium-rich foods can block the absorption of the hormone. Take them several hours before or after you take the hormone.

Find a Holistic Doctor to Help You

As you can see, the Real Cure Regimen for hypothyroidism is a partnership between patient and physician, requiring a lot of attentive care and calibration. I highly recommend you find a holistic doctor to guide you in the treatment of the problem. Holistic physicians are usually more knowledgeable about hypothyroidism than conventional doctors are, and are open to a variety of treatment strategies (such as using desiccated thyroid or a compounded medicine rather than Synthroid).

In fact, I'd go so far as to say that most conventional doctors don't know how to effectively diagnose or treat hypothyroidism. For example, they're trained to stop increasing the dose of thyroid hormone once your thyroid tests are in the normal range—even if the dose is grossly inadequate to treat your symptoms.

Resources on page 360 has a list of organizations that help you find a holistic practitioner at their websites.

Nonprescription Treatments for Hypothyroidism

Thyroid hormone is the best way to treat hypothyroidism. But if for some reason taking the prescription medication is not an option, there are several nonprescription treatments that can help the problem. *They include…*

• **Thyroid glandular supplements.** These supplements—formulated from the thyroid glands of animals—provide raw materials for your body to manufacture thyroid hormone. I recommend BMR Complex from Integrative Therapeutics, which contains not only extracts from thyroid glands, but also other thyroid supporting nutrients, such as the amino acid L-tyrosine, and the minerals iodine, zinc, and copper.

• **Thyroid-supporting nutrients.** I recommend that anyone with the symptoms of hypothyroidism—whether they're taking thyroid hormone or not—take the nutrients that are a must for optimal thyroid functioning. (Many of these are found in BMR Complex and the Energy Revitalization System, so if you take those two products, you won't need to take them separately.) *They include…*

• Iodine: 200 micrograms daily. For women with the symptoms of fatigue, a daytime body temperature below 98.3°F, and breast tenderness and cysts, I find that an iodine tablet of 12.5 milligrams (12,500 micrograms) taken daily, for two to four months, is very effective. *Caution:* Do not take over 6.5 mg (6500 µg) without a doctor's supervision, and usually for no more than four months. Long-term use can suppress thyroid function. Many people do like to take tri-iodine (a daily dosage of 6.25 mg) for three months to totally replete iodine stores and flush out fluorides from the body.

• Selenium: 50 micrograms to 100 micrograms daily (but not more than 300 micrograms to 400 micrograms daily).

• Tyrosine: 1,000 milligrams daily. This amino acid helps regulate the thyroid.

Infertility

Real Causes

- **Nutritional Deficiencies.** In women, a deficiency of iron, vitamin B_6, and dietary fat can cause or contribute to infertility, as can many dietary habits, such as drinking coffee. In men, studies link low blood levels of antioxidants and the omega-3 fatty acids in fish oil to a lower sperm count (page 3).
- **Hormonal Imbalances.** In women, low levels of thyroid hormone can cause infertility. In men, low levels of testosterone can contribute to the problem (page 84).

Infertility is common, affecting about six million American women, and 15 percent of couples who try to have a baby. (Male infertility is the main cause in about 10 percent of these couples, and plays a role in about 50 percent.) Many infertile couples see a fertility expert, who hopefully discovers a correctable problem, such as ovulatory difficulties, blocked fallopian tubes, or a low sperm count. When the problem is corrected, the couple conceives.

Many others, however, find out that there *is* no correctable (or even diagnosable) problem. And, in spite of treatment with assisted reproduction techniques such as in-vitro fertilization, they are unable to get pregnant.

Real Cure Regimen

I favor an approach to infertility that uses what I call comprehensive medicine: the best of both conventional and natural therapies. It can often succeed where conventional therapy alone fails.

And any infertility treatment needs to address both the woman and the man: 40 percent to 50 percent of infertility is caused by the man having sperm problems such as a low sperm count (too few sperm), sperm that are less active (poor motility), and misshapen sperm (poor morphology). In fact, raising even a normal sperm count can increase the odds of conceiving.

For the Woman

There are many habits and decisions that can either worsen or improve a woman's fertility.

- **Don't drink coffee.** Having more than four cups a coffee a day (and possibly any coffee) can result in infertility, perhaps because it reduces blood supply to the uterus. In fact, some fertility researchers joke that drinking coffee is a good form of birth control. (Don't rely on it, though!) Tea is okay.
- **Ditto for caffeinated soda.** Drinking caffeinated soda (even one a day) is linked to a 50 percent decrease in conception rate.

•**And for alcohol.** Alcohol boosts prolactin, a hormone that can worsen ovulatory infertility. Researchers from Denmark found that even one drink a day of alcohol can increase ovulatory infertility by 30 percent, and two drinks can increase it by 60 percent. Alcohol can also worsen endometriosis (a common cause of infertility), a disease in which the endometrial tissue that grows inside the uterus is found growing outside the uterus.

•**Don't take melatonin.** High doses of this over-the-counter hormone also can raise prolactin levels.

•**Don't eat an Atkins-type high-protein diet.** Research from scientists in the Department of Nutrition at the Harvard School of Public Health linked a diet rich in animal protein to impaired pregnancy. Instead, favor a diet rich in vegetables, fruits, whole grains, beans, nuts and seeds (a handful a day), and four to five servings a week of salmon or tuna. Fatty fish are loaded with DHA, an omega-3 fatty acid that is a must for brain development in the growing baby, and that can also help prevent postpartum depression.

•**Eat one serving a day of a full-fat dairy food.** A study of more than 18,000 women by researchers at Harvard School of Public Health showed that those who ate one or more servings a day of a *full-fat* dairy food had a 27 percent decreased risk of infertility, while those who ate at least two servings a day of *low-fat* dairy foods had an 85 percent increased risk of infertility.

•**Take a multivitamin/mineral supplement.** A good multivitamin-mineral nutritional supplement can increase fertility.

•**Take extra B$_6$.** Approximately 50 milligrams daily can increase the likelihood of pregnancy. This nutrient is especially important if you have irregular or absent periods, or abnormal (non-pregnant) production of breast milk after your period—signs of a hormonal imbalance (excess prolactin) that B$_6$ can help correct.

•**Test for adequate blood levels of iron.** In one study, women with low levels of ferritin (stored iron) became pregnant within seven months of taking an iron supplement.

To find out about an accurate test for iron levels (most aren't), read "The Right Way to Test for an Iron Deficiency" in Nutritional Deficiencies on page 23. Basically, if you're having trouble getting pregnant, ask your doctor to check your level of blood ferritin to be sure it's over 60. (The doctor may say it's normal if it's over 12, which is absurd!) If it's not over 60, take an iron supplement until it is. (*Warning*—this may result in pregnancy!)

I recommend 30 milligrams of iron daily. Take it on an empty stomach, with at least 200 milligrams of vitamin C, which aids absorption. If you develop side effects such as constipation, it's fine to take the 30 milligrams of iron every other day.

If you're taking thyroid hormone for hypothyroidism, do not take the iron within six hours of the hormone; iron (and calcium) can block the absorption of thyroid hormone.

•**Don't take too much vitamin C.** In women (but not in men), taking more than 1,000 milligrams a day may cause infertility. If you're taking vitamin C, cut the dose to a maximum of 900 milligrams daily. Infertility caused by the higher dose should resolve in a couple of weeks after stopping the vitamin.

Optimize Timing for Intercourse

Research shows that having intercourse even one day after ovulation is unlikely to result in a pregnancy.

Intercourse more than six days before ovulation is also unlikely to result in pregnancy. Also, the more frequently you have intercourse in the three or four days before ovulation, the more likely you are to get pregnant. (Research has overturned the misconception that frequent intercourse within this three- to four-day time span decreases the chance of pregnancy.)

To time ovulation, use an ovulation thermometer, a special, large-scale, easy-to-read thermometer that registers only from 96 to 100° F.

•**Consider taking prescription thyroid hormone.** If you have the symptoms of thyroid deficiency (constipation, cold intolerance, dry skin and hair, body temperature that runs under 98.2°F during the day), there's a good chance your thyroid is underactive. A very low dose of thyroid hormone might result in pregnancy.

If you don't have heart disease, talk to your doctor about a trial of either desiccated thyroid (a natural product containing the thyroid hormones T3 and T4), at ½ grain (30 milligrams) daily, or Synthroid, 50 to 100 micrograms each morning. You might have to fight with your doctor a bit to get this treatment, but it's worth it.

If you have the symptoms I listed, but your thyroid tests are "normal," remind your doctor that the best endocrinologists emphasize the importance of treating the patient, not the blood test. (To read more about the inaccuracy of thyroid tests, see Hormonal Imbalances on page 88.)

•**Check for anti-TPO antibody.** Make sure your doctor checks an important blood test called an anti-TPO antibody. If levels are high, you may have a type of thyroid inflammation called Hashimoto's thyroiditis, the most common cause of an underactive thyroid—and it's more evidence that low thyroid levels are contributing to your infertility despite a normal thyroid test.

If your anti-TPO antibody levels are high and you do become pregnant, it's critical that you be on thyroid hormone. Otherwise, the risk of miscarriage increases fourfold.

•**If you have polycystic ovary syndrome (PCOS), consider taking metformin (Glucophage XR).** Ten percent of American women have PCOS—a condition characterized by high levels of testosterone and blood sugar (glucose) problems—and it's a common cause of infertility. Research from Finland shows that taking 1,500 milligrams to 2,000 milligrams a day of the glucose-controlling drug metformin increases fertility in women with PCOS and decreases the risk of birth defects in their babies. PCOS also causes acne and darkening of the facial hair.

For the Man

Sperm counts are plummeting throughout the industrialized world. And fewer sperm means fewer pregnancies. A sperm count is the number of sperm per milliliter of semen, with at least

15 million to 30 million considered normal. But according to a study in *Human Reproduction Update*, in the last 40 years that normal level has decreased by an astounding 58 percent, in large part because of environmental toxins that oxidize fragile sperm. (Interestingly, studies show that organic farmers have had an increase in their sperm counts, compared to a decrease among conventional, chemical-using farmers.)

And there's not only *fewer* sperm. In many cases, the remaining sperm are less active (poor motility) and misshapen (poor morphology). *To reduce your load of toxic chemicals…*

•**Eat meat from grass-fed, hormone-free beef and drink milk with no added hormones.** I think this is important for any man whose wife is having trouble getting pregnant. Grass-fed beef is rich in omega-3s, which are linked to healthier sperm. And hormone-free beef and milk without added hormones are lower in estrogens, which can decrease sperm count. This type of meat is available at natural foods supermarkets, and even many conventional supermarkets and big box stores such as Costco.

•**Minimize exposure to toxins.** For example, don't have a heyday with a bottle of Roundup and your dandelions. Favor nontoxic products for house cleaning and personal hygiene. Above all, use common sense.

Ask yourself: Is this activity likely to be good or bad for my sperm?

Other ways to help reverse male infertility…

•**Take 500 milligrams to 1,000 milligrams of vitamin C.** Research shows that this antioxidant can increase sperm count and motility, and cure infertility in 20 percent of infertile males. It also protects the sperm from genetic damage, reducing the risk of inherited disease or cancer in the baby.

•**Take vitamin E.** Research shows that infertile men have lower blood levels of vitamin E than fertile men do and that men with higher vitamin E intake have greater sperm motility. And in a study of infertile men, published in the *Archives of Andrology,* taking 270 IU of E daily increased sperm motility (400 IU is the maximum amount to take: more can be counterproductive). Take a brand that says "natural vitamin E with mixed tocopherols" on the label. It provides the range of vitamin E compounds (tocopherols) found in foods.

•**Take zinc.** Studies show a correlation between blood levels of zinc and healthy sperm. The higher the blood level of zinc, the higher the sperm count and motility; the lower the blood level, the lower the count and motility. I recommend 25 milligrams to 50 milligrams daily for three to four months; then stop the zinc.

•**Take selenium.** In one study, published in the *Journal of Urology,* "all semen parameters [count, motility, morphology] improved" in men taking 200 micrograms of selenium daily.

•**Take fish oil.** A study published in the journal *Andrology* reviewed 16 studies on omega-3 and sperm quality, involving more than 1,000 infertile men and men in couples seeking fertility treatment. The researchers found that taking omega-3 supplements and having a diet rich in omega-3 was linked to healthier sperm—more sperm, more active sperm, and more normally shaped sperm.

To get more omega-3, eat three to four weekly servings of fish rich in omega-3s, such as wild salmon, tuna, sardines, anchovies, and trout. Also take an omega-3 supplement. I recommend

10 Tips for a Healthy Pregnancy

Mothers tend to make sacrifices during their lives to meet their children's needs—and those sacrifices start with pregnancy: A mother's body will give up its own essential nutrients to provide health and growth for her developing baby. Unfortunately, the Standard American Diet (SAD) is often so nutritionally deficient that even this sacrifice does not guarantee adequate nutrition for the unborn baby.

Fortunately, there are a number of tips that, if followed during pregnancy, can help both baby and mother stay healthy and vital!

Here are my top recommendations for ensuring a healthy pregnancy. They include recommendations on nutrition, vitamins, minerals, and other commonsense tips—all of which can lead to a happier, healthier and more vital pregnancy. (For example, try to eat more of the foods I list under "Richest Food Sources" below.

An important point: Powdered vitamin formulas are available that can markedly decrease the number of supplements a mother has to take to follow my recommendations. For example, the Energy Revitalization System multinutrient powder, which contains the nutrients in tips #1 to 4 below, plus vitamin D—and and much, much more.

Another tip: Check the prenatal vitamin recommended by your OB-GYN, and make sure it contains the nutrients I recommend. If it doesn't, talk to your doctor about taking a better supplement.

1. Take zinc. Inadequate zinc intake is the most common (and problematic) deficiency during pregnancy. Zinc is critical to the baby for two reasons: proper growth, and developing a healthy immune system. Studies suggest that inadequate zinc intake during pregnancy may even cause immune deficiency in the next generation (i.e., your grandchild). Be sure to get at least 15 milligrams per day of zinc in a supplement. Richest food sources: high-protein foods, such as meat and beans.

2. Take folic acid. Getting enough of this B vitamin is critical before and during pregnancy to help ensure proper growth and to prevent birth defects. Women should take a supplement that contains at least 800 micrograms per day. Richest food sources: deep green, leafy vegetables, such as spinach and kale.

3. Take magnesium. The Standard American Diet has low levels of magnesium, and low magnesium intake is common. This deficiency increases the risk of high blood pressure and seizures during pregnancy, a condition known as eclampsia. To prevent magnesium deficiency, take 200 milligrams of magnesium daily, in the glycinate form (which is highly absorbable). Taking the proper amount of magnesium a day also helps to decrease the leg cramps and constipation often experienced during pregnancy. In addition, magnesium is critical for more than 300 other body functions and will generally help you to feel a lot healthier. Richest food sources: whole grains, green leafy and other vegetables, and nuts.

4. Take the other B vitamins, too. While folate plays a unique role in pregnancy, all of the B vitamins are important. They're critical for energy, mental clarity, and to prevent depression (which affects up to 20 percent of pregnant women) and postpartum depression (which affects up to 15 percent). B vitamins have also been found to improve pregnancy-related complications such as gestational diabetes. In fact, taking 200 milligrams a day of vitamin B_6 can improve the health of pregnant women suffering from this form of diabetes. But please note that only women who develop gestational diabetes during pregnancy should take this high level of B vitamins, and they should decrease intake to 100 milligrams per day during the last month of pregnancy to avoid inhibiting the production of breast milk. For all other soon-to-be moms, take a dose of approximately 25 milligrams to 100 milligrams a day of B vitamins—and choose a supplement that includes plenty of vitamin B_{12} (in micrograms) for normal nerve function. Richest food sources: whole grains, beans, seeds and nuts, dark leafy green vegetables, beef, poultry, fish, eggs, dairy products, citrus fruits, avocados, bananas.

5. Take fish oil. The human brain is made predominantly of DHA, an essential fatty acid found in fish oils. But in spite of its importance to human health, DHA deficiency is very common. It is critical that pregnant women get adequate fish oil so the baby can develop optimal brain tissue. Fish oil also decreases the risk of postpartum depression. Unfortunately, though, the FDA has raised concerns about high mercury levels in the deep sea fish (salmon and tuna) that have the highest levels of these oils. An excellent alternative for those who'd rather not risk the mercury is to take fish oil. I recommend Vectomega, from Terry Naturally, a unique form of fish oil that supplies the equivalent of eight to 16 capsules of fish oil in one to two tablets, and has been tested to make sure that it doesn't contain mercury or other toxins.

6. Take calcium. Ideally, pregnant women should get 1,500 milligrams of calcium per day, plus 400 IU to 600 IU of vitamin D, and 200 milligrams to 400 milligrams of magnesium. (*Best*: all three in the same supplement, or taken at the same time.) I favor taking calcium at night (it helps with sleep), and in a liquid, powdered, or chewable form to maximize absorption. (Many calcium tablets are simply chalk and don't dissolve in the stomach, inhibiting absorption.) Richest food sources: Each cup of milk or yogurt contains 400 milligrams of calcium.

Caution: Don't take calcium or iron supplements within six hours of taking thyroid hormone, or they will block absorption of the hormone.

7. Take iron. Pregnant women who don't get enough iron are at risk for anemia, fatigue, poor memory, and decreased immune function. (Iron deficiency can also cause infertility.) Take 18 milligrams to 36 milligrams daily. Rich food sources: red meat, turkey, shellfish, beans, pumpkin seeds, spinach.

8. Drink plenty of water. When pregnant, blood volume can increase about 30 percent—and it's easy to become dehydrated. If your mouth or lips are dry, drink more! Adequate salt is also helpful in preventing dehydration. (But go easy on the salt if you have problems with fluid retention.)

9. Check your thyroid. Millions of women have undiagnosed hypothyroidism, which accounts for over six percent of miscarriages, and is associated with learning disabilities when the child is born. Treating a low thyroid is both safe and easy during pregnancy. And the earlier it's treated, the better. *So...*

As soon as you know you're pregnant (or trying to get pregnant), have a TSH blood test to check your thyroid. Most doctors don't understand that any TSH result three or over is a sign you need treatment—so make sure to see the result for yourself. (To learn more about this test, read "Unreliable thyroid tests" on page 88.)

One more important point about your thyroid: If you were on thyroid hormone, before getting pregnant, it's normal to need to increase the dose during pregnancy. (As a rule, TSH should be between .5 and 2.0 during pregnancy.)

In addition, check an anti-TPO antibody blood test (positive in one out of every eight pregnant women, which shows thyroid inflammation). If positive, taking thyroid hormone (even if the other thyroid tests are OK) decreases the risk of miscarriage from 13.8 percent to 2.4 percent, and decreases the risk of premature birth from an abnormally high 22 percent to the general average of 10 percent.

10. Avoid these risk factors. During pregnancy, it's not only what you do but what you don't do that counts. *My advice...*

Avoid taking more than 8,000 units of vitamin A per day. Don't engage in any activity that raises your body temperature too high, such as hot tubs, saunas, or steam rooms. These have been implicated as possibly increasing the risk for birth defects. Don't smoke, drink, or take recreational drugs. On the other hand (or leg), *do* exercise, which has been shown to be very beneficial and results in babies and moms that are quite healthy.

Best wishes on a healthy baby and mom!

Getting the Postpartum Support You Need

Did you know that one in seven moms and one in 10 dads suffer from postpartum depression? Postpartum Support International (postpartum.net or call 800-944-4773) provides peer support and professional connections for new parents who need it. This site features over 14 online specialty support groups, including grief counseling and volunteer opportunities.

Whatever the parenting and postpartum questions and problems you have, they will connect you to online experts. Quickly and effectively. Got questions? Get answers! You don't have to be alone anymore.

Vectomega from Terry Naturally, which is absorbed 50 times more effectively than other fish oils. One to two tablets a day deliver all the omega-3 you need. Other good brands of fish oil include products from Nordic Naturals, with a daily intake of 1,000 mg to 2,000 mg of combined EPA/DHA.

• **Take coenzyme Q10.** Studies show this antioxidant improves sperm count, motility, and morphology. I recommend 200 milligrams daily, using the Nature's Way chewable wafers (Smart Q10), which supply the amount of coenzyme Q10 listed on their label and are well absorbed—not always a sure thing with other coenzyme Q10 supplements.

• **Take L-arginine.** Studies show supplementing with this amino acid can help male infertility: Four grams a day for low sperm count; nine grams a day for poor sperm motility.

• **Take acetyl-L-carnitine.** This compound, which helps generate cellular energy, can increase sperm quality, according to several studies. Take 1,500 milligrams to 3,000 milligrams daily for four months.

• **Take astragalus.** Three studies show this herb can increase sperm motility. Reliable brands of astragalus include Herb Pharm, Douglas Laboratories, and Gaia Herbs. Follow the dosage recommendation on the label.

• **Talk to your doctor about vitamin B_{12} shots.** A study from Japanese researchers shows that high doses of intramuscular vitamin B_{12} (the shots are very safe) can increase sperm count in 50 percent of men with low sperm counts. The dose used in the study was very high: 1,500 micrograms to 6,000 micrograms daily. Talk to your doctor about this treatment. (If you can't get the shots, you take a 5,000 microgram sublingual (dissolved under the tongue) B_{12} tablet.

• **Don't take melatonin.** As in women, this over-the-counter hormone can contribute to male infertility.

• **Don't drink in excess.** More than two alcoholic drinks a day can damage sperm.

• **Skip the soy.** Soy products of all kinds (soy milk, tofu, miso, tempeh, etc.) can increase estrogen production and may significantly decrease sperm counts.

• **Avoid cottonseed oil.** It may contain gossypol, a compound that inhibits sperm function.

•**Don't overheat your sperm.** Sperm do poorly at temperatures over 96°F—that's why testes hang below the 98.6°F body.

To avoid heating up your sperm: Wear boxer shorts instead of tight-fitting underwear. Don't wear skintight jeans. And avoid long stays in hot tubs, jacuzzis, saunas, hot showers, and hot baths. You might also want to avoid long periods of high-intensity exercise, such as rowing or skiing machines, unless the testes can hang free. A study in the *American Journal of Men's Health* reviewed all the scientific literature on exercise and sperm quality and found that long periods of high-intensity exercise might *impair* sperm. But one type of exercise stood out as a no-no: cycling. It's "one of the most troublesome activities for fertility" write the researchers, because of "the mechanical impact sustained from sitting on the saddle, gonadal overheating, and wearing tight clothes."

•**Don't take nonsteroidal anti-inflammatory drugs (NSAIDs) such as *ibuprofen* (Motrin) and aspirin.** They block prostaglandin hormones, which assist in the formation of sperm. *Acetaminophen* (Tylenol) is okay, in moderation.

•**If you're taking *verapamil* or *nifedipine*, talk to your doctor about alternatives.** *Nifedipine* (Procardia) and *verapamil* (sold under many brand names) are calcium channel blockers used to treat high blood pressure and heart disease. They damage sperm—and stopping taking them has reversed infertility, according to many studies, summarized in a scientific paper in *Advances in Experimental Medicine and Biology*.

Inflammatory Bowel Disease

Real Causes

•**Digestive Difficulties.** Food allergies may contribute to diseases such as Crohn's (page 98).

•**Nutritional Deficiencies.** Because digestion is interrupted, nutrient deficiencies can occur that limit healing and worsen complications (page 3).

•**Chronic Inflammation.** Autoimmune issues may be prominent and trigger inflammation, which then triggers symptoms (page 118).

Inflammatory bowel disease (IBD) affects an estimated three million Americans. It's one of the more than 100 autoimmune diseases, in which the immune system mistakenly attacks a part of the body—in this case, the small or large intestine. The results of that attack include persistent diarrhea, crampy abdominal pain, fever, and intermittent rectal bleeding. (The last two of these symptoms distinguish IBD from the more common and benign irritable bowel syndrome, or IBS.)

IBD takes two main forms: Crohn's disease and ulcerative colitis. Crohn's disease most commonly affects the end of the small intestine (the ileum) and the beginning of the large intestine (the colon), though it can affect any part of the intestines. Ulcerative colitis affects only the colon and the rectum. Crohn's disease occurs in patches of inflammation on the lining of the intestine; in between the patches, there's healthy bowel. Ulcerative colitis occurs as a continuous sheet of inflammation, usually beginning at the anus and spreading up into the colon.

Doctors diagnose IBD by performing a colonoscopy and a tissue biopsy. Once IBD is confirmed, the pattern and location of the inflammation can usually distinguish between Crohn's and ulcerative colitis.

Real Cure Regimen

Standard medical therapy for IBD consists of one or more of the following treatments: anti-inflammatory steroids (prednisone); *mesalamine* (Asacol), an anti-inflammatory drug; antibiotics; immune suppressants and modifiers, such as *infliximab* (Remicade); and surgery to remove diseased sections of bowel and treat complications. The good news is that natural therapies are often very effective in treating the cause of the inflammation and the inflammation itself.

Treat Bowel Infections

I've found that a yeast (fungus) overgrowth called *Candida albicans* is common in IBD, worsening symptoms. Since no test can distinguish normal from abnormal levels of *C. albicans*, I consider it reasonable to treat candida in everyone with IBD. *Those treatments include...*

•**Take *fluconazole* (Diflucan).** This is a very effective antifungal medication. Take 200 milligrams daily, for six weeks.

•**Take probiotics.** Probiotics are friendly intestinal bacteria in a nutritional supplement, and they work in part by crowding out candida. In a recent analysis of 22 studies on probiotics and IBD, UK researchers found that probiotics were just as effective as drugs in preventing flare-ups of IBD, lowering risk by 26 percent.

Start with a one-month regimen of VSL #3 from Alfasigma, or Visbiome from ExeGi Pharma, superpotency probiotics formulated specifically to help control IBD. After one month,

---

Treat Food Allergies

After you've addressed bowel infections and nutritional deficiencies, I recommend detecting and eliminating food allergies, which can complicate IBD. For two effective food allergy detection and elimination methods—NAET and the multiple food elimination diet—see page 227.

Biological Modifiers: Best as a "Rescue Therapy"

If you're diagnosed with IBD, many doctors will recommend you take one of a class of drugs called biological modifiers, such as *infliximab* (Remicade). These injected drugs work by turning down your immune system—and they're very expensive, costing as much as $1,000 to $3,000 per month.

They're also potentially dangerous: Since they suppress immunity, you're vulnerable to other types of bacterial, viral, and fungal infections. And they may increase the risk of cancer in those who take them.

These aren't their only downsides. They typically work for less than two months, at which point you need another injection. And after a year of treatment, the drugs lose their effectiveness in about four out of five people. So why are they the drug of choice? Because they're very profitable and marketed intensively to physicians.

I recommend keeping these powerful drugs in reserve as a "rescue therapy" to be tried if and when all else fails. (They're definitely a better option than surgery.) And by using the natural treatments in this chapter, you may avoid the need for these costly and sometimes toxic medications.

switch to a maintenance dose of probiotics, such as Pearls Elite from Nature's Way, taking one pearl daily.

•**Test for other intestinal infections.** Other types of gut infections can complicate IBD, such as bacterial and parasitic infections. The best labs for these tests are Genova Diagnostics or DiagnosTechs. If any of the tests are positive, your doctor can treat you for that specific infection. Even if the tests are negative, a trial of *albendazole* (Albenza), an anti-parasitic medication, may be reasonable to try anyway to see if the treatment reduces symptoms.

Treat Nutritional Deficiencies

Because of absorption problems from a damaged intestine, nutritional deficiencies are common in both Crohn's and ulcerative colitis. Supplying the missing nutrients helps ease the disease.

•**Take zinc.** Low levels of zinc are linked to increased rates of a common complication of IBD: fistulas, in which the inflammation spreads to the skin or other organs. But lab tests for blood levels of the mineral are not reliable. If you have IBD, take zinc. I recommend 25 milligrams to 30 milligrams a day for three months, and then 15 milligrams a day as a maintenance dose.

•**Take vitamin D.** Studies show that low vitamin D levels may play a role in IBD. In a study from Denmark of 94 people with Crohn's, taking a daily vitamin D supplement of 1,200 IU reduced the recurrence rate by 56 percent, compared with people taking a placebo. Another study showed that people with Crohn's had vitamin D levels that were 34 percent lower than those of people who didn't have the disease—and the lower their vitamin D levels, the more severe the symptoms of Crohn's. I recommend 2,000 IU to 4,000 IU daily for six months.

Use Natural Anti-Inflammatory Compounds

Inflammatory bowel disease calls for natural anti-inflammatory herbs and food extracts.

•**Boswellia serrata—a must-take herbal for colitis.** One of the best natural anti-inflammatory agents is the herb boswellia (also known as frankincense). It's very helpful in IBD, costs only a few cents a day, is safe, and is well tolerated. In fact, several studies show that it's more effective for ulcerative colitis than many prescription medications.

In one study from researchers in India of people with ulcerative colitis, four out of five of those taking boswellia went into remission (no symptoms)—a much higher rate of remission than in those taking *sulfasalazine* (Azulfidine), a standard medication for the disease. And in an Italian study of 43 people with ulcerative colitis, those who took boswellia had less intestinal pain, less blood in their stools, less anemia, fewer cramps, fewer bowel movements and watery stools, took less drugs, and visited the doctor less often.

I recommend using BosMed, from Terry Naturally. Take one capsule, two or three times daily, for six to eight weeks, and then lower the dose to one or two capsules a day as needed to control symptoms.

•**Eat more fatty fish.** They are rich in anti-inflammatory omega-3 fatty acids. I recommend eating salmon or tuna three or four times a week—or more.

Consider Cortef

A standard treatment for IBD is the powerful anti-inflammatory drug prednisone, a synthetic version of cortisol, an adrenal hormone. However, long-term intake of high doses (more than five milligrams daily) is toxic, with side effects that can include osteoporosis, ulcers, diabetes, and weight gain. These side effects are not caused by treatment with natural (bioidentical) cortisol—the prescription drug Cortef, at a daily dose of 20 milligrams or less, taken first thing in the morning. I usually start my patients on doses lower than 20 milligrams, and quickly increase to 20 milligrams. But I do so on a case-by-case basis, closely monitoring the patient and their response. Ask your doctor about this option.

Insomnia and Other Sleep Disorders

Real Causes

•**Hormonal Imbalances.** Sleep is controlled by the hypothalamus in the brain, and it takes energy for the hypothalamus to function normally. Because of this, anything that depletes energy can disrupt sleep. Low levels of estrogen, thyroid, and adrenal hormones also disrupt sleep (page 84).

•**Happiness Deficiency.** Chronic stress is a major energy robber, interfering with deep sleep (page 55).

•**Nutritional Deficiencies.** Low levels of magnesium and iron can cause restless legs syndrome. A nutrient-poor, high-calorie diet can also cause excess weight and obesity, which causes sleep apnea (page 3).

If you want to find out about the problem of insomnia—what it is, how many Americans aren't sleeping well, and the health conditions it causes—please read Poor Sleep on page 33. *There you'll discover that...*

•**More than 100 million Americans struggle with sleep.**

•**Around 70 million have a sleep disorder,** such as sleep apnea or restless legs syndrome.

•**Insomnia is a little-recognized risk factor for dozens of conditions and diseases,** from anxiety, burnout, and depression, to big killers such as heart disease, stroke, and diabetes.

Real Cure Regimen

Sleeping pills are a popular solution, but they're not a cure. For one thing, they're not intended for long-term treatment. For another, they're potentially addictive. And they can cause a lot of side effects, including short-term memory problems and next-day drowsiness.

But this chapter isn't about the *problem* of insomnia. It's about the *solutions*—the easy-to-form habits and natural remedies that can almost guarantee you'll get a good night's sleep.

Good Sleep Starts with Good Sleep Hygiene

You know about "dental hygiene" because your dental hygienist always bugs you about it: Brush your teeth and floss at least twice a day and see your hygienist every six months for a cleaning. The purpose of good dental hygiene is healthy teeth. By forming those regular habits, you prevent gum disease and decay.

But there's no "sleep hygienist" to tell you about good sleep hygiene. And that's too bad. Good sleep hygiene—the daily (and nightly) habits that can prevent and reverse insomnia—is the best cure for insomnia. *Here are the habits that can help you write your own ticket to dreamland...*

•**Give caffeine a curfew.** The caffeine in coffee, tea, cola, and chocolate stimulates your nervous system, and jumpy nerves aren't very conducive to falling asleep. Stop ingesting caffeine seven or eight hours before your regular bedtime; 4:00 p.m. or so is a good cutoff point. Even better, reserve caffeine-containing food and beverages for the morning.

•**Exercise early.** Exercise is stimulating, too. Try to schedule your workout early in the day—at the latest, right after dinner.

•**Bedtime is a good time for snacks.** Hunger causes shallow sleep in all animals, and we humans are no exception. Have a light, high-protein snack before bedtime. A particularly good choice: foods rich in the amino acid tryptophan, which soothes the brain. Snack on a slice of turkey, a hard-boiled egg, or a chunk of cheese or soy cheese. This is especially important if you often find yourself wide awake in the middle of the night (which often occurs from a drop in blood sugar).

• **It's not a good time for a nightcap.** Alcohol boosts blood sugar, which drops a couple of hours later, in the middle of the night, which might wake you up. Having one or two drinks in the early evening is okay, but if you wake up or have restless sleep later in the night, try cutting back on alcohol to see if your sleep improves.

• **Limit fluids before bed.** If you wake up more than once each night to urinate, stop drinking fluids an hour or two before bedtime.

• **Prop up your feet on a pillow.** While sitting and relaxing in the evening, keep your feet propped up on a pillow. This allows fluid that normally pools in your legs to drain out of your legs and be urinated before you go to sleep.

• **Take a hot bath before bed.** It will soothe your mind and relax your muscles, allowing you to slip into sleep.

• **Keep your bedroom cool.** The ideal temperature for deep sleep is on the cool side, around the mid-60s.

• **Make your bedroom a sanctuary for sleep.** If you use the bedroom as a place to work… and pay your bills…and problem solve…it's less likely you'll find it easy to relax and sleep there. So don't use your bedroom for work you've brought home from the office, for household tasks, or for personal problem solving.

• **Head on pillow, mind on rainbows.** If your mind is racing when it's time to sleep, there are ways to shift it to a lower, sleep-friendly gear. After turning out the light and putting your head on the pillow, focus your thoughts on things that feel good and don't require concentration or problem solving. A happy moment with your children or grandchildren. Your dog romping joyfully in a field. The peaceful face of a spiritual figure. A double rainbow.

• **Make a list of your problems—and then forget about them!** If you're tossing and turning and worrying, trying to solve your problems, keep a pad and pen on your bed stand, and write down all your problems on a piece of paper until you can't think of any more. Then go back to sleep. Do this as often during the night as you need to. (You might also find it helpful to schedule 30 minutes of "worry time" in the afternoon or evening, when you can update your checklist of concerns.)

• **Wear earplugs.** If your partner snores, get yourself a good pair of earplugs. I like the silicone plugs that mold to the shape of the ear. But earplugs might not do the trick. The average snore is 60 to 90 decibels (90 is the same as a passing train), and the best earplugs reduce noise by only about 30 decibels. Another solution: Sleep in another bedroom. Tuck your partner in, give him or her a sweet kiss goodnight, and give yourself a night of sweet dreams.

Other helpful technology for blocking out noise or getting to sleep are sound machines, and apps such as Sleep Genius (AdvancedBrain.com/sleep-genius), which is based on technology that helped NASA astronauts get better sleep. Whatever works for you is the best way to achieve restful, refreshing sleep.

• **Limit your time in bed.** If you have insomnia, you probably think that increasing the amount of time you spend in bed will increase the amount of time you sleep. But that's not what

A Simple Strategy for Worry-Free Living

Worry and anxiety are common causes of insomnia. If you're awake at 2:00 a.m. and can't get back to sleep, you're probably also worrying about what you have to do, what you haven't done, and the problems you think you'll never, ever be able to solve. I've been there and done that! And here's a simple strategy I've devised to help me let go of worry and relax, particularly when it's time to sleep.

1. I create a page with three wide columns: #1, problems and projects; #2, plans; #3, "my" column.

2. I list my problems and projects in the left-hand column, column #1.

3. In the middle column, column #2, I write what (if anything) I plan to do soon about each of those problems and projects.

4. I consider those columns #1 and #2 to be what I leave in the hands of God or the Universe or Spirit (or whatever name or idea is meaningful to you).

5. Every so often, I move an item from the "Spirit" columns #1 and #2 over to the right-hand column—"my" column. The items in the third column are the one or two things that I want to work on—right now.

I am constantly amazed at how the problems and projects in the "Spirit" columns move forward (on their own) as quickly as the items in "my" column. On a separate piece of paper, I also keep a list of everyday errands and put a star next to those that must get done soon. I do the other items on that list if and when I feel like it.

And I sleep very deeply every night.

happens. When you routinely stay in bed longer than you need to, you develop a classic pattern of insomnia. You sleep deeply in the beginning of the night; you have shallow sleep in the middle of the night, with long periods of being awake; and you sleep soundly when it's time to wake up.

You can break that pattern by limiting the amount of time you spend in bed to no more than eight or nine hours. This will gradually squeeze out those long, middle-of-the-night waking periods, restoring a full night's sleep.

•**Get out of bed at the same time every morning—even after a poor night's sleep.** This resets your body's internal sleep/wake cycle (circadian rhythm), helping you fall asleep faster and sleep throughout the night. If you find that you're sleepy during the day, you can nap for up to 90 minutes. When you nap, set the alarm for 60 to 90 minutes of nap time. If you feel groggy when you wake up, splash cold water on your face. (Try not to nap after 2:00 p.m., which can interfere with the next night's sleep.)

Natural Sleep Aids Help Z's

Most natural sleep aids aren't sedating like sleeping pills, but they very effectively help you fall asleep and stay asleep. At the same time, they can help relieve pain, because they're muscle relaxants.

The first six sleep aids listed below—my favorites—are available in a single product called the Revitalizing Sleep Formula, from Nature's Way. I routinely recommend it to my patients with sleep problems.

•**Suntheanine: 50 milligrams to 200 milligrams at bedtime.** Theanine is an amino acid found in green tea. It not only improves deep sleep, but also can help you stay alert during the day. It works by assisting in the production of gamma-aminobutyric acid (GABA), an "inhibitory" brain chemical (neurotransmitter) critical for sleep (and the neurotransmitter stimulated by many prescription sleep medications). It also helps produce alpha waves, the type of electrical activity in the brain during relaxed, alert awareness, such as during meditation. In a study from Korean researchers, a theanine-containing supplement helped people fall asleep faster and sleep longer.

The only form of theanine that I use and recommend is Suntheanine (pure L-theanine), and it's the only form that reputable companies use. Other brands contain inactive forms of the amino acid that actually block its effectiveness.

•**5 HTP: 50 milligrams to 200 milligrams at bedtime.** This amino acid raises your natural serotonin levels, which helps sleep. It also improves mood and decreases pain. Three studies support the use of 5 HTP for insomnia, according to a scientific paper on the amino acid in *Alternative Medicine Review.*

•**Lemon balm extract: 20 milligrams to 80 milligrams at bedtime.** A study by French researchers show this herbal compound is synergistic with passionflower, valerian, and other herbs for improving sleep quality, including falling asleep faster, sleeping longer, and clearing up daytime fatigue from poor sleep. (As a side benefit, it can help relieve anxiety, and prevent or ease viral infections.)

•**Hops: 30 milligrams to 120 milligrams at bedtime.** This herb is familiar to most of us as an ingredient in beer, but it has a long history of use as a mild sedative for insomnia and anxiety. One study from India showed that it was as effective as benzodiazepine drugs (such as Valium) in inducing sleep, but much safer.

•**Passionflower (*passiflora*): 90 milligrams to 360 milligrams at bedtime.** This herb is used widely throughout South America as a folk remedy for insomnia and anxiety, and a number of scientific studies have validated its effect. For example, Korean researchers studied 110 people with insomnia, giving half of them passionflower and half a placebo. After just two weeks, those taking passionflower had dramatically longer sleep times, and woke up less frequently during the night.

•**Valerian: 200 milligrams to 800 milligrams at bedtime.** Calming, relaxing valerian is a classic herbal remedy for insomnia. A number of studies show that it can shorten the time it takes to fall asleep and lengthen the amount of time spent sleeping. And in moderate doses, it doesn't produce any next-day grogginess, a common problem with sleep medications. (High doses of 450 to 900 milligrams of valerian can cause next-day sedation.)

"Valerian is a safe herbal choice for the treatment of mild insomnia," concluded a team of doctors in the journal *American Family Physician*, after reviewing the many scientific studies on the herb. "Most studies suggest that it is more effective when used continuously rather than as an acute sleep aid," they added. In other words, though you can use it intermittently, it's more effective when used regularly.

Caution: About one in 10 people who take the herb finds it energizing rather than calming. If that's your experience, use this herb for daytime anxiety rather than insomnia.

The Restful Power of Essential Oils

The oral intake of essential oils add a whole new dimension to natural therapies for sleep problems. They can decrease brain fog and pain while improving immune function. Let's take a look at four outstanding essential oils, all of which you can find in the supplement Terrific ZZZZ, from Terry Naturally.

•**Lemon balm (*Melissa officinalis*).** As I discussed earlier in this chapter, this lemon-scented herb is both an effective calming agent and a mild sedative. (In a study from England, lemon balm significantly improved calmness and cognitive function.) Research from Japan suggests that it optimizes the function of the GABA (gamma-aminobutyric acid) receptors in the brain, which calms the nervous system. Optimizing these receptors also decreases pain. Lemon balm also strengthens the immune system, helping to keep viral infections in check.

•**Lavender (*Lavandula angustifolia*).** Long recognized in France for improving people's sense of well-being—even the smell of lavender is calming—lavender flowers were commonly placed in pillows to help promote sleep. Science fully supports this folk remedy: research shows that lavender oil—either taken orally or used topically—is sedating, relieving anxiety and improving deep sleep. Not surprisingly, people who use lavender also experience more energy and alertness in the morning. Research from Japan also shows that lavender supports the production of endorphins, molecules in the brain that tell your body to decrease pain. (They also trigger the "runner's high" in athletes.)

•**Mandarin (*Citrus reticulata*).** In Traditional Chinese Medicine, this herb is used to calm the nervous system and induce sleep.

•**Ravensara (*Ravensara aromatica*).** The leaves, bark, and nuts of this rainforest tree have a long history of being used by the indigenous people Madagascar for their powerful effects in supporting sleep, improving mood, and calming anxiety.

Terrific ZZZZ is synergistic with the other natural products discussed in this chapter, as well as sleep medications—that is, they work very well *together*.

Experiment with These Slumber Helpers

Below are a few other natural remedies that may help relieve insomnia. Try a few of them to find the remedy or remedies that work best for you.

•**Magnesium (200 milligrams).** Taken at bedtime, this muscle-relaxing, nerve-calming mineral can help you sleep.

Caution: If magnesium causes diarrhea (a possible side effect), lower the dose. Or use a magnesium supplement called MagSRT (for "sustained-release technology") from Jigsaw Health—it's highly effective, and it won't cause the runs. (Magnesium is also very safe for insomnia during pregnancy.)

•**Melatonin 5 milligrams.** Although a lot of research supports the use of melatonin for insomnia, I have been unimpressed with the effectiveness of most melatonin products. The exception is a mixed immediate- and sustained-release product called Dual Spectrum Melatonin 5 Mg, from Nature's Bounty.

●**Ashwagandha, magnolia, and phosphatidylserine.** If you find that you're wide awake and your mind is racing when your head hits the pillow, this mix of two herbs and a nutrient is for you. Together, these three compounds can lower levels of *cortisol,* an adrenal hormone that's a must for dealing with stress during the day but can keep you awake at night. All three are in the product Sleep Tonight from Nature's Way. If needed, you can safely take Sleep Tonight with any of the other supplements discussed in this chapter. You'll know within one week if it's helping enough to make it worth continuing.

If, over time, you start waking during the night (because your cortisol and blood sugar are now too low), lower the dose or eat a bedtime snack rich in protein.

●**Chamomile tea: good for pregnant women and children.** Chamomile tea is a very mild sedative, and won't treat moderate to severe insomnia as well as the other natural remedies in this chapter. But it's safe for pregnant women and children to use for insomnia.

●**Sleep medications.** If natural sleep aids don't work, consider medications. I think the safest sleep medications are *zolpidem* (Ambien), *trazodone* (Desyrel), taken in the range of 25 milligrams to 50 milligrams, and *gabapentin* (Neurontin), taken in the range of 100 milligrams to 300 milligrams. Avoid most benzodiazepines, such as Valium—they worsen sleep quality and are addictive. *Clonazepam* (Klonopin) and *alprazolam* (Xanax) are also addictive, but might be useful for a few weeks for a person who has insomnia and a severe anxiety disorder such as post-traumatic stress disorder (PTSD).

A Real Cure for Restless Legs Syndrome

Are your sheets and blankets scattered around the bed when you wake up? Does your spouse complain of being kicked at night? Do you notice that your legs are uncomfortable and restless when you're trying to fall asleep?

If you answered yes to one or more of those questions, you may have a nighttime subset of restless legs syndrome (RLS): periodic limb movements in sleep (PLMS), which bothers about 80 to 90 percent of people with RLS. RLS is a condition characterized by strange and unpleasant feelings in your legs (and possibly your arms) during the day—variously described as itching, tingling, burning, aching, creeping, crawling, or electric shocks—and the urge to move them.

If you have PLMS (which I'll abbreviate as RLS/PLMS, since the two conditions are usually found together), you probably wake up exhausted. Although you may be asleep at night, your legs are running a marathon!

The cause of RLS/PLMS is suspected to be a deficiency of the "pleasure/reward" brain chemical dopamine. Iron is critical for producing dopamine, and iron deficiency is a key trigger for RLS/PLMS. A deficiency of the mineral magnesium can also aggravate RLS/PLMS, as can a deficiency of adrenal and thyroid hormones.

The drug often prescribed for the problem is a very expensive medication called *ropinirole* (Requip). I never prescribe it. I don't think it's as effective as natural (or even other prescription) therapies for RLS/PLMS, and I'm concerned about its safety. Common side effects include nausea (in up to 40 percent of people who take it), excessive tiredness or somnolence (12 percent), vomiting (11 percent), dizziness (11 percent), and sore throat (9 percent). There's also a risk of addiction—not to the drug, but to impulsive activities such as gambling, shopping, and sex, because the drug may interfere with the inhibitory functions of the brain.

I think Requip is being prescribed mostly because it's expensive and profitable and therefore well publicized by drug companies—and *not* because it's uniquely effective.

Here are the remedies for RLS/PLMS that I think *are* effective.

•**Eat a sugar-free, high-protein diet, with a protein snack at bedtime.** Low blood sugar during the night can worsen the problem.

•**Take iron—it works better than Requip.** In a three-month study, RLS patients who were treated with iron had an 89 percent greater improvement than people taking a placebo—a level of improvement twice that usually seen with Requip. If your blood test for ferritin (the stored form of iron) is lower than 60, iron deficiency may be triggering your RLS/PLMS. (Some labs still ridiculously consider a ferritin level over 12 to be "normal." It's not.)

For RLS/PLMS, I recommend an iron supplement containing 25 milligrams to 30 milligrams of iron and at least 100 milligrams of vitamin C (which is also good for RLS/PLMS, and aids in the absorption of the iron). Take the iron and vitamin C combo on an empty stomach. Also take them six hours before or after you take thyroid medication (iron blocks its absorption). If you develop side effects from the iron, such as constipation, take the iron and C every other day.

•**Take magnesium.** A 200-milligram dose at bedtime can settle restless legs and help sleep.

•**Take vitamin E.** Vitamin E can help RLS, but it takes six to 10 weeks for the treatment to work. I recommend 400 IU daily of a natural "mixed tocopherol" form, which delivers many types of vitamin E compounds, and is more effective.

•**Consider folic acid.** Some cases of RLS (in which numbness and lightning stabs of pain are relieved by movement or local massage) are helped by five milligrams of folic acid, three times a day (an amount available by prescription). It didn't help people without those specific symptoms.

•**Consider the amino acid L-tryptophan.** Several case studies suggest that supplementing the diet with this amino acid may help, possibly because it boosts neurotransmitters that calm the nervous system.

•**Try 5-HTP.** I also recommend this tryptophan-boosting supplement for people with RLS/PLMS.

Caution: If you're taking antidepressants, talk to your doctor before taking 5-HTP. In rare cases, the two together could lead to dangerously high levels of the brain chemical serotonin.

•**Try medications.** If after two to three months these natural remedies don't work for RLS/PLMS, consider the medications *zolpidem* (Ambien), *gabapentin* (Neurontin), or *clonazepam* (Klonopin), all of which are highly effective for the problem. (Klonopin, however, can be addictive.)

If one of my patients with RLS/PLMS is taking Neurontin for insomnia, I work with them to increase the dose not only to get adequate sleep, but also to keep the bedcovers in place and stop kicking their partners.

•**Watch out for antidepressants and antihistamines.** They can worsen RLS/PLMS. If you're taking them, talk to your doctor about alternatives.

A Real Cure for Sleep Apnea

This condition is also called obstructive sleep apnea. That's because the soft tissue at the back of your throat (the soft palate) obstructs the airway during sleep, repeatedly cutting off your breathing and rousing you to a semi-awake state. As the sagging soft tissue vibrates, you snore. In severe sleep apnea, you can have more than a dozen episodes of breathlessness every hour throughout the night. Needless to say, you're exhausted during the day.

Sleep apnea is common among older, overweight men. And it's linked to a higher risk of heart disease, stroke, type 2 diabetes, depression, and erectile dysfunction—and a five-times-higher risk of dying from any cause. In fact, there's probably not a single condition that's not worsened by sleep apnea.

My recommendations...

•**Videotape yourself while you sleep.** A test for sleep apnea in a sleep lab is uncomfortable and time-consuming. (Though, on the upside, Medicare and most insurance companies cover the cost which is approximately $2,000.) An alternative is to simply videotape yourself for an hour or two while you sleep. Because if you're snoring and you stop breathing, you have sleep apnea. Or just ask your spouse. If you snore, are overweight, and fall asleep easily during the day—and your spouse says you stop breathing during the night—you have sleep apnea.

•**Ace apnea with a tennis ball.** If the video showed that you snore and that you stop breathing mostly when on your back, you can wear a tight pajama top or T-shirt at night with a tennis ball sewn into the area at the small of your back. This may help stop you from sleeping on your back, which may eliminate the problem.

•**Lose weight.** Overweight is the main cause of sleep apnea, and losing just 10 to 15 pounds may be enough to make it go away.

•**Ask your dentist about an oral appliance.** This mouthguard-like device, worn during sleep, adjusts your mouth and jaw in a way that helps keep your airway open. Over-the-counter versions are unlikely to work.

•**Ask your doctor about using a continuous positive airway pressure (CPAP) machine.** This small machine—typically about eight by six by three inches—generates a constant flow of pressurized air into a flexible tube connected to a strapped-on breathing mask. Studies show that for people with moderate or severe apnea (15 or more episodes of breathlessness per hour), CPAP cuts the episodes by about 75 percent. *A few science-proven tips to help make CPAP a more pleasant experience (many people who start using the device don't stick with it because of discomfort)...*

  •Humidify the bedroom.
  •Choose a nasal pillow mask rather than a full-mouth mask.
  •Consider an APAP (a device that pumps out air only when you're having an apnea episode).
  •Follow up with your sleep specialist in the first few weeks of CPAP therapy to help you make any needed adjustments in air pressure and the use of the mask.

Though folks with sleep apnea tend to take off the mask because it's uncomfortable, stay with it if you can. Your body will get used to it—and using CPAP at night will have you feeling much better during the day.

●**Ask your doctor about surgery.** A 20-minute outpatient surgery called Inspire, which internally stimulates airway muscles to keep them open, has been shown to be very effective for permanent relief of sleep apnea. Two other outpatient surgeries that can help with the problem include turbinate coblation, a 20-minute procedure that relieves breathing obstructions in both the soft palate and the nose; and laser tonsillectomy, a 20-minute procedure that reduces the size of the tonsils, which can obstruct breathing.

Relief from Night Sweats

Waking up with night sweats? *Consider these causes in addition to low estrogen or progesterone…*

1. Acid reflux. When this occurs during sleep, it can wake you with a sweat. To diagnose this, take a Pepcid at bedtime for two or three nights (no longer, because acid blockers are addictive and long-term use is dangerous). If the sweats stop, get a pillow wedge, and add ½ teaspoon of baking soda to four ounces of water and drink before bedtime to turn off stomach acid. (You don't need it during sleep.)
2. Low blood sugar. Eat a one-ounce protein snack at bedtime.
3. Candida or other infections. Clear any sinusitis (page 315), candida (page 181), or other infections.

Irritable Bowel Syndrome (Spastic Colon)

Real Causes

●**Digestive Difficulties.** Several different digestive problems can cause spastic colon. They include bowel infections, such as an overgrowth of the fungus *Candida albicans*; the inability to digest the sugars fructose and/or lactose; an infection with an intestinal parasite or small intestinal bacterial overgrowth (SIBO); food allergies; and gluten sensitivity and celiac disease (page 98).

●**Hormonal Imbalances.** Low levels of thyroid hormone can lead to an overgrowth of bacteria in the small intestine, which can cause symptoms mimicking spastic colon (page 84).

●**Happiness Deficiency.** Buried feelings—suppressed and unexpressed feelings about things that a person "can't stomach" or that are a "pain in the butt"—can surface as digestive ailments, including spastic colon (page 55).

An estimated 25 to 50 million Americans—two-thirds of them women—struggle with irritable bowel syndrome (IBS). A syndrome is a specific collection of symptoms with no known cause. Conventional medicine calls this problem "irritable bowel syndrome" because it doesn't have a clue as to the causes (though there's a lot of guesswork).

I prefer to call IBS by its older name, spastic colon, which I think is an accurate description of the condition, in which the muscles of the intestines spasm and cramp, causing abdominal pain, bloating, and gas. You might also be bothered in the bathroom, with either constipation or diarrhea, or an alternation of both.

Real Cure Regimen

The good news is that spastic colon has real causes—detectable and treatable causes. *The most common are…*

1. Food sensitivity to the lactose in milk or to the sugar fructose

2. Intestinal overgrowth of the yeast *Candida albicans*

3. Undiagnosed infection with an intestinal parasite or bacteria

4. Underactive thyroid, leading to a condition called SIBO (small intestine bacterial overgrowth)

5. Food allergy

6. Celiac disease, an autoimmune disease of the small intestine

7. Burying feelings in your gut

In my patients with spastic colon, I systematically test for and treat the possible causes of IBS. Let's look at those causes one by one. I start with a common and easily treatable cause: food sensitivity.

•**Food sensitivity: Cut out milk and fructose for 10 days.** In many people with spastic colon, the cause is not having enough of the enzymes needed to digest lactose in dairy products and/or fructose, the sugar that is a common ingredient in processed foods and beverages (particularly soda). To find out if you're sensitive, cut out lactose- and fructose-containing foods for 10 days. If your symptoms improve, drink two glasses of milk. If symptoms recur in the next one to two days, you're sensitive to lactose. If they don't, drink 16 ounces of orange juice or (ugh) non-diet soda. If symptoms recur, you're sensitive to fructose.

If lactose is the cause, cut down on or eliminate dairy products or add the enzyme lactase (for example, Lactaid) prior to eating or drinking them. If fructose is the cause, switch to fructose-free and stevia-sweetened diet sodas and other fructose-free foods.

•**Treat candida overgrowth.** If your symptoms don't resolve when you cut lactose and fructose out of your diet, the next step is finding out if you have an intestinal overgrowth of the yeast (fungus) *Candida albicans*, a common cause of spastic colon.

Unfortunately, there's no accurate test to distinguish a normal level of candida from an overgrowth. If a patient of mine with spastic colon also has other signs or symptoms of candida overgrowth, I treat this problem first (before testing for lactose/fructose sensitivity). *Signs include…*

●**Chronic sinusitis or nasal congestion** (which is usually caused by yeast overgrowth)

●**Food allergies** (a result of leaky gut syndrome, in which candida overgrowth damages the lining of the intestinal tract, allowing large, undigested food proteins into the bloodstream, where the immune system attacks them)

●**Chronic fatigue syndrome/fibromyalgia** (If you have either of these health problems, you can assume you also have candida overgrowth.)

●**Sugar addiction** (Sugar is yeast's favorite food, and cravings for sugar and other refined carbohydrates are often a sign of candida overgrowth.)

●**Recurrent canker sores** (inside the mouth, lasting for about 10 days)

●**A history of recurrent or long-term antibiotic use** (especially tetracycline for acne)

●**A history of long-term use of prednisone,** a corticosteroid used for inflammatory conditions such as asthma or rheumatoid arthritis

For the Real Cure Regimen, see Candida Overgrowth on page 181.

●**Test for and treat intestinal parasites.** Intestinal parasites are another little-recognized but surprisingly common cause of spastic colon. If the problem isn't food sensitivity or candida overgrowth, I test for parasites. If the test is positive, I treat with an antiparasite medication specific to the parasite. Parasite testing at standard laboratories is incredibly unreliable. It should be done at mail-away labs specializing in this, such as Genova or the Parasitology Center.

●**Check for SIBO (small intestine bacterial overgrowth).** In this condition, the relatively "sterile" small intestine (with billions of intestinal bacteria, rather than the trillions that live in the large intestine) is overgrown, with more than 10 times the normal number of bacteria.

The symptoms of SIBO are similar to spastic colon: abdominal pain and bloating, diarrhea and/or constipation, and excess gas. Achy muscles, fatigue, and hypothyroidism are also common among people with chronic SIBO.

If other tests and strategies haven't detected the cause and cleared up spastic colon, I may conduct a hydrogen breath test (HBT), which can detect SIBO.

A simpler approach? Remember in grade school, there would always be this one little kid who would pass "Silent-but-deadlies?" This smell is caused by bacterial overgrowth digesting the dietary protein in the small intestine, splitting off the sulfur. This is what causes the "rotten egg" smell. (Although candida can cause enough fermentation for you to fill up a hot air balloon, the gas usually doesn't have much of a smell. The sulfur smell usually suggests SIBO or parasites.)

Whether relying on smell or the HBT, if I diagnose a patient with SIBO, I begin treatment by putting them on an herbal mix called Ultra MFP Forte, from Douglas Labs. (The dose is two capsules, twice a day for one month, or one bottle's worth.) If this treatment doesn't clear up the smell and symptoms after a month, I next treat with the antibiotic *rifaximin* (Xifaxan), at a dose of 550 milligrams, three times a day, for 10 days. (Unfortunately, this is a ridiculously expensive

Is It IBS—Or a Bigger Problem?

Sometimes spastic colon is a symptom of a larger health issue. If you also have chronic fatigue or widespread muscle achiness and insomnia, it's likely you have chronic fatigue syndrome or fibromyalgia. (For more information on this, see Chronic Fatigue Syndrome and Fibromyalgia on page 189.) If your abdominal pain is worse around your period, you may have endometriosis, a condition in which the lining of the uterus starts growing outside the uterus; see your ob-gyn for an accurate diagnosis. In some cases, ovarian cancer is misdiagnosed as IBS (spastic colon) because the two share symptoms such as abdominal pain and bloating. However, in IBS those symptoms are intermittent while in ovarian cancer they are chronic and get worse over time. If your IBS symptoms don't come and go, see your ob-gyn for further testing, such as a pelvic exam and ultrasound.

---

drug, with the treatment costing well over $1,000.) I also look for and treat an underactive thyroid, a common cause of SIBO. (You can find the Real Cure Regimen for hypothyroidism on page 254.)

●**Detect and treat food allergies.** Maybe you've tried eliminating lactose and fructose… and treating candida infection…and testing for parasites…and testing for and treating SIBO—and none of them has worked. Your next step is to test for and eliminate *food allergies*. I recommend two methods: NAET and the multiple food elimination diet. (You can find a full discussion of these two methods in Food Allergy on page 227.)

●**Test for celiac disease.** In celiac disease, the protein gluten (found in wheat, rye, barley, and bulgur) triggers the immune system to attack and damage the lining of the small intestine. About one in 100 people in the general population has this genetic condition. But a study found that four in 100 people with IBS have it.

Your doctor can order a simple, insurance-covered test to diagnose celiac disease: an anti-transglutaminase IgA and IgG antibody blood test. If the test is positive, avoiding wheat and other gluten-containing foods should clear up the symptoms of spastic colon and also dramatically improve your general health.

Ask yourself: Am I burying my feelings? If you don't fully feel your feelings (a process I describe at length in Happiness Deficiency on page 55) they can bubble to the surface in the form of spastic colon. For an easy process to feel and release your feelings, see Happiness Deficiency on page 59.

Simple Symptom Relief

While you and your doctor are figuring out the cause of your spastic colon, use natural and over-the-counter remedies to relieve your symptoms.

●**For abdominal pain and gas: Take a peppermint oil supplement.** In a scientific paper titled "Peppermint Oil in Irritable Bowel Syndrome" in the journal *Phytomedicine*, researchers evaluated 16 studies on the remedy, involving 651 people. Some of the studies compared peppermint oil with a placebo; others compared peppermint oil with a conventional drug for IBS. Peppermint oil was very effective.

"Taking into account the currently available drug treatments for IBS, peppermint oil may be the drug of first choice in IBS patients with non-serious constipation or diarrhea to alleviate general symptoms and to improve quality of life," concluded the researchers. They recommend one or two 0.1-milligram capsules of enteric-coated peppermint oil, taken three times a day, for six months.

•**For bloating: Chew simethicone tablets.** This safe, effective drug changes the surface tension on gas bubbles, making it much easier for gas to pass, easing symptoms. It is available over the counter, under the brand names Mylanta One, Gas-X, Mylicon, Flatulex, and Phazyme. (Want to see it in action outside the body? *A fun trick*: Place a few drops onto the head of a glass of beer and see how quickly the beer loses its foam.)

•**For constipation: Take magnesium.** If constipation is a predominant symptom, this mineral is a natural laxative that can help relieve the problem. I recommend 200 milligrams to 300 milligrams daily.

•**Soothe your stress.** Researchers at the University of Washington in Seattle studied 229 women with and without IBS, tracking their stress levels and IBS symptoms for one month. Among women with IBS, higher levels of stress were linked to worsening IBS symptoms. "Gastrointestinal symptom distress is associated with self-reported stress in women with IBS," wrote the researchers in the journal *Nursing Research*. "The IBS treatment protocols that incorporate strategies that decrease stress and psychological distress (anxiety and depression) are likely to reduce GI symptoms." For more ways to relieve acute and chronic stress, see Happiness Deficiency (page 55).

Kidney Stones

Real Cause

•**Nutritional Deficiencies.** Low levels of magnesium and vitamin B_6 (*pyridoxine*) can increase the risk of kidney stones. So can low fluid intake. Other nutritional factors linked to an elevated risk of kidney stones include a high-sugar diet and a low intake of fruits and vegetables. Obesity is also a risk factor (page 3).

Your kidneys are filters—they pull toxins and other substances out of blood for disposal in the urine. But when some of those substances become too concentrated, they can crystallize and form kidney stones. Oftentimes, the stones just sit there. But if they begin to slide from the kidney into the ureter (the tube connecting the kidney to the bladder), they can cause excru-

Preventing the First Stone

Several studies show that there are many ways to decrease your risk of forming a first kidney stone. Not surprisingly, the recommendations are also good for overall health. (*Note*: Although some of this research was done solely with women or solely with men, I think it applies to both sexes.)

• **Reduce fructose.** Researchers from Harvard Medical School analyzed diet and health data from more than 200,000 people and found that those who had the highest intake of fructose—the sugar found in sodas and other foods with high-fructose corn syrup—had the highest risk of developing kidney stones. Fructose intake "may increase the urinary excretion of calcium oxalate, uric acid, and other factors associated with kidney stone risk," concluded the researchers in the medical journal *Kidney International*.

• **Cut sucrose, too.** In another study, the same researchers found that women with the highest intake of sucrose—sugar—had a 31 percent higher risk of stones.

• **Eat more whole grains, beans, nuts, and seeds.** These foods are rich in a plant compound called phytate, and the Harvard researchers found that women with the highest intake of phytate had a 37 percent lower risk of stones. "Dietary phytate may be a new, important, and safe addition to our options for stone prevention," they concluded in the *Annals of Internal Medicine*.

• **Drink plenty of fluids.** Drinking more fluid of any kind is linked to a 38 percent reduction in stone risk, reported researchers in the *Annals of Internal Medicine*. For every eight-ounce daily serving, the researchers found a 10 percent lower risk with caffeinated coffee, a nine percent lower risk with decaffeinated coffee, an eight percent lower risk with tea, and a 59 percent lower risk with wine. "An increase in total fluid intake can reduce the risk of kidney stones," they concluded.

• **Maximize magnesium-rich foods.** Men with the highest magnesium intake had a 29 percent lower risk of stones, reported Harvard researchers in the *Journal of the American Society of Nephrology*. Leafy green vegetables such as spinach, Swiss chard, and mustard greens are among the richest sources of magnesium.

• **Consider trying the DASH diet.** The DASH (Dietary Approaches to Stop Hypertension) diet is used to treat high blood pressure. It includes eight to 10 servings of fruits and vegetables a day, several servings of low-fat dairy products, and minimal red meat. Research showed that those who followed a DASH diet—rich in calcium, potassium, magnesium, and vitamin C—had up to a 40 percent reduced risk of forming stones, compared with those who didn't follow the diet. "Consumption of a DASH diet is associated with a marked decrease in kidney stone risk," concluded the researchers in the *Journal of the American Society of Nephrology*.

• **Don't gain weight.** Obese men had a 33 percent higher risk of kidney stones than normal-weight men, and obese women had more than double the risk, reported researchers from Harvard Medical School in the *Journal of the American Medical Association*. "Obesity and weight gain increase the risk of kidney stone formation," they concluded.

ciating pain, usually in the midback on the left or right side, radiating to the front of the body in the pelvic area. (Some women say it's worse than the pain of childbirth.)

Real Cure Regimen

If you've had one kidney stone, you definitely don't want another. But 40 percent of people who've had a first stone do have another symptom-causing stone within 15 years.

Many doctors prescribe potassium citrate, which alkalinizes the urine, making it slightly less likely for stones to form. But the treatment can cause nausea and diarrhea—not exactly ideal for long-term use. The good news: Prevention of a second kidney stone is simple.

Take magnesium (200 milligrams to 400 milligrams daily) and vitamin B_6 (10 milligrams to 25 milligrams daily). In several studies, this nutritional regimen decreased the recurrence of new calcium-based kidney stones (which most are) by an astounding 90 percent.

A good way to get these two nutrients is with the Energy Revitalization System multinutrient powder, discussed in Nutritional Deficiencies on page 30. It supplies 200 milligrams of magnesium and 85 milligrams of B_6. Take another 200 milligrams of magnesium with dinner. The stone-preventing power of the mineral may increase when you take it with a meal.

●**Drink plenty of water.** This keeps your urine diluted, making it less likely that calcium and oxalate (the two compounds that form most stones) will crystallize.

●**When life hands you a kidney stone, make lemonade.** You might want to add some lemon juice to that water. Lemons contain the chemical citrate, which inhibits the formation of stones. In fact, when researchers at the Comprehensive Kidney Stone Center at Duke University Medical Center studied people with chronic stone problems on nearly four years of "lemonade therapy," they found that their average level of stone formation dropped from one stone per year to 0.13, according to a study in the *Journal of Urology*.

●**Don't worry about calcium.** Many doctors tell their patients with kidney stones to cut their intake of calcium. After all, most stones are partly made of calcium, so reducing dietary intake of the mineral seems to make sense. But it's wrong-minded advice.

When researchers at Creighton University in Nebraska analyzed worldwide data on diet and stone risk, they found that "most of the studies show no increase in stone risk with high calcium intake (from either diet or supplements)." In fact, they pointed out, there is a lot of scientific evidence showing that high calcium intake decreases stone risk (probably by decreasing the amount of oxalate in the urine).

●**As a last resort, pay attention to oxalates.** If you have chronic stone problems, you may want to reduce your intake of high-oxalate foods and beverages: tea, coffee, beans, nuts, chocolate, red meat, spinach, kale, collard greens, beets, and rhubarb. However, because these foods (except red meat) are otherwise so healthful, limit them *only if* all the other treatments in my Real Cure Regimen for kidney stones have failed and stones have recurred.

Macular Degeneration

Real Cause

- **Nutritional Deficiencies.** Several nutritional compounds—such as the pigments lutein and zeaxanthin, found in colorful vegetables and eggs; and the omega-3 fatty acids, found in fish oil—have been shown to help prevent and treat the disease (page 28).

Macular degeneration is the number-one cause of vision loss and blindness in seniors, dimming the eyesight of 20 percent of Americans ages 65 to 74, and 35 percent over 75. It's not hard to see why.

The retina is the gatekeeper of vision—the lining of cells at the back of the eyeball that first translates light into electrical signals, and then funnels those signals into the optic nerve for transmission to the brain. In the center of the retina is the macula, the retinal cells that are responsible for your ability to focus, to see precisely and with detail.

As you age, the arteries that supply the retina and macula with oxygen and nutrients can begin to harden. The result is a condition called age-related macular degeneration (ARMD): the gradual destruction of the cells of the macula. Symptoms range from blurry, darkened vision in early-stage ARMD, to the loss of all central vision (while still retaining peripheral vision) in advanced ARMD. ARMD can strike slowly (some people notice very little change in their vision) or quickly (which can then lead to a loss of vision in both eyes).

Top risk factors for ARMD include aging (increased risk starts around the age of 55); having blue, green, or hazel eyes (which allow in more macula-damaging ultraviolet rays from the sun); frequent exposure to sunlight without sunglasses; and smoking.

Wet and Dry ARMD

Ninety percent of cases of ARMD are *dry* ARMD—the gradual destruction of the macula and loss of central vision. But 10 percent are *wet* ARMD. The body sometimes responds to macular degeneration by growing new and fragile blood vessels behind the retina. These flimsy vessels can leak blood (hence the name wet), causing rapid loss of central vision in one eye.

Symptoms of wet ARMD include: The sudden and worsening development of distorted vision, such as wavy or crooked lines; objects appearing lopsided or smaller than they are; and blurry or blind spots. If you suddenly develop any of these symptoms, see an eye doctor immediately. Laser surgery can repair the leaking blood vessels. However, it's much more effective to prevent this problem before a severe retinal bleed occurs, by using the Real Cure Regimen in this chapter.

Real Cure Regimen

As we said above, ARMD is an arterial problem, like heart disease. And as with heart disease, you can use a whole-foods diet and nutritional supplements to prevent and slow the cellular oxidation and chronic inflammation that are damaging the arteries that feed the eyes. *There are many nutritional and natural strategies that can help prevent or slow ARMD...*

●**Eat more fruits and vegetables.** People who eat three or more servings of fruit a day are 36 percent less likely to develop ARMD, reported researchers at Harvard Medical School in the *Archives of Ophthalmology.* Colorful, antioxidant-rich berries—blueberries, strawberries, blackberries—are best. In another study, Dutch researchers found that eating two to three servings of vegetables a day, and two daily servings of fruit (along with eating fish twice a week) lowered the risk of ARMD by 42 percent.

●**Eat eggs.** They supply plenty of lutein and zeaxanthin, two carotenoids that act like internal sunglasses, protecting the cells of the macula. And make sure you eat the yolks! That's where the nutrients live. Research from the 10-year Blue Mountains Eye Study of nearly 4,000 people showed that those with the highest intake of lutein and zeaxanthin had a 65 percent lower risk of ARMD. The two nutrients are also found in dark green, orange and yellow vegetables, including broccoli, Brussels sprouts, carrots, corn, green beans, green peas, kale, mustard greens, parsley, pumpkin, spinach, squash, and yams.

Important: Studies show that eating eggs every day has no effect on blood cholesterol levels, yet the myth persists that eggs cause high cholesterol. Eat eggs without guilt. They're nature's perfect protein and protect your eyes.

●**Eat fatty fish (salmon, albacore tuna, sardines, mackerel, herring, lake trout) or take fish oil.** These are rich in omega-3 fatty acids, which calm inflammation and boost circulation. (The omega-3 fatty acid DHA is also a major component of retinal cells.) A study in the *Archives of Ophthalmology* involving nearly 89,000 people linked a high intake of omega-3s with a 38 percent reduction in advanced ARMD; eating fish twice a week was linked to a 24 percent reduction in early-stage ARMD. And when researchers at the National Eye Institute of the National Institutes of Health studied 12 years of diet and health data from nearly 2,000 people with macular degeneration, they found that those with the highest intake of omega-3s were 32 percent less likely to develop the advanced form of the disease. (You can read more about fish oil in Nutritional Deficiencies on page 28.)

●**Reduce sugar and white flour.** Researchers at the Laboratory for Nutrition and Vision Research at Tufts University in Boston found that people who ate more refined carbohydrates had a higher risk of developing ARMD. "Many cases of ARMD could be prevented if individuals ate a diet rich in unrefined carbohydrates," said study author Allen Taylor, PhD.

●**Take an eye-protecting supplement.** I recommend OcuDyne II, from NutriCology, a multivitamin-mineral supplement that also supplies a range of nutrients that may help prevent or slow the disease, such as lutein and zeaxanthin.

I also recommend that people with newly diagnosed ARMD take the following nutrients. (Some of them are in lower dosages in OcuDyne II.)

•Bilberry (25 percent extract): 40 milligrams to 80 milligrams, three times daily. (Ocu-Dyne II supplies 20 milligrams.)

•Zinc: 25 milligrams to 50 milligrams daily. (OcuDyne II supplies 25 milligrams.) (Research published in the *Archives of Ophthalmalogy* links high zinc intake to a 25 percent lower risk of ARMD. And in a six-month study from researchers at the Retinal Institute of New Orleans of 40 people with ARMD, those who took 25 milligrams of zinc twice daily had clearer vision, according to results in the journal *Current Eye Research*.)

•Vitamin C: 1,000 milligrams, three times daily. (OcuDyne II contains 200 milligrams.)

•Vitamin E: 600 IU daily, of natural mixed tocopherols. (OcuDyne II contains approximately a total of 170 IU of mixed tocopherals.)

•Selenium: 200 micrograms daily. (OcuDyne II contains 100 micrograms.)

•B complex: 50 milligrams daily. (In a study of more than 5,000 women, taking a daily supplement containing 50 milligrams of B_6, along with 2.5 milligrams of folic acid and 1 milligram of B_{12}, lowered the risk of developing ARMD by 34 percent; the results were in the *Archives of Internal Medicine*.) (OcuDyne II supplies a range of B vitamins. To reach the optimal therapeutic levels, take a "B50" supplement. The two together will supply the levels I'm recommending.) Note that regular doses of vitamin B_6 over 45 mg a day can aggravate neuropathy. You can avoid this by using the pyridoxal 5 phosphate (P5P) form of the vitamin.

•Ginkgo biloba (24 percent extract): 40 to 80 milligrams, three times daily. (OcuDyne II supplies 30 milligrams.)

•**Avoid heavy drinking.** A study from the University of Wisconsin School of Medicine shows that men who have four or more alcoholic drinks a day have a nine-times-greater risk of developing ARMD. Moderate drinking—no more than one drink a day for women and two a day for men—does not increase risk. If you drink moderately, red wine is protective, but beer can worsen ARMD.

•**Quit smoking.** A study by researchers at the Jules Stein Eye Institute of the David Geffen School of Medicine at UCLA showed that smokers in their seventies and eighties have more than a five times (549 percent) greater risk of developing ARMD. This study "reinforces recommendations to quit smoking, even for older individuals," concluded the researchers in the *American Journal of Ophthalmology*.

•**Protect your eyes.** Ultraviolet (UV) rays from the sun can damage the macula. Protect your eyes with sunglasses that have UV protection—look for lenses with a UV400 rating, which blocks out most of the damaging rays.

•**Make reading easier.** If you have ARMD, these two tips will help you read…

•Shine the light directly on your reading material. This improves the contrast and makes the print easier to see.

•Use a handheld magnifier. A cheap drugstore magnifier dramatically increases print size. If you're reading on a computer or tablet, increase the print size there, too.

Male Menopause
(Testosterone Deficiency)

Real Cause

• **Hormonal Imbalances.** A decrease in testosterone is normal in aging men, but in some men the drop causes a wide range of physical, mental, and emotional problems (page 92).

Testosterone is practically synonymous with manhood. Manufactured by the testes, it endows a man with muscles, strength, a deep voice, a beard, the ability to have erections and the sex drive to use them, and even what I would call "life drive"—the enthusiasm, energy, and interest to encounter and enjoy every day.

I discuss the health-enhancing powers of testosterone at length in Hormonal Imbalances on page 92. There, I describe how testosterone levels in men can decline in middle age, producing symptoms such as fatigue, depression, loss of motivation, irritability, poor concentration, memory loss, vague aches and pains, extra fat around the middle, low libido, and erectile dysfunction. Low testosterone can also increase the risk of heart disease, high blood pressure, high cholesterol, and diabetes. It can even shorten life.

I also describe how the standard medical test for testosterone levels is inaccurate—with so-called normal ranges that are often absurdly low—and how to make sure you get an accurate, actionable test result.

And I debunk the mistaken but widely held notion that testosterone treatments increase the risk of getting prostate cancer. The scientific literature is clear on this point: Testosterone does not increase the risk.

In this chapter, I'll describe how I treat middle-aged men who have too-low testosterone, using a natural, bioidentical, safe form of the hormone.

Real Cure Regimen

If your testosterone level is low, I recommend talking to your doctor about using a topical testosterone cream or gel, applying 25 milligrams to 100 milligrams to your skin daily. You can get the medication (AndroGel or Testim, one percent gel) from a regular pharmacy. It is expensive ($6 a day for a 50-milligram dose) but is often covered by prescription insurance.

The good news: You can get a testosterone cream from a compounding pharmacy, which creates customized medications on-site. A compounded version of the drug is much less expensive but just as effective. This is an excellent option for those without prescription insurance that covers testosterone. (You can find a list of compounding pharmacies I trust in Resources on page 360. I usually use Women's International Pharmacy, which has excellent quality and lowest prices for customized hormone prescriptions; and yes, they do serve both men and women.)

Caution: Wash your hands after applying the gel or cream to your skin. If you don't wash them before touching someone else—such as your spouse—she can develop a high, unsafe blood level of testosterone.

It's best to apply the testosterone in an area that's least likely to come in contact with anyone else, such as your thighs, and use a different spot each day. And apply it at a time of day when that area is likely to be covered, such as in the morning before you get dressed. Allow it to dry before putting on your clothes. Don't shower for five to six hours after applying it or you may wash it off. A simple approach would be to apply it at bedtime and put on your pajamas.

Why don't I recommend taking a testosterone pill or capsule by mouth? Because oral testosterone goes straight to the liver, where cholesterol is made, and can increase cholesterol levels. Injections are another option. But this delivery method causes testosterone to shoot up for a few days after the injection and then plummet a week later. (Riding a hormone like a roller coaster is no fun.) All in all, I consider topical skin cream to be the best approach. In fact, rather than increasing cholesterol, it decreases it—lowering the risk of heart disease.

Adjusting the Dose

Stay in touch with your doctor after beginning treatment with testosterone, adjusting your daily dose to the level that feels best—the level that gives you the most energy, brightest mood, clearest thinking, level of sexual desire that feels right to you, etc. Most men feel best with a blood level around the 70th percentile of normal range, and that's what I aim for in my patients, if it can be achieved with a dose no higher than 100 milligrams a day.

Caution: Too high a dose can initially cause a bit of a "libido high," but your body adapts to the extra testosterone by increasing a type of protein that binds to testosterone and makes it inactive. Sometimes, men then try to "chase the feeling" by pushing the dose higher and higher—*not* a good idea! Over time, doctors who treat their patients with bioidentical hormones (including bioidentical testosterone) are finding that lower doses may be more effective than higher doses. For testosterone, I now usually aim for a dose of 25 milligrams to 50 milligrams a day, quite a bit lower than the 75-milligram to 100-milligram doses used in the past. Once you're at the 50-milligram dose, if your blood level of testosterone is not too high (in which case the dose should be lowered), it's reasonable to stay at this dose and go no higher.

Starting with a lower dose is also prudent for the heart. Like exercise, testosterone is *very* heart-healthy—and addressing testosterone deficiency lowers the risk of high blood pressure, high cholesterol, and diabetes, a major risk factor for heart disease. But also like exercise, starting testosterone can "unmask" hidden heart disease—which is perhaps one reason why a study in the *Journal of the American Medical Association* found an increased risk of heart attack and stroke in men using testosterone (although other studies have shown the opposite). I address this potential "risk" by starting with a low dose of 25 to 50 milligrams daily, and increase it as is comfortable for my patient.

If I start seeing a patient who has been using the higher dose—to which his body has adapted over time—I counsel him to slowly lower the dose, if he comfortably can. If he can't, I leave him at the 75- to 100-milligram dose.

Similarly, you and your doctor want to make sure your blood levels don't exceed the upper limit of normal, which can cause problems such as acne. Fifty may be the new 30, but I don't think you want to be a teenager again! I suggest seeing a holistic practitioner for treatment with bioidentical testosterone, as they are usually the doctors most familiar with bioidentical hormones and the most up-to-date treatment recommendations.

As I just wrote, I like to begin treatment with the cream, to make sure I find a dose that feels good to the patient. But if the cream works well, I recommend my patient change delivery methods—to testosterone pellets, which are inserted under the skin every four to six months. This delivers a very stable level of testosterone, with less risk of prostate enlargement.

Many holistic doctors are qualified to treat with pellets. You can find one near you at Biote.com, using the "Find A Provider" function on the home page.

Monitoring Side Effects

As with any drug, testosterone isn't risk free, but those using it properly are likely to be healthier. In fact, I suspect the main "side effect" of using testosterone properly (along with the overall approach to health described in this book) will be that you die very "young"—very late in life!

Nonetheless, side effects can occur. These are usually from dosing at too-high levels. They are uncommon, and when they do happen, they are easily managed. High blood levels of testosterone can cause elevated blood counts (hematocrit) in a complete blood count (CBC) test; liver inflammation; and a decreased sperm count and male infertility (usually reversible). So, if you're taking testosterone, your doctor may monitor not only your testosterone level, but also your CBC (a hematocrit over 48 suggests lowering the testosterone dose) and perhaps liver enzyme tests.

At the same time, your doctor may order a PSA (prostate-specific antigen) test to check for elevated levels, which could indicate prostate cancer. As I point out in "Testosterone Doesn't Increase the Risk of Prostate Cancer" in Hormonal Imbalances on page 93, supplemental testosterone is *not* a risk factor for prostate cancer (as is mistakenly thought by many doctors). In fact, men with low testosterone have a *higher* risk of prostate cancer. However, if prostate cancer is present, I don't prescribe testosterone, and would certainly stop the treatment if my patient were diagnosed with the disease.

Your body can convert testosterone to two other hormones: DHT (dihydrotestosterone) and estrogen. Your doctor may also monitor the levels of these hormones. If DHT levels rise too high (an uncommon result), they can cause prostate enlargement and a worsening of male-pattern baldness. If estrogen levels rise too high, breast size can increase and erections may decrease. Both elevated DHT or elevated estrogen may suggest the need to lower the testosterone dose. If lowering the dose doesn't work, these problems can also be addressed with medications. If DHT is high, talk to your doctor about taking the DHT-blocking medication *finasteride* (Proscar) at a dose of 2.5 milligrams to 5 milligrams daily. If estrogen is high, talk to your doctor about adding the medication *anastrozole* (Arimidex) at a dosage of 0.5 milligram, every other day.

If you're taking thyroid supplements, testosterone can cause elevated thyroid hormone levels. If you develop a racing heart or anxious and "hyper" feelings after starting to take testosterone, stop the testosterone and consult your physician immediately. The doctor can restart the testosterone at a lower dose while adjusting your thyroid hormone dose if levels are high. (This isn't an issue unless you're taking the thyroid hormone; testosterone on its own won't raise your thyroid hormone levels.)

Menopausal Problems

Real Cause

- **Hormonal Imbalances.** Menopause is a natural phenomenon, but falling estrogen levels can cause uncomfortable symptoms that a woman may want to address (page 94).

If you've turned to this chapter looking for solutions to the most common problems of menopause—such as hot flashes, night sweats, insomnia, depression, mood swings, memory loss, low libido, and painful intercourse—please begin by reading the relevant section in Hormonal Imbalances on page 94. *There you find information about…*

- **The many distressing symptoms of perimenopause** (when the length of the menstrual cycle starts to change and there are missed menses) and menopause (12 months after your final period)

- **Why falling levels of estrogen cause those symptoms,** and the role played by progesterone

- **The deadly toxicity of conventional treatment for menopausal problems:** synthetic versions of estrogen and progesterone

- **The safety and effectiveness of natural, bioidentical estrogen and progesterone, exact replicas of the chemical structure of your own hormones**

- **The regimen of bioidentical hormones I prescribe for most of my perimenopausal and postmenopausal patients seeking relief from menopausal symptoms**

- **The many benefits of taking bioidentical hormones,** from relief of menopausal symptoms to protection against heart disease

Real Cure Regimen

In this chapter, I'll present a summary of the regimen presented there, along with a few more ideas for dealing with the discomforts of menopause.

Remember, however, that menopause is not an illness, any more than puberty is. If you feel comfortable weathering the change, it's fine to simply ignore the symptoms or live with them. The time to consider addressing symptoms is if they are uncomfortable. Some women also find that they feel and look younger on the bioidentical hormones, and prefer them for this reason as well. Whether you prefer to simply add more edamame to your diet (a rich source of phytoestrogens, as discussed on page 293)…or take a hormone-balancing herb…or take bioidentical hormones…or simply live with the changes…it's always a personal preference. There is no right or wrong answer for the process of menopause. Choose the options that feel best to you, for as long as they feel best to you. Trust your feelings, and what your body is telling you.

Take Bioidentical Hormones

The main treatment I use in my perimenopausal and menopausal patients is the bioidentical estrogen hormone Biest, along with natural progesterone. (Progesterone is like your body's natural Valium, helping you to stay calm and fall asleep.) These hormones are compounded into a cream by a compounding pharmacy, which makes customized medications on-site. I find that Women's International Pharmacy, which supplies bioidentical hormone creams by prescription, has excellent quality and lowest prices. You can find their contact info in Resources on page 360.

(Of course, you can use a regular pharmacy. The pharmaceutical companies have found that women prefer bioidentical hormones, so bioidentical estrogen is now also available from your regular pharmacy, and may be covered by insurance. These are delivered in estrogen patches, all of which now have bioidentical estradiol. Unfortunately, the patch has only one of the two major estrogens found in Biest—estradiol; in the future, I hope the patches will combine both. The biggest problem with the patches: they tend not to stay on when you sweat. Now, back to the compounded cream…)

If you're comfortable doing so, I strongly recommend you use the vaginal cream rather than the skin cream. Why? In my patients, I'm finding that after about a year of treatment the skin stops absorbing the cream—and it stops working. (Make sure to read the product insert—and follow the directions and cautions. They include precautions such as washing your hands before and after application, and not having sexual intercourse right after using the medicines so you won't expose your partner to estrogen.)

If you find your body likes the hormones, then consider switching to estrogen pellets (often combined with testosterone), which are inserted under the skin three to four times a year. These work wonderfully, and give very stable blood levels. You can take the progesterone by mouth. Bioidentical progesterone is now available from regular pharmacies under the name Prometrium 100 mg. If you're on estrogen, it's critical to take daily progesterone to prevent uterine cancer. You can take doses of up to 400 milligrams a day, although for most women the

New Research on the Natural Treatment of Menopause

Although I would begin your personal treatment with bioidentical hormones and edamame, if more hormonal support is needed, you can consider any of the following remedies…

●**Omega-3s—for hot flashes.** Canadian researchers studied 91 women with hot flashes (an average of 2.8 a day), giving half the women a supplement of the omega-3 fatty acid EPA (eicosapentaenoic acid). Those taking EPA had an average decline of 1.6 hot flashes a day; there was an average decline of 0.5 in the placebo group.

●**Red clover extract—for anxiety and depression.** In a three-month study of 109 menopausal women, a red clover extract (with phytoestrogen-rich isoflavones) of 80 milligrams decreased anxiety by 76 percent and depression by 78 percent, reported Austrian researchers in the journal *Maturitas*.

●**Hops extract—for hot flashes and other symptoms.** In a four-month study of 36 menopausal women, a standardized extract of hops—also rich in phytoestrogens—reduced hot flashes and other menopausal symptoms, reported Finnish researchers in the journal *Phytomedicine*. "Phytoestrogen preparations containing standardized hops extract may provide an interesting alternative to women seeking relief of mild" menopause symptoms, they wrote. Take between 30 and 120 milligrams of hops flower extract (6.6:1) each night.

●**Black cohosh—for hot flashes, mood swings, depression, and low libido.** In a three-month study of 122 menopausal women, those who took 40 milligrams a day of black cohosh had improvements in a wide range of menopausal symptoms, reported Spanish researchers in the journal *Gynecological Endocrinology*. Use only the Remifemin brand (others don't work).

●**St. John's wort (Hypericum)—for hot flashes.** In a two-month study of 100 perimenopausal and menopausal women, those who took the herb St. John's wort (often used for depression) had a significant decrease in the daily number of hot flashes, reported Iranian researchers in the journal *Menopause*. A combination product that contains black cohosh, hops, and St. John's wort that I like is Woman's Passage Menopause Support, from Vitanica (at Vitanica.com, or call 800-572-4712).

●**Chasteberry (Vitex) and St. John's wort—for PMS-like symptoms of perimenopause.** In a four-month study of 14 women in "late perimenopause" with PMS-like symptoms (including bloating, carbohydrate cravings, anxiety, and depression), this herbal combination significantly reduced symptoms, reported Australian researchers in the *Journal of Alternative and Complementary Medicine*.

●**Soy isoflavones—for hot flashes and night sweats, fatigue, low libido, and painful intercourse.** In a study of 93 menopausal women, with an average age of 56, those who took 160 milligrams a day of phytoestrogen-rich soy isoflavones had significant improvements in hot flashes and night sweats, fatigue, low libido, and painful intercourse. "The use of isoflavones, as an alternative to estrogen therapy, may be potentially useful and seemingly safe in…women who are looking for relief from menopausal symptoms," concluded researchers from the Johns Hopkins University School of Medicine in the *Journal of Endocrinological Investigation*.

100-milligram dose is fine. (100 milligrams of oral Prometrium equals 30 mg of progesterone cream.)

When should you begin taking these hormones? Standard blood testing doesn't detect estrogen or progesterone deficiency until you've been deficient for five to 12 years. If you have decreased vaginal lubrication, and your sleep, energy, and mental clarity are worse around your periods, there's a good chance that your hormones are low and that bioidentical hormones will help. As I often say: Treat the patient, not the test.

Consider Testosterone, Too

I've found that a deficiency of testosterone in perimenopausal and menopausal (and other) women can cause problems similar to those caused by low testosterone in middle-aged men: fatigue, depression, osteoporosis, weight gain, muscle achiness, and low libido. As with men, I test for low free-testosterone levels (not total testosterone, which measures the inactive, storage form of the hormone). If levels are low, I treat with a testosterone cream made by a compounding pharmacy. The usual dose is 0.5 milligrams to 2 milligrams a day. (As with estrogen and progesterone, we are finding that lower doses than those used in the past are equally effective.) With this dosing, most menopausal women notice they have more energy, thicker hair, younger skin, and an improved libido.

If you also are taking estrogen and progesterone, the compounding pharmacy can combine the three hormones in one cream, for ease of application and lower cost. (As I pointed out above, if you're taking estrogen and testosterone, consider pellets. Their downside is that they're more expensive than the cream. But if the cost isn't prohibitive for you, explore this option with your doctor.)

Natural Relief for Symptoms

In addition to bioidentical hormones, you can try these herbal and dietary approaches to soothing menopausal symptoms.

•**Try black cohosh.** Black cohosh stabilizes the functioning of the autonomic nervous system, which regulates temperature, and can decrease hot flashes and night sweats. I prefer Remifemin, from Nature's Way, a black cohosh product that has been proven effective in dozens of studies. Take two capsules, two times daily, for two months (it takes two months to see the full effect). After that, you can usually lower the dose to one capsule twice daily.

•**Eat more edamame.** More commonly known as soybean pods, this tasty food is a standard appetizer in Japanese restaurants. You can find it in the frozen food section of most supermarkets and health food stores. Edamame is rich in phytoestrogens, a weaker, plant-based version of estrogen. Eating a handful a day raises your estrogen levels naturally. It's the dietary approach traditionally used by Japanese women to manage menopause symptoms. (Eat the pea-like beans that are inside the pod, not the pod itself.)

Nerve Pain (Neuropathy)

Real Causes

- **Nutritional Deficiencies.** Low levels of vitamins B_6 and B_{12} can damage nerves, causing pain (page 12).

- **Prescription Medications.** Chemotherapy for cancer can injure nerves (page 70).

- **Hormonal Imbalances.** Low levels of thyroid hormone can hurt nerves (page 87).

- **Diabetes.** It's the leading cause of neuropathy—because chronically high levels of blood sugar destroy nerves (page 210).

One of the most torturous types of chronic pain—and one of the most poorly treated by most physicians—is nerve pain, or neuropathy.

Those who have nerve pain describe it as burning, stabbing, and shooting (often to distant areas, as in sciatica, where pain from the back shoots down the legs). It has an "electric" quality, like a shock. There might be numbness and tingling. In some cases, the pain is constant—it doesn't go away, no matter what you do or don't do. The chronic pain can also trigger a problem called central sensitization, in which the "wiring" of the nerves and brain becomes overstimulated and the pain is amplified in the brain. In other cases, even the slightest touch—for example, the pressure of clothes on the skin—causes pain, a phenomenon called allodynia.

The good news is that nerve pain is very treatable! Just because your doctor hasn't helped you doesn't mean you can't be helped.

And that's good news for a lot of people. An estimated 33 million Americans suffer from neuropathic pain, according to a study in the *Journal of Pain Research*. Why so many of us? Because so many different health problems can damage nerves.

Let's start down the road to relief by looking at the most common causes of nerve pain—each of which is either preventable or treatable.

- **Diabetes.** The decreased circulation, high blood sugar, nutritional deficiencies, and toxic by-products of diabetes damage the nerves of an estimated 50 percent of people with the disease, a complication called diabetic neuropathy. This is the most common kind of nerve pain. (You can read more about treatments for diabetes and diabetic neuropathy in Diabetes on page 210.)

- **Shingles.** Herpes zoster, the virus that causes chickenpox, never exits the body: It hibernates in your nerves. Later in life, it can cause the rash known as shingles, damaging nerves and leading to postherpetic neuralgia (PHN). This type of nerve pain will strike one in three Americans during their lifetimes, most of them over the age of 60. (You can read more about treatments for shingles and PHN in Shingles on page 313.)

Testing for the Causes of Nerve Pain

It's important for your doctor to determine if your nerve pain has a treatable cause. *Any medical workup for nerve pain should include...*

- **A complete blood count and an inflammation/sedimentation rate**
- **Thyroid testing, with Free T4 and TSH tests**
- **A blood test for vitamin B$_{12}$ levels**
- **Screening for diabetes, with a morning fasting blood sugar and a glycosylated hemoglobin (HgBA1C)**

The medical history should find out if there is excessive alcohol use (which can cause a nerve-damaging B vitamin deficiency), treatment with medications that can cause nerve injury, or a family history of neuropathy.

With test results and a medical history in hand, the doctor can put together a strategy for addressing and correcting any underlying causes of nerve pain.

- **Pinched nerve.** A ruptured disk in your spinal column can pinch a nerve in your back, causing the radiating pain called sciatica. In another condition, tissues can swell in your wrist, pinching a nerve and causing the hand and arm pain called carpal tunnel syndrome. (You can read more about treatments for these in Back Pain on page 167 and Carpal Tunnel Syndrome on page 186.)

- **Chemotherapy and radiation.** An estimated 40 percent of cancer patients suffer pain from nerves damaged by chemotherapy and/or radiation. In some cases, the cancer itself can also compress nerves. (You can read more about cancer and supportive therapies for people undergoing chemotherapy and radiation in Cancer on page 174.)

- **Hypothyroidism.** Low levels of thyroid hormone can hurt your nerves. (You can read more about accurate tests and effective treatments for hypothyroidism in "Hypothyroidism: Millions of Missed Diagnoses" in Hormonal Imbalances on page 87, and in Hypothyroidism on page 254.)

- **Nutritional deficiencies.** Healthy nerves depend on B vitamins. Deficiencies, particularly of B$_6$ and/or B$_{12}$, can cause neuropathy. Other nutritional deficiencies can also play a role. (On the other hand, regular doses of vitamin B$_6$ over 45 milligrams a day can aggravate neuropathy. You can avoid this by using the pyridoxal 5 phosphate (P5P) form of the vitamin.)

- **Drug side effects.** Various drugs can cause neuropathy, including the antibiotic *metronidazole* (Flagyl) and drugs used to treat AIDS.

Real Cure Regimen

With so many causes of nerve pain and so many people afflicted by the problem, you'd think doctors would have a handle on how to control it. Unfortunately, most physicians aren't trained to treat the problem effectively.

Controlling Side Effects

Some people feel they can't tolerate any pain medications because of the side effects. What's happening? Well, in their understandable hurry to achieve pain relief, people often start at too high a dose too quickly, get side effects, and stop the medication.

Here's the amazing physiological fact that can help you stop those side effects: Your body usually "adapts" to eliminate the side effects from most nonnarcotic pain medications, while still allowing them to achieve their pain-relieving benefits. So if you get side effects from a pain medication, simply lower the dose to a level at which they subside, and then slowly raise the dose to a level at which the pain is relieved. You'll find you can do so without the side effects. To achieve this type of effect, I often mix lower doses of several pain medications, allowing more benefit with fewer side effects.

You might receive a prescription for an anti-inflammatory medication such as *ibuprofen* (Motrin, Advil), which probably won't work. Or the doctor might prescribe a narcotic, which will work but probably not very well.

But as I said earlier, just because doctors aren't trained in managing nerve pain doesn't mean you have to be in pain. It's worth repeating: Nerve pain is very treatable! The very first thing to do for any type of nerve pain is to start the process of healing your damaged nerves. The way to do that: Optimize your intake of nerve-protecting, nerve-repairing nutrients.

Nerve-Healing Nutrients

Yes, these nutrients can actually help heal nerves (not just temporarily mask nerve pain). But nerves don't heal overnight. You'll need to take these remedies for three to 12 months to see their full effect. Hang in there: I think you'll be amazed at how much relief they provide over time—and sometimes even fairly quickly!

•**Alpha-lipoic acid: 300 milligrams, twice daily.** This powerful antioxidant protects nerves from damage and can help relieve nerve pain. In one of many studies on the nutrient's ability to reverse nerve pain, people with diabetic neuropathy who took a daily dose of alpha-lipoic acid had "significant reductions" in neuropathic symptoms, according to Greek researchers. The patients also felt better able to work, spend time with family, and socialize. As an additional benefit, the supplement also lowered triglycerides, a heart-hurting blood fat.

•**Acetyl-L-carnitine: 500 milligrams to 1,500 milligrams, twice daily.** This nutrient helps generate the energy that can heal nerve cells. Studies show it is effective in both diabetic neuropathy and chemotherapy-induced nerve pain.

•**Vitamin B$_6$: 30 milligrams daily.** In a scientific paper published in the *Journal of Clinical Neuromuscular Disease*, Canadian researchers point out that B$_6$ can prevent peripheral neuropathy. Use the pyridoxal 5'-phosphate form.

•**Vitamin B$_{12}$: 500 micrograms to 5,000 micrograms daily.** Researchers at Harvard Medical School conducted a two-year study of 581 people with polyneuropathy—nerve damage in several areas of the body (such as the hands and feet), causing symptoms such as burning, tingling, weakness, and numbness. They found that up to 32 percent of the study participants had a possible vitamin B$_{12}$ deficiency as the "sole contributing cause of their polyneuropathy." Of those treated with the vitamin, 87 percent improved. In a patient with nerve pain, I give B$_{12}$ injections if the B$_{12}$ blood test is under 540 picograms per milliliter. After 15 injections, a 500-microgram daily dose is often enough. In one study, B$_{12}$ shots relieved nerve pain four times more effectively than a pain-relieving medication. If you can't get the shots, consider a daily 5,000-microgram sublingual (under the tongue) tablet of methylcobalamin, a special form of B$_{12}$ used in several studies on nerve pain.

•**Vitamin D: 2,000 IU daily.** In a study published in *Diabetes/Metabolism Research and Reviews*, people with diabetes with low levels of vitamin D were 2.6 times more likely to develop diabetic neuropathy. And in a study in *Diabetes and Metabolic Syndrome*, regular supplementation with vitamin D significantly decreased pain in diabetics with peripheral neuropathy.

•**Vitamin E: 400 IU daily.** Cisplatin, a widely used chemotherapeutic drug, causes severe side effects, including neuropathy. Italian researchers treated 108 cancer patients receiving cisplatin with either vitamin E (545 IU daily) or a placebo. Only six percent of those in the vitamin E group developed neuropathy, compared with 42 percent in the placebo group. And in patients taking vitamin E who developed neuropathy, the severity of the problem was 66 percent less.

Easing Pain—Today

Long-term healing of nerves using the treatments above is a must. But relief of pain—as soon as possible—is also a big priority: You should not remain in pain! Strategies for pain relief differ, depending on the cause of the pain. You might find, for example, that treating low levels of B$_{12}$ or thyroid hormone quickly eliminates nerve pain.

•**Hemp oil.** In my experience, natural remedies can be very effective for nerve pain. I often start my patients on hemp oil, which delivers an array of pain-soothing cannabinoids, including CBD. Unfortunately, many brands are low quality and don't deliver cannabinoids. My favorite product is Hemp Select hemp oil, from Terry Naturally (50 milligrams). Each of these 50-milligram capsules contain 10 milligrams of CBD, along with 10 other critically effective cannabinoids. Get the product without curcumin; it's more cost-effective for pain relief (any hemp oil is going to be pricey). You can also find good hemp oil at licensed marijuana dispensaries. Optimal dosing is three to five of the 50-milligram Hemp Select capsules, three times daily. It may be four to six weeks before you see the full effect of this regimen, although relief is usually much quicker.

For localized areas of pain, it's worth trying hemp oil, rubbing it over the areas of nerve pain three times a day, for six weeks. You can use the capsules and topical oil together.

The Worst Nerve Pain of All

One of the most severe kinds of nerve pain is Complex Regional Pain Syndrome (CRPS). (The older term for this problem is Reflex Sympathetic Dystrophy, or RSD.) It's so horrific, I've seen people have amputations to try to get rid of the pain. (Tragically, it didn't.) I have spent 20 years asking researchers at the pain conferences where I lectured if they had any new answers for this illness—and they didn't. However, there have been several recent breakthroughs in effectively treating CRPS, although describing them is beyond the scope of this chapter. If you have the problem, please visit my website and download the free "CRPS and Reflex Sympathetic Dystrophy: Approach to Treatment—an Overview," which you should share with your doctor. You can find it at: Vitality101.com/health-a-z/key-articles, under the "Pain" section.

For many, taking pain-relieving medications is also necessary, and it's a reasonable form of support while you are using nutrition to heal your nerves. The way to figure out which medications work for you is to try several and see which work best—a lot like trying on different pairs of shoes to see which fit best. The good news: There are a lot of helpful shoes to try on!

When I treat patients with nerve pain, I typically prescribe the medications in the order in which they're listed below. For most people, using one or two medications does the trick. I'm providing this long list of medications so that you have a lot of options to choose from and can work with your doctor to achieve pain relief.

Many who prefer a natural approach to health and healing are leery of medications and their side effects. Let me make this simple observation: The chronic pain is much more toxic to your body (and mind) than the medications.

•*Lidocaine* **patch (Lidoderm).** If only a small area is painful, it makes sense to begin with this topically applied patch of lidocaine (5 percent), a prescription product that delivers an anesthetizing, Novocain-like medication. Apply the patch directly over the spot where there's pain. The best use of the patch is in a small area of pain, under four by eight inches. But you can also apply it over the most painful part of a larger area of pain.

You can cut a single patch to fit a small area or several small areas (this also lowers the cost). Or you can use up to four patches simultaneously (though the package insert says up to three). You can use the patches on a schedule of 12 hours on, 12 hours off (although research suggests that 18 hours on, six hours off is also safe and effective).

You should see results within two weeks, often much quicker. The most common side effect is a mild skin rash in the area of the patch. But it's rarely experienced. The patches (like many other topical medications) are remarkably free of side effects. The downside of the patches: They're expensive. But they're usually covered by prescription insurance.

Caution: Don't use the lidocaine patch if you have an allergy to Novocaine or lidocaine.

•*Gabapentin* **(Neurontin).** This antiseizure drug wasn't formulated for nerve pain, but it can be very helpful in relieving it. Studies show, for example, that gabapentin is effective in reducing the pain of diabetic neuropathy and PHN. Common side effects include sedation, dizziness, and sometimes (when first starting treatment) mild swelling in the ankles. To avoid these side effects, begin with a low dose and increase it slowly. (This is true of all the medications discussed in this chapter.)

•**Tricyclic antidepressants.** This is an older class of antidepressants that have been largely replaced by the newer selective serotonin reuptake inhibitors (SSRIs). But tricyclics work wonderfully to help relieve nerve pain. There are more than 20 tricyclics, including *amitriptyline* (Elavil), *imipramine* (Tofranil), *nortriptyline* (Pamelor, Aventyl), and *doxepin* (Adapin, Sinequan). For nerve pain, very low dosing—for example, 10 milligrams to 25 milligrams of Elavil at bedtime—may be all you need.

•**Topical gels.** Compounding pharmacies (pharmacies that formulate customized medications on-site) can now make well-absorbed creams and gels that combine multiple pain-relieving medications in low doses of each medication. The creams/gels maximize effectiveness while minimizing side effects. Rubbed on the painful area, they can be very effective in relieving pain after one to two weeks of use.

For example, a gel called the Nerve Pain Lotion, available by prescription from ITC pharmacy (ITCpharmacy.com), includes *ketamine* (10 percent), Neurontin (6 percent), *clonidine* (0.2 percent), *ketoprofen* (5 percent), lidocaine (5 percent), *amitriptyline* (4 percent), and *doxepin* (2 percent). Apply a pea-size amount of the lotion to the painful area three times a day, though larger amounts can be used for bigger areas. For severe or persistent pain, you can also put some of the lotion on a line going from the pain area traced back to the spine, which will help soothe the nerves that are conducting the pain. I think this class of topical drugs is a wonderful addition to the treatment of nerve pain (and many other types of pain). It provides the benefits of pills, but without their cost and side effects.

Think about it this way: Why take enough medicine to saturate your body in order to saturate only a small, painful area, when you can achieve the same effect by putting a tiny amount on the skin over the pain? Topical is better.

•**Other medications.** If needed for additional relief, several other medications have been found effective for nerve pain. *They include…*

•Neuropathy medications: *pregabalin* (Lyrica), *tiagabine* (Gabitril)

•SSRI antidepressants: *duloxetine* (Cymbalta), *venlafaxine* (Effexor)

•Antiseizure medications: *Topiramate* (Topamax), *lamotrigine* (Lamictal), *levetiracetam* (Keppra), *oxcarbazepine* (Trileptal), *phenytoin* (Dilantin)

•Capsaicin: Used topically in a cream, usually for the relief of postherpetic neuralgia

•Antihistamines: Over-the-counter *diphenhydramine* (Benadryl). No one knows why it sometimes works, but it does, even in people who haven't been helped by high doses of narcotics. Start with 25 milligrams every six to eight hours and adjust the dose to a maximum of 50 milligrams, four times daily, to achieve the optimum effect. Like many pain medications, it may be sedating.

•Intravenous ketamine. This drug has shown itself to be very promising for easing intractable nerve pain. However, it can cause a very dramatic, dissociative "high," which lasts for a few hours. So the first few doses of ketamine need to be administered under medical supervision, until the patient is comfortable with this effect. Unfortunately, ketamine costs as much as $400 to $800 per dose. *The good news*: It's now available as a prescription nose spray for treating depression. So once the patient is comfortable with the psychological experience of using ketamine, some physicians will allow the patient to use it at home. *The bad news*: Drug companies are now charging $600 to $800 per dose for the nose spray! But let's end this discussion with more good news: Compounding pharmacies can make the ketamine nose spray for about five dollars per dose.

•Narcotics, which are only modestly helpful, but are medically considered an acceptable treatment for nerve pain. I prefer using nonaddictive treatments when possible.

Nighttime Leg Cramps

Real Causes

- **Nutritional Deficiencies.** Low levels of muscle-relaxing minerals such as magnesium, calcium, and potassium can cause muscle cramps (page 3).
- **Hormonal Imbalances.** Low levels of thyroid hormone can fatigue muscles, leading to cramping (page 87).

How did that monster in my nightmare get hold of my legs? That's how you might feel when you have nighttime leg cramps—when your calf and other leg muscles (and sometimes your foot) go into spasm while you're sleeping, waking you up. What's causing those nighttime leg and foot cramps? There are five main causes, and you can have more than one of them.

•**Tight calf muscles.** When you shift position during sleep, you further contract those muscles and stretch their tendons. This sends a signal back to the spinal cord that tells the calf muscles to contract even more, triggering spasms and cramps. It's an exaggeration of a muscle's normal reflex—like a shout when it would be fine to talk in a normal tone of voice.

•**Nutritional deficiency.** Low blood levels of muscle-relaxing minerals such as magnesium, calcium, and potassium can contribute to muscle cramps.

•**Hormonal imbalance.** Low levels of thyroid deprive your entire body of energy, and a low-energy muscle is more likely to cramp. (Hypothyroidism can cause leg cramps and other types of muscular cramps.)

•**Circulatory problem.** Peripheral artery disease—blocked arteries in your legs—can cause nighttime leg cramps, just as it causes calf pain when you walk (a condition called intermittent claudication).

•**Fibromyalgia.** If you have tight calf muscles and tight, painful muscles all over your body, you may have fibromyalgia. (For more information on this problem, see Chronic Fatigue Syndrome and Fibromyalgia on page 189.)

Real Cure Regimen

What to do about the cramp? You can always walk it off, of course—though who wants a painful stroll in the middle of the night? No, it's better to prevent the problem. And prevention is easy. Start with nutrition.

•Potassium. You can ask your doctor for a prescription supplement. *Better:* Boost your daily intake of potassium by eating a potassium-rich banana every day, and drinking a daily 12- to 16-ounce glass of potassium-packed V8, tomato juice, or coconut water.

•Calcium. Take 500 milligrams to 1,000 milligrams at bedtime (with the magnesium described below).

•Magnesium. Take 200 milligrams daily. (If diarrhea isn't a problem when you take this laxative mineral, higher doses might be more helpful.)

•B complex. Take a high-potency B complex. Or, for your magnesium and B vitamins, simply take the Energy Revitalization System multinutrient powder (more about it on page 30), which includes 200 milligrams of magnesium and high levels of B vitamins. Take the powder at bedtime rather than in the morning.

•**Warm your calves at bedtime.** Apply a heating pad to your calves for 10 minutes before you go to sleep. And wear socks to bed—cold feet sometimes trigger the problem.

•**Stretch at bedtime and during the day.** Stretch your calf muscles before you go to sleep: Just sit on the bed with your legs out in front of you and pull your toes toward you. As for a daytime stretch, here's an easy one that really works: the wall pushup. Stand eight inches away from a wall. Put your palms on the wall. Now, lean your chest into the wall. You will feel your calf muscles stretch. Push yourself away from the wall. That is one pushup. Do three to six pushups, three times a day. Do them slowly and deliberately. Take about 10 seconds with each. Over time, as your muscles release and lengthen, you can get more stretch by starting the pushup a bit farther from the wall—up to 16 inches.

•**Consider quinine.** The antimalarial medication quinine is very effective in preventing and treating nighttime leg cramps. Quinine should never be used during pregnancy, and too much is toxic for anybody. Work with a holistic practitioner to determine safe dosing. Another option: At bedtime, drink four ounces to eight ounces of tonic water, which contains quinine.

Osteoporosis

Real Causes

- **Nutritional Deficiencies.** Many nutrients contribute to strong bones, and low levels of these nutrients—particularly of vitamin D, vitamin K, and magnesium—can play a role in osteoporosis (page 3).

- **Hormonal Imbalances.** Low estrogen and testosterone and elevated thyroid hormones can cause bone loss (page 84).

- **Inactivity.** Weight-bearing exercise, such as walking, preserves and builds bone (page 40).

More than fifty-four million—that's the number of Americans, most of them over 50, and two-thirds of them women, with low bone mass, causing thinning and weakening bones.

There are two stages of low bone mass: the earlier stage, osteopenia; and the later stage, osteoporosis. Osteopenia and osteoporosis are usually diagnosed using a DEXA (dual energy x-ray absorptiometry) test to measure the bone mineral density (BMD) in your hip, spine, and wrist. If your score is -1 to -2.5 below the normal bone mass for healthy women or men in their twenties, you have osteopenia; if your score is -2.5 or more, you have osteoporosis.

Every year, millions of people diagnosed with osteoporosis end up with an osteoporotic fracture—usually a broken hip, collapsed vertebra (also called a compression fracture), or snapped wrist. In all, 50 percent of women will have an osteoporotic fracture in their lifetime.

The medical approach to treating osteoporosis is bisphosphonate drugs that increase BMD, such as *alendronate* (Fosamax), *ibandronate* (Boniva), *risedronate* (Actonel), and *zoledronate* (Zometa). If you've been diagnosed with osteoporosis, it's reasonable to take a bisphosphonate. But these drugs are not without significant risks and side effects, as I describe in "Osteoporosis Drugs: Building or Wrecking Bones?" in Prescription Drugs on page 82.

Real Cure Regimen

I think natural remedies are much safer and far more effective than these medications. But if you decide to take a bisphosphonate, I recommend that you take it with the natural remedies featured in this chapter. If a future DEXA test shows you're no longer osteoporotic, talk to your doctor about stopping the bisphosphonate—while continuing to take the bone-building, bone-protecting natural remedies. *Here is what I recommend to my patients diagnosed with either osteopenia or osteoporosis, usually saving the medications for when these remedies aren't adequate...*

- **Take a multivitamin-mineral supplement.** Calcium gets the most press for its role in protecting bone, but there are many other nutrients that are critical for bone production. In fact,

> ## Three Tips for Taking a Bisphosphonate (Fosamax)
>
> **1. Fosamax and other bisphosphonates can irritate the stomach.** To prevent or minimize this side effect, it's best to take your dose immediately upon waking and then stay upright for 30 minutes. That way, gravity helps move the medication quickly past the stomach.
>
> **2. Some people take 35 milligrams a week of Fosamax as a preventive dose.** The 35-milligram and 70-milligram tablets cost exactly the same. So, if you're on 35 milligrams a day, I recommend asking for the 70-milligram tablets and cutting them in half with a pill splitter to save yourself money.
>
> **3. If you've been on a bisphosphonate for five years or more,** it's time to stop the drug, as studies show long-term use may actually weaken bone. Talk to your physician.

calcium has minimal benefit compared to these other nutrients, which include magnesium, silica, boron, vitamin K, vitamin D, folic acid, copper, manganese, zinc, and vitamins B_6, B_{12}, and C. You can find all these nutrients (except silica) in the Energy Revitalization System multinutrient powder, which I discuss at length in Nutritional Deficiencies on page 30. Another good multivitamin-mineral supplement is Clinical Essentials, from Terry Naturally.

• **Take calcium: 400 milligrams to 600 milligrams daily.** I recommend taking a chewable, powdered, or liquid form of calcium, because it will dissolve better in your stomach. On the other hand, plain calcium carbonate tablets (aka chalk) don't always dissolve—they often go in your mouth and out the other end, doing you no good along the way. (To see what I mean, take a calcium tablet and put it in some vinegar for an hour. If it doesn't dissolve—and chances are it won't—it won't dissolve in your acidic stomach, either.)

Calcium blocks the absorption of thyroid medication, so if you're taking thyroid hormone, take the calcium two to four hours before or after the medication.

Caution: It's important not to take calcium by itself. Research shows it may increase the risk of heart disease and heart attack. But combined with magnesium and vitamin D, calcium is safe and helps build bone.

Bottom line: Take it at the same time you take the multinutrient powder. But here's an even better strategy: Get your daily calcium by drinking a glass of milk or calcium-fortified, unsweetened plant-based "milk"—whenever you like!

• **Take strontium: 340 milligrams to 680 milligrams daily (elemental strontium).** This is by far the most important nutrient for improving bone density. In fact, research shows that it is nearly twice as effective as Fosamax. And it's very safe, even in big doses.

There have been more than 50 clinical studies showing the effectiveness of strontium in osteoporosis. In a two-year study published in the *Journal of Clinical Endocrinology and Metabolism*, 353 people with osteoporosis took 680 milligrams of daily elemental strontium (from 2,000 milligrams of strontium ranelate). The mineral increased BMD in the lower spine by 15 percent. The same team of French researchers then conducted another study on 1,649 women with osteo-

Breakthroughs in Nutritional Healing: Osteopenia and Osteoporosis

Many studies show that there are a range of nutrients crucially important for protecting and building bone.

●**Vitamin D.** When scientists from the Centre on Aging and Mobility in Switzerland analyzed bone mineral density (BMD) in nearly 10,000 Americans over the age of 20, they found that a high calcium intake was linked with higher BMD only in people with low blood levels of vitamin D. In other words, if you're getting plenty of vitamin D, you don't need extra calcium to build bone. "Correcting inadequate levels of vitamin D is more important than increasing dietary calcium for better bone density," concluded the researchers in the *Journal of Bone and Mineral Research*.

●**B vitamins.** A high blood level of the amino acid homocysteine is a risk factor for osteoporosis. In two studies published in the *New England Journal of Medicine*, researchers from the United States and the Netherlands found that a high homocysteine level was a greater risk factor for hip fractures than was low bone mineral density, the standard indicator of risk. The researchers theorize that excess homocysteine may weaken collagen, the protein fibers that form a structure for calcium crystals to build bone. The researchers recommend supplemental folate, B_{12}, and B_6 as one way to help prevent hip fractures.

●**Vitamin K.** This vitamin plays a key role in the formation of osteocalcin, a protein that helps secure calcium to bone. When researchers at Harvard Medical School studied more than 70,000 women, they found that those with the highest intake of vitamin K had a 30 percent decreased risk of hip fracture compared to those with the lowest intake. And when English researchers analyzed 13 studies on vitamin K supplementation and osteoporosis, they found that the vitamin reduced spinal fractures by 40 percent and hip fractures by 13 percent.

●**Magnesium.** Researchers from the University of Tennessee studied more than 2,000 people 70 to 79 years old and found that those with the highest dietary intake of magnesium also had the greatest bone mineral density. And researchers at the Yale University School of Medicine found that supplementing the diet of healthy girls eight to 14 years old with 300 milligrams of magnesium improved their bone mineral density.

porosis. Compared with a placebo group, those taking strontium had 49 percent fewer first-time fractures, a 14.4 percent increase in BMD in the lower spine, and an 8.9 percent increase in hip BMD. And in another study, taking strontium for three to 36 months markedly reduced bone pain in people with osteoporosis.

Another way to look at those results: Strontium is 70 percent more effective than Fosamax, but without the toxicity.

Take it on an empty stomach (preferably at night) and at a different time of day than calcium or vitamin D (both of which can block strontium absorption).

●**Consider taking the herb horsetail, which is rich in silica.** Horsetail is a unique plant that has remineralizing and regenerating effects. It is a rich and highly bioavailable source of silica—an ingredient that you need if you want healthy tissue, including bone, skin, hair, and nails. Unfortunately, the level of silicon in your body decreases with age, which results in weaker bones, and in nail and hair brittleness. I recommend 800 mg daily, which delivers 20 mg of silica (a form of silicon). My favorite brand is Silica-20 from Terry Naturally.

●**Optimize hormone levels.** Optimizing estrogen levels in perimenopause and menopause with natural, safe, bioidentical hormones can powerfully help protect against osteoporosis. In fact, I think that most women with loss of bone density should be on bioidentical hormones, usually including testosterone along with the estrogen and progesterone. (For more on using bioidentical estrogen, see Hormonal Imbalances on page 94 and Menopausal Problems on page 290.)

In men, testosterone deficiency is a major cause of osteoporosis, and improving levels can improve bone density. (For more on testing for and treating low testosterone, see Hormonal Imbalances on page 92 and Male Menopause [Testosterone Deficiency] on page 287.)

●**Get your omega-3s.** Although less important than the other nutrients I've been discussing here, a deficiency of omega-3 fatty acids can contribute to osteoporosis. Add a fish oil supplement to this regimen if you have dry eyes, dry mouth, or depression—all signs of a deficiency of omega-3s. I recommend an excellent brand of fish oil called Vectomega, which supplies the equivalent of eight to 16 capsules of fish oil in one to two tablets. You don't need a supplement if you eat a serving of fatty fish (such as salmon, tuna, or sardines) at least four times a week.

●**Walk regularly.** Weight-bearing exercise such as walking protects and builds bone density. I recommend walking 30 to 60 minutes daily.

Best: Walk outside, so you get your exercise and a dose of sunshine, which provides vitamin D. If you have bone pain, you can walk in a warm pool, which provides the resistance that helps build bone but spares you the pain. Other good weight-bearing exercises for osteoporosis include strength-training, yoga, dancing, aerobics, and tennis and other racquet sports.

●**Cut out excess alcohol.** Imbibing more than two to three alcoholic drinks a day for many years can contribute to bone loss.

Overweight

Real Causes

●**Nutritional Deficiencies.** A diet loaded with sugar and other refined carbohydrates—nearly a third of the typical American diet—is a set-up for overweight (page 33).

●**Inactivity.** Calorie-burning physical activity helps prevent weight gain, or regain after successful weight loss (page 40).

●**Hormonal Imbalances.** Overweight is not always a lifestyle issue. Metabolic causes—such as low levels of thyroid hormone, adrenal hormone imbalances, and low testosterone—also can cause the problem (page 84).

- **Digestive Difficulties.** An intestinal overgrowth of the fungus *Candida albicans* triggers weight gain in many people (page 98).

- **Poor Sleep.** Sleep helps regulate leptin, the key appetite-controlling hormone (page 33).

You don't need a statistician to tell you that a lot of Americans are overweight. Just look around. Still, the numbers are startling.

Research shows that 30 percent of Americans are overweight and 40 percent are obese—in other words, seven out of 10 Americans are above normal weight! (For a precise definition of the terms "*normal weight*," "*overweight*," and "*obese*," read the box "Defining Overweight" below.) That's nearly four times the rate of overweight and obesity 40 years ago.

A few more statistics graphically convey the health impact of those extra pounds. A person who is overweight at 18 has double the risk of dying prematurely, compared to an 18-year-old of normal weight. An 18-year-old obese person has triple the risk—about the same risk as a person who smokes 10 cigarettes a day. Not surprising, really, when you consider that overweight increases the risk for heart disease, cancer, and stroke, three of the biggest killers of Americans. (It also increases the risk of bladder problems, depression, gallbladder disease, gout, infertility, liver disease, menstrual irregularities, osteoarthritis, pregnancy complications, sleep apnea, and type 2 diabetes.)

Defining Overweight

Medical experts use specific terms when defining normal weight and degrees of overweight, based on "body mass index" (BMI), a number derived from a complex formula that divides weight by height. *The terms...*

- **Normal weight.** 24.9 or lower BMI. *Examples*: a 5' 4" woman is normal weight at 144 pounds or less; a 5' 10" man is normal weight at 173 pounds or less.

- **Overweight.** 25 to 29.9 BMI. *Examples*: a 5' 4" woman is overweight from 145 to 173 pounds; a 5' 10" man is overweight from 174 pounds to 208 pounds.

- **Obese.** 30 to 39.9 BMI. *Examples*: a 5' 4" woman is obese from 174 pounds to 231 pounds; a 5' 10" man is obese from 209 pounds to 277 pounds.

- **Extremely obese.** 40 or higher BMI. *Examples*: a 5' 4" woman is extremely obese at 232 pounds or more; a 5' 10" man is extremely obese at 278 pounds or more.

To figure out your BMI, use the BMI calculator at the website of the Centers for Disease Control and Prevention, CDC.gov (search "BMI calculator").

But it's not as if we Americans aren't trying to lose weight—we are! Every year, 45 percent of us go on a diet, according to the government's Centers for Disease Control and Prevention. But if all of us actually managed to shed our excess weight, research presented at the annual meeting of the Endocrine Society shows that eight out of 10 of us will gain it all back!

What's going on? Why do we have so much trouble staying thin, losing weight, and maintaining weight loss? There are a lot of reasons, some known and some still to be discovered. Appetite and weight regulation are complex. But I think one very important reason for our epidemic of extra pounds is this: Doctors and their patients don't understand, detect, and correct the real causes of overweight and obesity.

Real Cure Regimen

Yes, there are several often-overlooked but important causes of overweight (the term I'll use throughout the rest of the chapter to indicate any level of weight above normal).

Detecting and treating those causes has led to substantial weight loss for many of my patients—without extreme, unsustainable, unhealthy dieting. For example, one patient I recently treated lost 50 pounds in four months. Needless to say, she was thrilled. As you'll see, several of the real causes of overweight are among the nine Real Causes covered in Part I of this book.

Fix Nutritional Deficiencies

When you're deficient in vitamins and minerals, your metabolism is sluggish (burning fewer calories) and your body craves more food than it needs (taking in more calories).

Two Crucial Nutrients for Weight Loss

There are two nutrients that may be particularly important for weight loss but are often overlooked…

•**Acetyl-L-carnitine.** In a study reviewing the use of the amino acid carnitine, published in *Obesity Reviews*, the researchers concluded that taking the supplement "resulted In weight loss." That's because if you're deficient in the amino acid carnitine, your body can't burn fuel effectively, and it's almost forced to turn calories into fat. But I've found that carnitine itself isn't easily absorbed in supplemental form. Instead, take acetyl-L-carnitine, which can raise carnitine levels. In my clinical experience, this nutrient won't increase weight loss on its own, but it will help you shed pounds with diet and exercise. The dosage: 1,000 milligrams daily, for four months, or until your weight has normalized.

•**Vitamin D.** In a study presented at a meeting of The Endocrine Society, doctors found a direct link between blood levels of vitamin D and weight loss: For every one nanogram per milliliter (ng/mL) increase in blood levels, women lost ½ more pound of fat. Since vitamin D supplements often increase blood levels by as much as 40 ng/mL, that's a very important finding for anybody who wants to lose weight. Important: Take a vitamin D_3 supplement and walk outdoors for plenty of D-producing sunshine. (*The key to healthy sun exposure*: Get sunshine, not a sunburn.)

Top 10 Weight Loss Tips

Along with addressing the real causes of overweight presented in this chapter, my patients have found these tips particularly effective in shredding pounds.

1. Don't go on a very low-calorie diet. Your body thinks there's a famine, your metabolism plummets, and you gain weight—while eating almost nothing. Then you give up your diet, resume eating normal, and gain ever more weight because your metabolism hasn't reset itself. Sound familiar? Don't eat less than 1,200 calories a day.

2. Eliminate sugar and grains. Following just this one dietary admonition—essentially, eating a low-carbohydrate diet—is very effective for weight loss. That's because sugars and carbohydrates trigger the release of the hormone insulin, which packs on the fat. The guidelines: NO sugars; NO fruit juices; NO wheat or grain products, including rice and pasta; NO potatoes or other very starchy vegetables (squash, beets, carrots).

3. Use sugar substitutes. The body has a natural craving for sweetness, and sugar substitutes satisfy it just as well as sugar. Stevia is the best sugar substitute, and a taste test conducted in my office chose brands from Body Ecology, SweetLeaf, and Stevia Select. (Many others have a bitter aftertaste—not what you want from a sugar substitute.) Saccharin is safe. But NutraSweet (aspartame) can be toxic for many people, causing migraines and other health problems. It also does not help weight loss.

4. Eat smaller portions. If you cut your portion size by 20 to 25 percent, you'll lose a lot of weight. But how to do it? Chewing a lot helps. So does using a smaller plate. And when you serve yourself dessert, take a very small portion and move the tempting goody away. You'll find that 80 percent of the pleasure comes from the first few bites (and most of the calories from the rest). Eating smaller portions is also easier if you know you can always go back for seconds—by following the next simple tip…

5. Wait 30 minutes to go back for seconds. It takes 30 minutes for the message "You're full" to move from your stomach to your brain. If you wait 30 minutes before going back for the seconds, you'll usually find that you don't want any more food because the appetite center in your brain has heard from your stomach.

6. In a restaurant, ask for half of your meal to go—before you eat it! That's right: when you order, tell the waiter that you want one-half (or even one-third) of your meal wrapped up to go. In the United States, restaurant portions are supersized. One-half of a typical restaurant meal will fill you and leave you feeling great, and by the time you've finished, your brain will have gotten the signal from your stomach that you're full. Eat the leftovers for tomorrow's lunch or dinner.

7. In the supermarket, shop the perimeter first. That's where you'll find the produce, meat, and other whole foods. The processed foods are typically in the center of the store.

8. Sleep seven to eight hours a night. Research shows that folks who get enough sleep weigh an average of six pounds less than folks who don't. If you wake up during the night and can't get back to sleep, try eating a brain-soothing snack of one to two ounces of protein (turkey, hard-boiled egg, cheese, etc.) to see if that helps.

9. Ease up while on vacation. If you're on vacation, enjoy yourself and ease up on your diet. Keep sugar intake moderate, and still get the one-half portion when you eat out (or split an appetizer or soup, salad, and the main dish with your mate or a friend).

10. Forget about the guilt! Feeling guilty about eating something is completely counterproductive—you won't even notice the good taste as the food goes down! Pick up your knife and fork, and put down your guilt. Eating is for good times and good health.

You can take individual doses of specific nutrients you need, or you can take the Energy Revitalization System multi-nutrient powder—one scoop provides top-level nutrition, and replaces the need for about 35 different supplements. (You can read more about nutritional deficiencies on page 3.)

Get Active

Just walking an hour a day can burn 25 pounds a year. A 13-year study, in the *Journal of the American Medical Association*, showed that the only people who were able to maintain normal weight over the course of the study were those who averaged an hour a day of moderate-intensity activity (such as brisk walking).

Stop Insulin Resistance

Tens of millions of Americans have insulin resistance: Muscle, fat, and liver cells don't respond normally to insulin, the hormone that ushers blood sugar (glucose) out of the bloodstream and into cells. Because insulin isn't working, the body pumps out more and more of it—and all that excess insulin in the blood turns sugar and other calories into fat!

To find out if you're insulin resistant, ask your doctor for a fasting insulin blood test, which is conducted first thing in the morning, before eating or drinking. If the result is over 10 microunits per milliliter (mcu/ml), you are insulin resistant (even though this level is in the "normal" range).

There are two lifestyle keys to preventing or reversing insulin resistance: (1) Eat a diet that emphasizes whole foods such as fish, vegetables, fruit, whole grains, beans, and nuts and seeds (see page 30) and minimizes refined carbohydrates (sugar and white flour), saturated fats in red meat and dairy products, and trans fats in processed and packaged foods; and (2) exercise regularly.

Optimizing levels of thyroid, testosterone, and adrenal hormones can also help curb insulin resistance (page 84).

Get a Good Night's Sleep

Deep sleep triggers the production of growth hormone. In turn, growth hormone stimulates the production of muscle, which burns more calories than fat, and improves blood sugar control (decreasing your tendency to make and store fat). Sleep also helps regulate leptin, the key appetite-controlling hormone. Studies show that people who don't get adequate sleep (about 105 million Americans!) have a 30 percent higher risk of becoming obese. (You can read more about the link between sleep and health in Poor Sleep on page 33).

Correct Hypothyroidism

More than 20 million Americans suffer with hypothyroidism (low level of thyroid hormones), and less than one-third of them are properly diagnosed and treated. Hypothyroidism slows down your metabolism, almost forcing you to gain weight. (You can read more about the accurate detection and effective treatment of hypothyroidism in Hormonal Imbalances on page 87 and in Hypothyroidism on page 254.)

Stop Yeast Overgrowth

Yeast (fungus) feed on sugar. When you have an internal overgrowth of the yeast *Candida albicans*, you have sugar cravings, a higher sugar intake—and weight gain. (You can read more about this on page 181.)

Limit Adrenal Exhaustion

An imbalance of adrenal hormones can cause weight gain, whether levels of cortisol (also called the stress hormone) are too high or too low. High cortisol causes more insulin resistance. On the other hand, when adrenal glands are worn out from chronic stress, they don't produce enough cortisol to keep blood sugar levels from dropping during stress. That low level of blood sugar deflates energy, driving you to eat sweets to boost blood sugar levels and restore energy—and the high sugar intake leads to insulin resistance and weight gain. (For more information on detecting and treating adrenal exhaustion, read Adrenal Burnout on page 90 and Adrenal Exhaustion on page 138.)

Premenstrual Syndrome

Real Causes

- **Hormonal Imbalances.** The symptoms of premenstrual syndrome (PMS) are mostly caused by a deficiency of progesterone (page 94).
- **Nutritional Deficiencies.** Low levels of vitamin B_6, magnesium, and essential fatty acids can play a role in PMS (page 3).

Ninety percent of women of reproductive age experience premenstrual syndrome (PMS). Twenty percent to 40 percent say the symptoms of PMS interfere with daily life. And that's not surprising, because PMS can cause a lot of symptoms. The list includes irritability, anxiety, mood swings, depression, headaches, bloating, weight gain, constipation, fatigue, sugar cravings, cramps, acne, breast tenderness, and backache.

What's behind all these pre-period problems? A low level of progesterone, the hormone that (along with estrogen) regulates the menstrual cycle, keeps reproductive organs healthy, prepares the body for pregnancy, and acts as our body's natural Valium, creating a sense of ease and calm. Because there are progesterone receptors throughout the body, a lack of the hormone can cause a wide range of symptoms.

Another cause is low levels of the prostaglandin PGE1. Prostaglandins are hormone-like compounds with many functions, including regulating other hormones, controlling levels of inflammation, and regulating calcium. A low level of PGE1 can play a key role in the irritability, anxiety, and mood swings.

Real Cure Regimen

Natural remedies can help boost pre-period levels of both progesterone and PGE1, easing the symptoms of PMS. Give them about three months to start working (though they often start sooner).

•**Take omega-3 fatty acids.** The omega-3 fatty acids in fish oil boost levels of PGE1. For my patients with PMS, I recommend one teaspoon to three teaspoons a day of fish oil for three months. (Taking fish oil in liquid form rather than via a capsule delivers a very high dose of omega-3s.) After three months, switch to one teaspoon (or about three capsules) a day. A unique fish oil product called Vectomega, from Terry Naturally, dramatically improves absorption of omega-3s, so one or two tablets are all you need. It's now my favorite omega-3 supplement. Carlson and Nordic Naturals also make excellent (and flavored) liquid fish oil. (For more information on fish oil, see Nutritional Deficiencies on page 28.)

•**Take evening primrose oil.** The evening primrose is a plant native to North America, and the oil from the seed is rich in gamma-linolenic acid (GLA), an essential fatty acid that boosts PGE1. Look for the word "Efamol" on the label: It's a top-quality oil used in several different brands. Barlean's makes an excellent evening primrose oil. Take 3,000 milligrams a day for three months. After that, take it daily the week before you expect to have your period. If this is too expensive, you can use borage oil instead, at the same dosage. (I've found evening primrose oil works best for my patients—probably because its GLA is better absorbed—but borage oil is still a good choice.)

•**Take vitamin B_6 (75 milligrams to 250 milligrams daily) and magnesium (200 milligrams to 400 milligrams daily).** In a study by UK researchers, women with PMS who took a combination of 50 milligrams of B_6 and 200 milligrams of magnesium had a lessening of "nervous tension," mood swings, irritability, and anxiety, according to findings in the *Journal of Women's Health & Gender-Based Medicine*. Vitamin B_6 helps regulate progesterone and estrogen levels. Magnesium calms nerves, relaxes muscles, and eases pain. To get your B_6 and magnesium, I recommend taking the Energy Revitalization System multinutrient powder, which supplies 200 milligrams of magnesium and 45 milligrams of B_6. Add 200 milligrams of magnesium and 100 milligrams of B_6 at bedtime for three months for intensive treatment; after three months, your symptoms should be under control. Use the pyridoxal 5 phosphate (P5P) form of vitamin B_6 for this to avoid the risk of nerve injury from high-dose B_6.

•**Take natural progesterone.** Talk to your doctor about natural progesterone (Prometrium). Take 200 milligrams at bedtime, starting a week before your period or when PMS symptoms begin.

Another option: Use 10 to 50 milligrams of prescription natural progesterone cream, applied to your skin at bedtime or twice daily during the 10 days before you expect your period. In some cases, I go as high as 800 mg a day of Prometrium.

Prostate Problems

Real Causes

- **Nutritional Deficiencies.** Low levels of many nutrients—particularly zinc—can play a role in prostate problems (page 3).

- **Hormonal Imbalances.** An excess of dihydrotestosterone (DHT), a by-product of testosterone metabolism, is a major factor in benign prostatic hypertrophy (BPH) (page 84).

Are you a man over 50 who has difficulty starting your urine flow? Once it starts, is it slow and slight? Do you wake up repeatedly at night to urinate?

If so, you probably have the problem called benign prostatic enlargement. (Doctors also call it benign prostatic hypertrophy or benign prostatic hyperplasia, both abbreviated BPH.) And you're far from alone.

Nine out of 10 men over age 40 end up with BPH. What's happening to all those prostates? The walnut-size prostate rings the urethra, the tube that transports ejaculate and drains urine. When you hit 40, the prostate can start to swell slowly, probably because of a drop in testosterone levels. The bulkier prostate squeezes and narrows the urethra, producing the symptoms of BPH. They can include urinary urgency, the feeling that you have to go to the bathroom now; straining to urinate; urinary frequency, including waking up several times a night to urinate; weaker stream; difficulty stopping the stream; dribbling at the end of urination; and incomplete emptying (the sense that your bladder hasn't emptied but you're unable to urinate any more).

Caution: If you have the symptoms of BPH, see your doctor for a prostate exam and a blood test, to rule out prostate cancer.

There are several medications doctors often prescribe to address these symptoms. *Tamsulosin* (Flomax)—an alpha-blocker—works by relaxing the muscles where the bladder and urethra intersect, allowing for easier flow. *Finasteride* (Proscar) and *dutasteride* (Avodart) work by decreasing the production of dihydrotestosterone (DHT), the compound that enlarges prostate cells.

Of all these medications, I consider Proscar to be the most helpful and reasonable. But instead of the standard daily dose of five milligrams, I usually recommend one-half tablet (2.5 milligrams). This lowers the risk of side effects while delivering most of the benefit.

However, if you have BPH and high blood pressure, talk to your doctor about taking *terazosin* (Hytrin), a medication that can control high blood pressure and the symptoms of BPH.

Although I consider Proscar to be a reasonable option, natural alternatives are also available—and you can always use them with the medication, for even greater effect.

Real Cure Regimen

Natural remedies for prostate enlargement are often as effective as—and sometimes more effective than—prescription medications. *My favorite remedies for the problem…*

•**Saw palmetto extract: 160 milligrams, twice daily.** This herb (also known as *Serenoa repens*) blocks DHT and treats the hormone imbalance. Give it six weeks to work. Over the years, there have been dozens of studies on saw palmetto, involving thousands of men, with varying results. Many have shown that the herb works to lessen the symptoms of BPH—often just as effectively as Flomax and other medications. Some studies, on the other hand, haven't produced positive results.

My bottom line: I've found the herb to be helpful for my patients with BPH and research agrees that it's very safe. In a paper in the journal *Complementary Therapies in Medicine,* researchers who conducted the Saw Palmetto for Treatment of Enlarged Prostates study reported no difference between herb takers and placebo takers in "serious adverse events" (study lingo for "bad reactions"), "non-serious symptomatic adverse events," sexual functioning, or laboratory tests of blood and urine. In other words, saw palmetto was extremely safe.

•**Add zinc and selenium.** Adding daily doses of 15 milligrams to 25 milligrams of zinc and 50 micrograms of selenium—two minerals that protect the health of the prostate—may boost saw palmetto's effectiveness. In one study, German researchers measured blood selenium levels in 21 men with BPH and found them "significantly lower than the recommended normal range." Their conclusion: "Our findings may support the recommendation of selenium supplementation" for BPH.

Shingles

Real Causes

•**Nutritional Deficiencies.** This disease is a reactivation of the chicken pox virus, which hibernates in the nerves. The virus is "awakened" by a weakened immune system, which can be caused by nutritional deficiencies (page 3).

•**Poor Sleep.** This is another underlying cause of a weakened immune system, which allows the virus to reactivate (page 33).

The virus that causes the itchy, fluid-filled blisters of chicken pox (varicella zoster) is a little bit like the shark in the movie *Jaws II. Just when you thought it was safe…*

If You're 50 or Older, Get the Shingles Vaccine

A landmark study of nearly 40,000 people age 60 and over showed that the shingles vaccine reduced the incidence of the disease by 51 percent, reduced the severity of the disease in those who did get it by 33 percent, and—most important—reduced the incidence of subsequent postherpetic neuralgia (PHN) by 66 percent.

"That means if you are 60 or older, the shingles vaccine reduces your risk of getting PHN by two-thirds," we were told by Michael N. Oxman, MD, the lead author of the study and a professor emeritus of medicine at the University of California, San Diego. "I recommend that anyone who is 60 and over, and has no contraindications, get the vaccine," he said. (Contraindications include an allergy to components of the vaccine, such as gelatin and the antibiotic *neomycin*.)

That recommendation was for Zostavax, a vaccine approved by the FDA in 2006. (They approved it for people 50 to 59 in 2011.) Then, in 2017, the FDA approved Shingrix, a new and more protective shingles vaccine, which the Centers for Disease Control and Prevention formally recommended in 2018. It offers better protection against shingles and PHN (for example, Zostavax cuts the risk of PHN by 67 percent, while Shingrix cuts it by 86 percent). You get the vaccine starting at age 50, so you're protected for longer. (Unfortunately, you need two doses rather than one, and the shot hurts more.) The CDC says those who've had Zostavax should now also get Shingrix. (Zostavax is no longer available for use in the U.S., as of November 2020.)

Caveat: Shringix is not recommended for people who are immunocompromised, such as someone undergoing chemotherapy. But do get a shingles vaccine when you can.

Varicella zoster hibernates for decades in nerve endings along your spinal cord and near your brain. When your immune system is weakened—by stress, nutritional deficiencies, or illness—the virus can wake up and migrate along the path of your nerves to your skin. There it causes a disease called shingles, or herpes zoster.

Shingles targets one side of your body along the route of a single nerve. It starts with painful, itchy bumps, which turn into fluid-filled blisters that, without treatment, take about a month to open, crust over, and heal.

Unfortunately, in up to 20 percent of those with shingles (including 50 percent of those 70 and older), the virus damages the nerves—a condition called postherpetic neuralgia (PHN). The pain of PHN is usually burning and electric or deep and aching. And for many people, it's also long-lasting, continuing for weeks, months, or even years, severely disrupting daily life.

Important: If you have a painful rash (and the pain may precede the rash by a few days) on only one side of your body, consider that it could be shingles, and get treatment quickly. The faster the rash is treated, the less likely you are to develop PHN.

That's the good news about shingles: Fast action when you have it can prevent PHN.

Real Cure Regimen

If I see a patient with a new and painful rash that fits the description of shingles, in addition to using natural therapies, I prescribe immediate treatment with the antiviral medication *valacyclovir* (Valtrex). This drug is very safe for short-term use, and taking it early in the outbreak (as soon as the first blisters are visible) is the best way to prevent PHN.

The recommended dose is 1,000 milligrams three times a day for the first week of shingles, though I frequently prescribe 1,000 milligrams four times a day for 10 days, which often stops the attack cold. The critical factor is starting the treatment early in the shingles attack, within the first 24 to 72 hours.

How do you know you're having an attack? The main symptom is a painful, blistering red rash, usually on the torso or the face. It's usually preceded by days of tingling, itching, burning or stinging in the area of the rash. You might also have a headache, fever and chills, nausea, and a general body ache.

So, if you're having the first symptoms of what might be shingles, see your doctor immediately (that day), specifically request this antiviral treatment—and don't take no for an answer! If you can't see your doctor, go to the emergency room and request the same.

You can also ease an acute attack of shingles with nutritional support, which you should use in addition to Valtrex. For more information on treating the pain of PHN, see Nerve Pain (Neuropathy) on page 294.

•**Vitamin B$_{12}$ injections.** Ask your doctor for B$_{12}$ injections for 10 days and then as needed for pain. Make sure each injection has 1,000 micrograms to 5,000 micrograms of B$_{12}$. An alternative: Take B$_{12}$ sublingually (a tablet dissolved under the tongue), at a dose of 5,000 micrograms a day for 10 days.

•**Lysine: 2,000 milligrams to 2,500 milligrams.** This amino acid can help heal the herpes zoster virus (cold sores or genital herpes), though it hasn't been tested for shingles.

•**B complex and magnesium.** Both of these nutrients support nerve healing. Look for a B complex with 25 to 100 milligrams of each B vitamin, and at least 250 micrograms of vitamin B$_{12}$. (*Caution*: A high level of B$_6$ is contraindicated for people with neuropathy because it can worsen the condition.) Take 200 milligrams of magnesium daily.

Sinusitis

Real Causes

•**Poor Diet.** Fungal overgrowth is the main underlying cause of sinusitis—and high-sugar diets feed the fungus.

- **Digestive Difficulties.** Dysbiosis—an overgrowth of candida (a yeast) that starts in the digestive system—is the main cause of chronic sinusitis (page 98).

- **Prescription Medications.** The antibiotics used to treat acute sinusitis or other bacterial infections kill the good bacteria that keep candida in check (page 70).

Sinusitis is an infection in the air-filled cavities located behind and around the nose and the eyes. The infection causes your nasal passages to swell shut, triggering symptoms such as headache, facial pain, and fatigue. The swollen, blocked sinuses can develop a secondary bacterial infection, generating a lot of yellow-green mucus.

There are two types of sinusitis. Acute sinusitis is a sudden-onset and often "postcold" infection, afflicting millions of Americans yearly. Chronic sinusitis is an ongoing, low-grade sinus infection, with runny nose, postnasal drip, and repeated flare-ups of acute sinusitis. About 30 million Americans have this problem. In all, 10 percent of Americans make a yearly visit to the doctor for sinusitis.

If you show up at your doctor's office with either acute or chronic sinusitis, you're likely to get a prescription for antibiotics—nine out of 10 patients with acute sinusitis are prescribed the drugs. (In fact, 15 to 20 percent of all outpatient, nonhospital antibiotic prescriptions are for acute sinusitis.) But it is dawning among doctors that antibiotics don't work for acute sinusitis.

For example, in a study in the *Journal of the American Medical Association*, acute sinusitis was treated with either (1) an antibiotic, (2) a nasal spray of a corticosteroid (an anti-inflammatory drug), (3) both drugs, or (4) neither drug. None of those treatments—including no treatment—was better than any other in lessening the symptoms of acute sinusitis or shortening the infection. And a Finnish study involving more than 15,000 people showed that people with acute sinusitis typically recover in two weeks—whether or not they take antibiotics. "Clinicians need to weigh the small benefits of antibiotic treatment against the potential for adverse effects for both individuals and the general population," they concluded.

The "adverse effects" those researchers are talking about: antibiotic resistance. Antibiotics don't slay 100 percent of bacteria. And those that survive quickly evolve into new generations of bacteria that can resist antibiotics. One example of those bacteria is the "multiple-resistant" bacteria called MRSA, which causes unstoppable staph infections of the skin and is now a major problem in hospitals and other healthcare settings. Worldwide, bacteria that cause many types of infections—from tuberculosis to bladder infections—are becoming antibiotic resistant.

I think there's another side effect that's overlooked when people talk about the failure of antibiotics to treat acute sinusitis: the fact that antibiotics actually cause chronic sinusitis. Here's what happens. Antibiotics don't specialize in bad bacteria. They target all the bacteria in your body, including the friendly bacteria that live in your colon, aiding digestion, manufacturing vitamins, disarming toxins, and lending the immune system a helping hand. When those friendly bacteria are decimated, the fungus (yeast) *Candida albicans*—normally a well-behaved denizen of your digestive tract—can multiply. And that overgrowth of candida doesn't confine itself to your intestines. It also ends up in your sinuses, causing chronic sinusitis and the bacterial infections that go with it.

Antibiotic-sparked fungal overgrowth is the main (but little-recognized) cause of the tens of millions of chronic sinus infections in the United States. It's also the reason why there are more and more of these infections, as the rampant use of antibiotics remains mostly uncontrolled.

I think it's important to note that I'm not alone in this perspective. A study on chronic sinusitis in the *Mayo Clinic Proceedings* reported that, although in the past "fungus...was thought to be involved in less than 10 percent of cases," their research showed that an inflammatory reaction to fungal overgrowth "is likely the cause of nearly all of these [sinusitis] problems." Unfortunately, it took a type of specialized testing available only in research labs to find the candida. There's an easier way.

Real Cure Regimen

If you have chronic sinusitis, assume you have fungal overgrowth and start curing your sinusitis today—by clearing up both the fungal overgrowth and the bacterial infection. The key treatments for acute sinusitis are the nasal rinses and sprays that I'm about to describe. For chronic sinusitis, adding in an antifungal medication for six weeks is an important part of clearing up the underlying problem. Here is what I recommend for my patients. For more on resolving candida overgrowth, see Candida Overgrowth (page 181).

Treating Acute Sinusitis

When you're in pain from acute sinusitis, you probably don't care much about the long-term problem. You just want the pain and swelling to go away! Here's the first and most important step.

•**Use this saltwater nasal rinse.** Why let your immune system face cell-to-cell combat with billions of bacterial invaders, when you can rinse 90 percent of them away? Here's how to do just that: Dissolve ½ teaspoon of salt in a cup of lukewarm water. (Some folks use just the lukewarm water, to make the rinse even simpler.) If you find this solution irritating to your nasal linings, make it gentler by adding a pinch of baking soda.

Inhale some of the solution, about one to three inches up each nostril, one nostril at a time. Do this by either using a baby nose bulb (also called a nasal bulb syringe) or sniffing the solution out of the palm of your hand while standing by a sink. Then gently blow your nose, being careful not to hurt your ears by blowing too hard. Continue to repeat with each nostril—left, right, left, right—until the nose is clear. Do this at least twice a day until the infection improves.

You can also use the premixed sinus rinses available in most drug and health food stores, such as NeilMed. Follow their directions for use. Or use a neti pot—the mother of all nasal rinse aids—a device from Ayurveda, the ancient system of natural healing from India.

Whatever method you use, each rinsing washes away about 90 percent of the infection, making it much easier for your body to heal itself. This is much more effective than an antibiotic, in most cases. After giving your nose a few minutes to dry, use the additional nasal sprays I'm about to describe, which address both acute and chronic sinusitis.

● **Use Sinusitis Nose Spray.** The bacteria that live in sinuses form what microbiologists call a biofilm: a sturdy, hard-to-destroy layer of organisms. Oral antibiotics can't break up that biofilm. You need to kill it with a special nasal spray and also wash out the infection.

I recommend a unique compounded nasal spray (made by a compounding pharmacy, which customizes medications on-site). The Sinusitis Nose Spray contains five key ingredients: (1) the topical antibiotic *mupirocin* (Bactroban); (2) the natural molecule xylitol, which kills bacteria and fights biofilm infections; (3) low-dose cortisol to shrink the swelling; (4) tiny amounts of the mineral bismuth to break up the biofilm; and (5) an antifungal.

I recommend patients use one or two sprays in each nostril, twice a day, for six to 12 weeks, while on Diflucan (which I'll mention in a moment). This combination is often enough to knock out the sinusitis, although some of my patients stay on the spray long term or use it intermittently for recurrent infections.

The spray is available by mail, with a prescription, from ITC Pharmacy. (You'll find contact info in Resources on page 360.) Simply have your physician ask for the Sinusitis Nose Spray.

● **Spray with colloidal silver.** Another treatment to consider is the over-the-counter silver-containing nose spray Argentyn 23. In low doses, silver is anti-infectious, killing both bacteria and viruses. You can also safely and repeatedly take oral liquid silver for chronic sinusitis (and other difficult-to-treat chronic infections). As with the compounded spray, you can use it intermittently or long term.

I've found that the Sinusitis Nose Spray and the silver spray are a wonderful combination. During sinus infections, use one to two sprays of the colloidal silver spray in each nostril. You can use it at the same time as the Sinusitis Nose Spray.

The use of colloidal silver is controversial, but that's more a matter of medical politics than medical science or sanity. Because it's cheap and can't be patented, colloidal silver hasn't been (and can't be) put through the FDA approval process, so conventional doctors take potshots at it, just as they do at most "unproven" natural remedies. Ignore the politics and try the remedy. (And like most natural remedies, there's science to support it, with a study out of Australia showing a colloidal silver spray reduced a biofilm in the sinuses by 99 percent.) Many of my patients have found it very helpful. Used in the proper dosing (as described here), it's also very safe.

Remedies to Take at the First Sign of a Cold

These sprays and rinses are often enough to help your body recover more quickly. Here are a few more tips that may help you prevent sinusitis if you take them for a day or two at the first sign of a cold.

● **Take ProBoost.** You can boost infection-fighting immunity by energizing your thymus gland, which plays a key role in early-life production of immune system cells. Try ProBoost, an all-natural thymus-supporting supplement. Dissolve one packet under your tongue, three times a day, until the infection is gone. (This remedy speeds healing of most infections and should be in everyone's medicine cabinet.)

● **Take vitamin C: 1,000 milligrams to 8,000 milligrams daily.** Vitamin C helps you fight off the bacterial infection. I recommend taking enough powdered vitamin C to cause (harmless) diarrhea (an indication that the body has all it needs to fight the infection) and then cutting back to a comfortable level.

Treating Chronic Sinusitis

Once you've dealt with acute sinusitis, it's time to go after the root causes of acute and chronic sinusitis so it stays gone. The key to eliminating chronic sinusitis is eliminating the underlying candida infection. Continue using the rinses and sprays, as described beginning on page 317, and add:

•*Lufenuron.* You can read all about this unique, little-known, but very effective fungal-killing drug in Candida Overgrowth on page 181.

•*Fluconazole* (**Diflucan**). This is a very effective and important antifungal medication. Take 200 milligrams daily, for six to 12 weeks, to clear up the underlying problem of candida overgrowth. It's a medication well worth taking. The other two treatments below that help restore healthy bowel bacteria in the long term are natural.

•**Pearls Elite.** This product from Nature's Way contains an effectively high amount of friendly bacteria (probiotics) that the Pearl coating protects from destruction by stomach acid. This remedy will restore a healthy balance of bacteria to your digestive tract, helping to keep candida at bay. Take one Pearls Elite a day.

If symptoms persist despite these treatments, consider allergy desensitization with NAET. (See Hay Fever and Other Airborne Allergies on page 231.)

Urinary Incontinence

Real Causes

•**Nutritional Deficiencies.** Low levels of magnesium can play a role in bladder spasm (page 20).

•**Hormonal Imbalances.** A drop in estrogen can cause the problem (page 94).

Urinary incontinence isn't talked about much, but that doesn't mean it's not a common problem. An estimated one out of every three women experiences stress urinary incontinence (SUI) every now and then. In SUI, you urinate a little when you cough, laugh, sneeze, exercise, or lift something heavy—any movement that increases pressure within your abdominal area, thereby increasing pressure on your bladder. (Cough right now, and you'll see exactly what we mean about that increased pressure.)

As a woman ages, SUI can turn from a rare embarrassment to a regular occurrence. That's because when estrogen levels decrease, there's also a decrease in the muscular tone and length of the urethra (the tube draining urine from the bladder), increasing the risk of leakage. One out of every six women between the ages of 40 and 65 has frequent SUI. Men also have the problem as their bladders age, but with an estimated incidence of three percent to 11 percent.

Good news: The natural remedies in this chapter can work for men, too!

Real Cure Regimen

Medical care is prudent if you have incontinence. A urologist can accurately identify the type of incontinence you have and suggest effective treatments. But before you see the doctor, try one or more of the treatments described here, for two or three months. They may work so well that your incontinence is well controlled or even cured.

Important: If your incontinence has developed suddenly rather than gradually, have your doctor order a urine culture and sensitivity test to see if you have a bladder infection. If you're positive for E. coli bacteria, use the supplement D-mannose to suppress the infection safely. Follow the dosage recommendations on the label.

Kegel Exercises

In baseball, a squeeze play is a bunt that scores a runner from third base, hopefully winning the game. In urinary incontinence, a squeeze is also a smart move that can help you beat the condition.

These squeezing exercises strengthen the pelvic floor and sphincter muscles, reducing stress leakage. In a review of 24 studies on Kegel exercise for urinary incontinence, researchers found the exercise cured women of SUI in 73 percent of cases and improved the situation in 97 percent of cases. (Kegels can also work for men, according to a six-month Italian study, in which 62 per-

---

The Five Types of Urinary Incontinence

1. Stress urinary incontinence. Discussed on page 319, this accounts for nine out of 10 cases of urinary incontinence.

2. Urge incontinence. The involuntary loss of urine while suddenly feeling the urge, or need, to urinate. The most common trigger for this less-frequent problem is an involuntary spasm of the bladder. Causes of that spasm can be an undiagnosed bladder or vaginal infection; nerve problems from stroke, Parkinson's disease, or multiple sclerosis; a spasm of the muscle attached to the top of the pubic bone; or nutritional deficiencies that weaken muscles. This is the most common type of incontinence in men.

3. Mixed incontinence. Incontinence with features of both stress and urge.

4. Overflow incontinence. Urine leakage occurring when the bladder is full but doesn't contract properly to push the urine out because of weak bladder muscles.

5. Total incontinence. The constant loss of urine.

---

cent men who had surgery for prostate cancer recovered their continence using the technique, compared to 12 percent in a group of men who didn't do Kegels.)

Pretty impressive results. So why do many doctors say Kegels don't work for their patients with SUI? "Kegels don't work because they usually aren't taught properly," Kathryn Burgio, PhD, director of the continence program at the University of Alabama in Birmingham, told us. Her instructions:

•**Know where the muscles are.** "Locate them by stopping or slowing the stream of urine the next time you go to the bathroom," she advised. "Another way to identify them is to tighten the same muscles that you use to stop yourself from passing gas in public. You can also find them by tightening the vaginal muscles."

•**Squeeze and hold.** "Several times a day, squeeze the muscles and hold the contraction for 10 seconds," said Dr. Burgio. "At first, you may not be able to hold for very long, but don't worry about that. Start by holding for a count of three—one Mississippi, two Mississippi, three Mississippi—then let go. Over time, build up to a count of 10."

•**Don't contract your abdominal muscles.** "You may have a tendency to contract these muscles by mistake," said Dr. Burgio. "Breathing normally and regularly while doing the Kegels will help you keep those muscles relaxed. You can also put one hand over your abdomen to double check that you're not tightening the muscles there."

•**How to know you're doing them correctly.** You're doing them correctly when you feel a lifting sensation in the area of your vagina or a pulling sensation in your rectum, said Dr. Burgio.

•**Do 45 a day.** That's the most effective number, Dr. Burgio told us. "It's best to do them 15 times in a row, three times a day."

•**Do them during other activities.** "The best way to remember to do your Kegels is to pick a few activities that you do every day—such as taking a shower or brushing your teeth—and do the exercise during those activities," she said.

•**Stop incontinence on the spot.** "Squeeze the muscles right before and during any activity that causes leakage, such as coughing and sneezing. This helps to close the opening to the bladder and prevent urine loss," said Dr. Burgio.

•**Let them become a habit.** "At first, you'll have to concentrate quite a bit to do the Kegels," she said. "After they become a habit, you'll do them automatically."

Other Helpful Advice...

Several other treatments are effective, particularly for urge incontinence.

•**Angelica.** Research shows this herb is very effective for incontinence. It's available as SagaPro Bladder Health, from Terry Naturally. Take one capsule, twice a day, for three days, and then one daily as a maintenance dose.

•**Take magnesium: 200 milligrams to 400 milligrams daily.** This muscle-relaxing, nerve-calming nutrient can help decrease bladder spasms after six weeks of use.

●**Go easy on the caffeine.** Drinking more than a few cups of caffeinated beverages a day can irritate the bladder, causing incontinence. If you think your caffeine intake is linked to the problem—cut back!

●**Use estrogen/progesterone cream daily.** Apply low-dose, bioidentical estrogen/progesterone cream vaginally, near where the urine exits. Give this treatment three months to work. It can be very helpful for any type of urinary incontinence. (For more information on bioidentical hormones, see Hormonal Imbalances on page 95 and Menopausal Problems on page 290.)

Vaginitis

Real Causes

●**Digestive Difficulties.** Eating a high-sugar diet can change the body's acid-alkaline balance, allowing an overgrowth of the yeast Candida albicans (page 98).

●**Prescription Medications.** Overuse of antibiotics can encourage the growth of candida (page 70).

●**Hormonal Imbalances.** Low estrogen is the cause of the dry, irritated vaginal tissue of atrophic vaginitis (page 94).

Ten percent of all visits by women to health care practitioners are for vaginitis, an infection or irritation of the vagina. But this common problem is also commonly misunderstood. In a telling study, only 26 percent of women who thought they had a yeast infection—one type of vaginitis—actually had one.

Here's a simple, straightforward guide to the most common types of vaginitis. First, I'll describe each type of vaginitis, and then present preventive and curative regimens for each.

●**Bacterial vaginosis (BV).** Forty to 45 percent of the time, vaginitis is BV—not an infection, but an overgrowth of the anaerobic (non-oxygen-requiring) bacteria that usually coexist peacefully in the vagina with aerobic (oxygen-requiring) bacteria. Typical symptoms include a thin, grayish discharge; slight irritation; burning during urination; and a fishlike odor.

The problem is triggered when the normally acidic pH of the vagina (3.8 to 4.2) becomes more alkaline (4.5 or higher), allowing the anaerobic bacteria to thrive. Common causes of increased alkalinity include menstruation (levels of hormones at menstruation make the vagina less acidic, and menstrual blood is alkaline); intercourse (ejaculate has an alkaline pH); douching; using heavily scented soaps and laundry detergents; and scented fabric softeners.

●**Yeast (fungal) infection.** Twenty to 25 percent of the time, vaginitis is a yeast infection—and 95 percent of the yeast organisms that do the infecting are *Candida albicans*. The most common symptom is itching. Other possible symptoms include a thick, white, cottage cheese–like discharge; burning; painful urination; painful sex; and a swollen vulva (the external part of the vagina) that has pinpoint red lesions, like a baby with diaper rash. It usually doesn't have a fishy odor, like BV.

Common causes include antibiotics (which kill friendly bacteria that keep yeast in check); unprotected intercourse (usually with a new or recent partner who has a yeast infection you don't know about); douching; excessive stress; a high intake of sugar and other refined carbohydrates (yeast feeds on sugar); diabetes; and a weakened immune system from chemotherapy or high doses of anti-inflammatory steroids.

•**Trichomoniasis.** This is a sexually transmitted disease (STD) caused by the trichomonad protozoa, an amoeba-like creature. In 20 to 50 percent of cases, there are no symptoms. When there are symptoms, they can include large amounts of a frothy, green-yellow discharge; pain with urination; itching; and bleeding after intercourse.

•**Atrophic vaginitis.** This is a common postmenopausal problem: drier, thinner, more easily irritated vaginal tissue, caused by a decrease in estrogen.

Real Cure Regimens

Yes, you can treat some types of vaginitis (BV, yeast infections, and atrophic vaginitis) yourself if they're a recurrence and you're absolutely sure you know what kind of infection or irritation you have.

But you should always see a doctor for vaginitis if it's your first episode; you're not sure what kind of infection or irritation it is; the symptoms are persistent; you have recurrences; you're pregnant; you have an underlying serious health condition, such as diabetes, cancer, or AIDS; or your sexual partner is also experiencing symptoms.

Also check out the chapters on the underlying real causes that contribute to various vaginal problems. Digestive Difficulties (page 98) will steer you away from a sugar-laden diet that yeast loves; Prescription Medications (page 70) will show you why it's bad for vaginal health to always be on antibiotics.

Bacterial Vaginosis (BV)

If you've never had vaginitis or BV, you need to see your doctor and receive an accurate diagnosis. If your doctor diagnoses BV, you'll receive the antibiotic *metronidazole* (Flagyl), taken twice a day for seven days.

But you should also take a probiotic, a supplement or suppository with friendly lactobacillus bacteria. This additional treatment doesn't kill the bacteria. Instead, it helps restore normal vaginal pH—and helps defeat BV—in several ways. They increase the cure rate of an antibiotic—in one study, from 50 to 87 percent. On their own, they reestablish normal bacterial balance and acidic pH, knocking out the BV. And they prevent recurrence of BV when taken daily.

"Lactobacilli were beneficial for the treatment of patients with BV," concluded researchers from the University of Wisconsin in a review of 25 studies on probiotics and BV. The probiotic product used in many BV studies is an over-the-counter product called RepHresh Pro-B. Its manufacturer also makes a vaginal gel that helps restore proper vaginal acid/alkaline balance.

You can preserve the acidity of the vagina by avoiding the products and habits that destroy it. *Here are recommendations from Cherie A. Lefevre, MD, director of the Vulvar and Vaginal Disorders Specialty Center at the St. Louis University School of Medicine…*

•**Wear all-white cotton underwear with a white crotch, not nylon with a cotton crotch.** Thong-type underwear is not recommended on a daily basis. Sleeping without underwear is advised.

•**Avoid full pantyhose.** If you wear them, cut out the diamond crotch (be sure to leave about ¼ to ½ inch of fabric from the seam to prevent running), or wear thigh-high hose.

•**Use a detergent free of dyes, enzymes, and perfumes.**

•**Don't use a fabric softener in the washer or dryer.** White vinegar can be used in the washer as a natural softener.

•**Limit stain-removing products.** Bleach or stain removers are not recommended for your underwear.

•**Avoid bath soaps, lotions, gels, etc., that contain perfume.** This includes many baby products and feminine hygiene products marked "gentle" or "mild." Use these soaps in a bar form: Dove-Hypoallergenic; all-natural olive oil soap; Neutrogena; Basis; or Pears.

•**Avoid all bubble baths, bath salts, and scented oils.** Instead, use a baking soda soak—soaking in lukewarm (not hot) bath water with four to five tablespoons of baking soda to help soothe vulvar itching and burning. Soak one to three times a day, for five to 10 minutes, when you have vulvar symptoms.

•**Use white unscented toilet paper.**

•**Avoid all feminine hygiene sprays, perfumes, and adult or baby wipes.**

•**Avoid deodorized pads and tampons.** Tampons should be used when the blood flow is heavy enough to soak one tampon in four hours or less. Use only pads that have a cotton liner that comes in contact with your skin (no dry-weave pads).

•**Do not douche.**

•**Keep dry by choosing cotton fabrics, not wearing pads daily, and keeping an extra pair of underwear handy and changing once during the day.**

Yeast (Fungal) Infection

You can tell if you *don't* have a yeast infection with the over-the-counter Vagisil Screening Kit. If the results are alkaline, you don't have a yeast infection and may have BV. However, it takes a visit to the doctor to confirm.

Many yeast infections resolve on their own, without treatment. To speed healing, cut out sugar and other refined carbohydrates and alcohol.

The safest, easiest, and most reliable treatment for a yeast infection is using an over-the-counter antifungal, such as *miconazole* (Monistat) or *clotrimazole* (Mycelex). As with BV, taking probiotics may help a yeast infection resolve. Taking a probiotic regularly can decrease recurrences. Other ways to help prevent recurrences are to avoid antibiotics and to reduce or eliminate sugar.

You could also try supplementing your diet with sea buckthorn berry extract. A study from Finland shows it can improve the moisture of vaginal mucous membranes, reducing susceptibility to infection. I recommend the product Omega-7, from Terry Naturally. Follow the dosage recommendations on the label.

Trichomoniasis

If diagnosed, trichomoniasis is treated with *metronidazole* (Flagyl): a two-gram, one-day dose. Your sexual partner also needs to receive Flagyl.

Atrophic Vaginitis

Bioidentical vaginal estrogen creams are very effective, and I generally recommend them for this problem. However, these creams may not be appropriate for women with breast cancer or a clotting disorder. (See Menopause Problems on page 290 for a complete discussion of bioidentical hormones for women.)

A wonderful natural alternative, recommended by Dr. Lefevre: vegetable-based oils, such as sunflower oil, canola oil, and olive oil, and solid vegetable shortenings, with a small amount applied twice a day, inside the vagina. The oils are completely safe for vulvar and vaginal tissues. "I have seen women who have suffered for five or more years with atrophic vaginitis and painful intercourse achieve complete relief within six weeks of starting this regimen," she told us. My late wife and live wife did and do this, without much muss or fuss, following the exact instructions here: applying a small amount inside the vagina twice a day. As long as you use a small amount, it's very straightforward—and very effective, just as the doc says. (And you quickly learn what a "small amount" is from direct experience.) Also, the Vulvar and Vaginal Disorders Center gives exactly this written advice, without any extra guidelines, so it's a good guess that the advice is working for their many patients without need for more detail.

Another excellent option to use as a lubricant during intercourse: coconut oil that is liquid at room temperature. Nature's Way makes an excellent product called Always Liquid Premium Coconut Oil. It is nonirritating and pleasant to use.

PART 3

The 28-Day Life-Change Cure

Don't Follow My Advice!

'm joking, of course. But not entirely. The key to success in following any health plan is to follow *your* plan—to do what feels right to you, at the pace that feels right to you.

As you may have read in Happiness Deficiency on page 55, I firmly believe that what *feels* good to you usually *is* good for you. That's because what feels good—deep down good—is usually in alignment with your deepest being: with your psyche, soul, or spirit (or whatever name you use to acknowledge your essential self). There is no authority—no parent, priest, politician, teacher, or doctor—who should (or can) replace your personal sense of what's right or wrong for you. And that includes me!

So consider these 28 days' worth of feel-better ideas to be recommendations, not requirements. They're like 28 tools in your life-change toolbox. Choose and use whatever tools you find are best for the daily "job" of optimizing your health and well-being.

That said, I do think that following the day-by-day tips and recommendations in the 28-Day Life-Change Cure *can* improve your health and happiness in only four weeks, boosting energy, enlivening and calming your mind and emotions, and helping prevent, control, or reverse many health problems you may have. If it feels good to you to implement this day-by-day plan just as it's described, from Day 1 to Day 28—go for it!

As you'll see, I've made it easy to figure out what to do on each day of the 28-Day program by presenting not only the new tip for that day, but a recap of all the tips you've already put into place. The recaps are at the end of each one of the 28 days, under the heading *Life-Change Checklist*.

Your life-changing 28-day journey begins with a single day...

Week 1

Nutrition:
Customize Your Curative Cuisine

DAY 1: Eat Whole, Fresh, Locally Grown Foods

Eating a healthful diet is a key to good health. And following one simple dietary guideline can make all the difference in helping you eat more good-for-you foods: Eat lots of whole, fresh foods, locally grown or raised. That includes fresh vegetables, whole fruits (fruit juices deliver too much sugar), whole grains, beans, fish, lean red meat, and low-fat dairy products. Just this one action can protect your heart, stabilize your blood sugar, boost your brainpower, balance your emotions, encourage weight loss, and generally buff up your health.

Let's call this the Day 1 Diet. A few tips can help you follow it.

•**Shop the supermarket perimeter first.** You'll find most of the whole, fresh foods in the outer edges of the market. That's where the produce section, dairy products, butcher, fish counter, and (if it's a naturally oriented store) bins with whole grains, nuts, and seeds are found. Only after you've strolled the perimeter should you venture into the interior aisles, where the shelves are mostly stocked with packaged and processed foods.

•**Be a localtarian.** Once upon a meal, the corn you ate was the corn that you, your friendly neighbor, or a local farmer grew—it was picked, cooked, and eaten in a matter of days or maybe even a matter of minutes. Now, you're probably getting that corn (and many of the other "fresh" foods you eat) at the end of a very long journey, from some faraway state or nation. And that "fresh" food has probably been bred not for better flavor but for better shipping—in other words, it's tough but not necessarily tasty (think supermarket tomatoes).

That's why I urge you to become what I call a localtarian. When you can, buy foods that are produced locally, perhaps by shopping at a farmers' market once a week. (A weekly trip to the farmers' market—where maybe you'll meet some friends and go out for a fun lunch after-ward—is a wonderful routine.) For fresh and healthy local produce in the off-season, emphasize super-nutritious root vegetables, such as carrots, sweet potatoes, yams, potatoes, pumpkin, tur-nips, and parsnips. Also look to cruciferous vegetables, that are in season over the winter, such as broccoli, cauliflower, kale, chard, Brussel sprouts, cabbage, and radishes as well as beets and winter squash.

•**Go organic, when you can.** When you see "organic" produce, it's reasonably certain that an effort has been made to produce a food that's relatively free of pesticides and chemical fertil-izers—and that's good.

Pleasure is permitted—in fact, it's encouraged! Trying to eliminate all foods that are "bad for you" is stressful (because it's no fun and most people can't do it) and counterproductive (a period of intense dietary deprivation almost always leads to a period of intense overeating). I'm in favor of pleasurable moderation, which, for me, includes indulging now and then in the foods I love to eat, even when they don't fit the description "whole, fresh, and local." For example, dark chocolate and coffee are two of my favorite health foods!

Day 1: Life-Change Checklist...

☐ Eat whole, fresh, locally grown foods.

DAY 2: Take a Vitamin/Mineral Supplement

Many Americans have an extremely low intake of the vitamins and minerals that are crucial for good health. The mineral magnesium is a good example. Most Americans fail to get the recommended daily allowance.

This mineral plays a role in more than 300 key biochemical reactions, regulating the function of muscles and nerves, and protecting the health of your heart and brain. In the Real Cure Regimens in this book, I recommend supplemental magnesium for dozens of different health problems, including anxiety-caused panic attacks, asthma, attention-deficit/hyperactivity disorder, constipation, depression, diabetes, dry mouth and dry eyes, epilepsy, fatigue—well, that's just the beginning of a long alphabetical list, so you get the idea. Magnesium is important for preventing and healing nearly every condition included in this book!

Magnesium is just one mineral among many minerals and vitamins. And if you're a typical American, you're deficient in a lot of them. In my opinion, those nutritional deficiencies are the leading cause behind the development of so many modern illnesses. Taking a high-quality multivitamin-mineral supplement can protect you from nutritional deficiencies.

You can obtain optimal levels of most nutrients by mixing just one drink each morning using the Energy Revitalization System multinutrient powder from Nature's Way. This supplement replaces 35 pills. If you're well and looking to prevent disease, ½ to 1 scoop per day is plenty. If you're ill and looking for optimum nutritional support in treating and reversing disease, take the full scoop. Adjust to whatever feels best to you. (I take ⅘ scoop each morning.)

Because the supplement is a powder, you can take it many different ways—add it to yogurt. ...add the orange-flavored form to two ounces of orange juice and two ounces of milk and blend it with four ounces of water, producing an orange smoothie. I favor the berry flavor and simply add water and stir. I add a 5-gram scoop of ribose, a key building block of cellular energy (Corvalen) or Smart Energy (a combination of ribose, magnesium, and energy-enhancing herbs) to the Energy Revitalization powder to turbo-charge my energy. (You can read more about the Energy Revitalization System on page 30, and ribose on pages 222–223).

If you hand-mix (as I do) rather than use a blender, put the powder in a dry glass and add two to three ounces of whatever liquid you're using, give it a few stirs until any lumps are gone, and then add the rest of the liquid. It's the most worthwhile 10 seconds you'll spend each day!

If you don't like powders, the best multivitamin tablet is Clinical Essentials. All of the supplements discussed here—the Energy Revitalization System, the Clinical Essentials multivitamin, and ribose (I recommend the SHINE brand, my own formulation)—are widely available online and in some retail stores where supplements are sold.

Day 2: Life-Change Checklist...

☐ Eat whole, fresh, locally grown foods.
☐ Take a multivitamin-mineral supplement.

DAY 3: Dress Up Your Breakfast with Berries

Studies show that, compared with folks who don't eat breakfast, those who regularly eat a morning meal are slimmer, have lower levels of insulin (too-high levels play a role in many diseases, including heart disease and diabetes), and have lower levels of "bad" LDL and total cholesterol (two risk factors for heart disease).

If you're headed to a day of heavy manual labor, you may need a protein-rich breakfast of eggs and bacon. If you're headed to the computer for a morning of mental work, you may find that a lighter breakfast is ideal.

But if you're eating a bowl of cereal at breakfast today or a cup of unsweetened yogurt, or making a fruit smoothie, I encourage you to turn boring into wow by adding berries. Berries—blueberries, strawberries, raspberries, blackberries—are loaded with super-powerful antioxidants that studies show can play a role in preventing heart disease, stroke, diabetes, cancer, and Alzheimer's disease. (In a study, folks in their seventies who upped their daily intake of blueberries improved their memory by 30 percent in just three months.)

So take a bowl of whole grain cereal (good choices include cholesterol-lowering cooked oatmeal or a dry cereal such as Original Life, Cheerios and Total) and add a sprinkling of fresh, luscious berries. You don't need to stop there, though. Add a sliced banana for a delicious dose of potassium, a mineral that helps normalize blood pressure. As you'll see throughout the 28-Day Life-Change Cure, it's simple actions that often take no more than a couple of extra seconds—like sprinkling some berries on your breakfast cereal—that add up to a life of good health.

Day 3: Life-Change Checklist...

☐ Eat whole, fresh, locally grown foods.
☐ If you're eating cereal or oatmeal for breakfast, add a sprinkling of berries and a sliced banana.
☐ Take a multivitamin-mineral supplement.

DAY 4: Declare Today Sugar-Free Day

For most of human history, the only sugar we ate was found naturally in food. Now, sugar-loaded processed foods such as sodas, doughnuts, and candy bars add 60 to 100 pounds of sugar per person to our diets each year. After you eat or drink a sugary food or beverage, your blood sugar level skyrockets, giving you an initial high. But you crash several hours later (or even sooner), which leaves you wanting more sugar. In short, you're addicted. And like any addiction, sugar addiction is hard on your health.

Excess sugar in the diet plays a role in many chronic health problems, including heart disease, diabetes, metabolic syndrome, anxiety and depression, chronic pain, chronic sinusitis, fibromyalgia and chronic fatigue syndrome, autoimmune diseases, and even cancer.

So declare today Sugar-Free Day—declare your independence from sugar addiction. However, I recommend you forgo *sugar*, not *sweetness*. For a healthy sugar substitute, use stevia, a sweet-tasting herb. My favorite brands are Now Food's Better Stevia and Stevia Select (which has an awesome line of flavored liquid stevias). Another good natural sugar substitute is erythritol. Stevia and erythritol are combined in the products Pure Via and Truvia. You can also use saccharin (Sweet'N Low), which has a long record of safety.

I don't recommend aspartame (NutraSweet), because some individuals experience severe reactions to it, including seizures, headaches, nausea, dizziness, and depression. It's surprising to me that it ever received FDA approval for use. And I think the jury is still out on the safety of sucralose (Splenda), with some people reporting side effects such as gut pain. Preliminary research shows it may decrease friendly gut bacteria and imbalance blood sugar.

Use the healthful sugar substitutes anywhere you'd ordinarily use sugar. For a sweet treat, enjoy up to an ounce a day of dark chocolate (65 percent cacao or more)—a healthy (though not low-calorie) food when eaten in moderation. Get the best-tasting one you can find, and savor!

Some people go through "withdrawal symptoms" when cutting out sugar—sugar cravings, fatigue, irritability—that last seven to 10 days. If that happens to you, reduce sugar intake more gradually. Allowing yourself a few pieces of that dark chocolate can help, as can a healthy snack of fruit. For more information, my book *The Complete Guide to Beating Sugar Addiction* can guide you on how to avoid these symptoms—while enjoying your sweet tooth.

Day 4: Life-Change Checklist...

- ☐ Eat whole, fresh, locally grown foods.
- ☐ If you're eating cereal or oatmeal for breakfast, add a sprinkling of berries and a sliced banana.
- ☐ Minimize sugar, using a natural sweetener instead, such as stevia.
- ☐ Take a multivitamin-mineral supplement.

DAY 5: Get a (Fish) Oil Change

Fats are made up of fatty acids, and the fats in our diet deliver two main types of fatty acids: omega-6 and omega-3. The omega-6 fatty acids are found in beef, pork, and chicken; in vegetable oils such as corn, peanut, safflower, soybean, and sunflower; in trans fats (found in many store-bought baked goods, chips, and other processed products); and in margarine. The omega-3 fatty acids are found in oily fish such as salmon and tuna; in some nuts (walnuts) and seeds (flaxseed); and in small quantities in leafy greens.

Your body processes omega-3s and omega-6s in very different ways. Omega-3s are *anti-inflammatory*: They douse the low-grade inflammation that fuels cardiovascular disease, the number-one killer of Americans. Many of the omega-6 fats, on the other hand, are *pro-inflammatory*.

Our hunter-gatherer ancestors consumed a diet with a very healthy 2:1 ratio of omega-6s to omega-3s. But the ratio of the average American diet, with its preponderance of processed foods, is now 15:1. You can bring that ratio back into healthy balance by increasing your intake of fish oil, which is loaded with two omega-3 fatty acids: eicosapentaenoic acid (EPA) and docosahexaenoic acid (DHA). You should also cut back on omega-6 foods—mainly vegetable oils (sunflower, corn, safflower, soy), and products containing them.

Fish with the most omega-3s include salmon, tuna, sardines, and trout. (White albacore tuna has three times more omega-3s than chunk light.) I recommend eating three to four servings of fatty fish every week. Have one of those servings today.

If you don't want to, or can't manage to, eat fatty fish a couple of times a week, I recommend an omega-3 supplement. I favor a unique omega-3 fatty acid from salmon called Vectomega from Terry Naturally. It contains phospholipids, a natural part of fish oil that increases absorption of omega-3s, 50 times more than other fish oils. One to two tablets deliver all the omega-3s you need, instead of the typical eight to 16 capsules.

Increasing fish oil intake is especially important for anyone with a disease that has an inflammatory component, such as heart disease, asthma, rheumatoid arthritis, or any other type of autoimmune disease. And since most of the brain is made up of fat—particularly DHA, one of the fatty acids in fish oil—fish oil is also critical for optimizing your mood and mental clarity.

Day 5: Life-Change Checklist...

- ☐ Eat whole, fresh, locally grown foods.
- ☐ If you're eating cereal or oatmeal for breakfast, add a sprinkling of berries and a sliced banana.
- ☐ Eat fatty fish such as salmon or sardines three to four times a week, or take a daily fish oil supplement.
- ☐ Minimize sugar, using a natural sweetener instead, such as stevia.
- ☐ Take a multivitamin-mineral supplement.

DAY 6: Hydrate for Health

Water is essential for good health. In fact, it's just as essential as the essential amino acids (components of protein), the essential fatty acids (components of fat), and other nutritional basics that your body doesn't make on its own and that you must regularly consume. It's critical for energy and detoxification. It transports crucial compounds around the body. It helps break up food into the nutrients you need.

But how much water should you drink today, and every day, to stay healthy? Eight 8-ounce glasses? Six 6-ounce glasses? Half your body weight in ounces? Those are all actual recommendations by one expert or another. If you ask me, keeping track of how many glasses of water (or worse, ounces of water) you drank today is a very annoying way to spend a day, especially if you plan to do it every day for the rest of your life. Instead, just check your lips and mouth. If they're dry, you need to drink more water. It's as simple as that!

Another simple method: Take a look at the color of your urine. If it's a dull yellow, there's not enough water diluting it, and you should drink more. (Urine can also turn bright yellow from an intake of B vitamins, but that's different from the murky yellow of overly concentrated urine.)

A third method: When you feel tired, drink a glass of cold water. If your energy improves in a couple of minutes, you were dehydrated.

Another method I often use: When I'm thirsty, I can easily chug a whole glass of water; when I'm not thirsty, I prefer to sip it. I favor filtered tap water to minimize your intake of possibly toxic chemicals in the water supply. If you're a senior—a time when your "thirst sensors" aren't working as well—keep water on hand and sip as you go.

Day 6: Life-Change Checklist...

- ☐ Eat whole, fresh, locally grown foods
- ☐ If you're eating cereal or oatmeal for breakfast, add a sprinkling of berries and a sliced banana.
- ☐ Eat fatty fish such as salmon or sardines three to four times a week, or take a daily fish oil supplement.
- ☐ Minimize sugar, using a natural sweetener instead, such as stevia.
- ☐ Stay hydrated—if your lips are dry or your urine is yellow, you need to drink more water. If you drink tap water, use a filter.
- ☐ Take a multivitamin-mineral supplement.

DAY 7: Go Nuts at Snack Time

There's nothing like a snack. It's a tasty treat between meals, a way to boost your blood sugar (glucose) midmorning and midafternoon, and a refreshing break from the duties of the day. But many people snack on sugary foods or beverages. They might taste good for a moment, but they aren't particularly good for you. Is there a yummy alternative?

Nuts! Nuts supply plenty of glucose-balancing protein. Many types of nuts deliver anti-inflammatory fatty acids. They're also rich in digestion-regulating fiber. And they are high in fat, so they satisfy appetite.

But maybe you don't snack on nuts because you think they're fattening. Not so. Studies show that adding a handful of nuts a day to the diet doesn't promote weight gain, even when you don't cut any other calories. In fact, studies show that nuts are incredibly good for you in lots of different ways. *In recent research, eating a handful or more of nuts a day...*

- Reduced DNA damage to cells (mixed nuts)
- Lowered LDL cholesterol (pistachios)
- Lowered total cholesterol and LDL cholesterol in people with high cholesterol (macadamia nuts)

- Decreased C-reactive protein, a biomarker of inflammation linked to cardiovascular disease as well as to diabetes and autoimmune diseases (almonds)
- Reduced insulin levels in type 2 diabetes, a sign of better blood sugar control (walnuts)
- Reduced the risk of diabetes by 50 percent when added to a Mediterranean diet (mixed nuts)
- Lowered the risk of cardiovascular disease (overall nut consumption)
- Improved blood levels of selenium—an important anticancer mineral—as effectively as 100 micrograms a day of a selenium supplement (two Brazil nuts daily)

Go nuts at snack time today…and every day!

Day 7: Life-Change Checklist…

☐ Eat whole, fresh, locally grown foods.

☐ If you're eating cereal or oatmeal for breakfast, add a sprinkling of berries and a sliced banana.

☐ Eat fatty fish such as salmon or sardines three to four times a week, or take a daily fish oil supplement.

☐ For snack time, choose a handful of nuts—walnuts, almonds, and macadamia are best.

☐ Minimize sugar, using a natural sweetener instead, such as stevia.

☐ Stay hydrated.

☐ Take a multivitamin-mineral supplement.

Week 2

Physical Activity:
Easy Really Does It

DAY 8: Plan Ahead—and Head Out!

A vast amount of evidence shows that moderate physical activity (such as brisk walking) can help prevent and ease a wide range of health problems, from anxiety to Alzheimer's disease, from cancer to cardiovascular disease, and from stress overload to stroke (see Inactivity on page 40). Researchers have calculated that if every American met the standard recommendation for moderate physical activity—150 minutes a week—there would be 250,000 fewer deaths every year. But most of us don't exercise. Less than five percent of American adults meet that standard recommendation, reported researchers from the National Institutes of Health. That's less than one in 20 people. What are the other 19 doing?

Well, they probably aren't planning to exercise, so it never happens!

I agree with the experts in exercise psychology who say that a lack of planning is the number-one reason why regular exercise doesn't become a part of a person's life. And that planning doesn't have to be complex. In fact, I've found that the best type of planning is super simple: Plan on meeting a friend for a session of mutually enjoyable exercise, whether it's a brisk walk or a game of tennis or a yoga class. If you've agreed to meet a friend for a workout, it's very likely to happen—because it's part of a routine and you don't want to disappoint or annoy your friend by not showing up, and because you're looking forward to a fun time of talking and socializing (particularly if you're walking).

Planning could also include making the following decisions in advance...

•**Where you will exercise** (Around the neighborhood? At the gym? In the basement?)

•**What exercise you will do** (A walk? An aerobics class? A ride on a stationary bike?)

•**When you are going to exercise** (First thing in the morning? At lunch? After work?)

•**How you will fit that exercise session into your busy day** (Keep your sneakers by the door. Ask your spouse to watch the kids while you go to the gym, or find a gym with child care. Dust off the exercise bike in the basement.)

Some find that putting the exercise machine in front of the TV works. The rule? As soon as the TV goes on, you go on the exercise machine for 15 to 45 minutes. So, starting today—and at the beginning of every week or every month—get out your calendar and pencil in your exercise sessions. And get a friend to pencil them in, too.

Day 8: Life-Change Checklist...

Nutrition

☐ Eat whole, fresh, locally grown foods—especially berries and fatty fish. Snack on nuts.

☐ Minimize sugar, using a natural sweetener instead, such as stevia.

☐ Stay hydrated.

☐ Take a multivitamin-mineral supplement.

Physical activity

☐ Plan on meeting a friend for a walk—in fact, meet up a couple of days every week, for 150 minutes worth of weekly exercise (30 minutes, at least five days a week) .

DAY 9: Put on a Pedometer

You'll find there is one type of exercise that more regular exercisers choose to do than any other, probably because it's easy, enjoyable, and cheap: walking. And one of the most reliable ways to make sure you walk more is by using a pedometer, a device that counts the number of steps you take. (There are many types of pedometers, from simple devices that clip to your waistband, to products such as Fitbit and Apple Watch that count steps and also provide many other measurements of health, to smartphone apps. Choose the one that works best for you.)

Exercise experts and behavioral scientists say a pedometer motivates people like no other device for a couple of reasons. You can set a goal (steps per day). You can monitor the goal yourself. And you feel satisfaction once you've reached the goal.

To help you set your goal, use your pedometer for three days (starting today). At bedtime, write down the number of steps you took that day. On the third day, calculate the average: the total number of steps divided by the number of days. (For example, 12,000 steps over three days equals an average of 4,000 steps.) That average is your baseline. For the next week, increase your baseline by 2,000 steps. If your baseline was 4,000, for example, try to walk 6,000 steps every day. Two thousand steps equals one mile, or 15 to 20 minutes of walking.

If you want to keep going, add 2,000 steps per day the next week (8,000 steps a day) and 2,000 steps a day the week after that (10,000 steps a day). Many experts recommend 10,000 steps a day as a good goal. I think your daily goal should be the number of steps you enjoy walking. That might be 6,000, 8,000, 10,000, or more.

Don't worry about your level of intensity. Brisk walking is moderate intensity, and almost everybody who is out for a walk is walking reasonably briskly. Enjoy yourself!

Day 9: Life-Change Checklist...

Nutrition
- ☐ Eat whole, fresh, locally grown foods—especially berries and fatty fish. Snack on nuts.
- ☐ Minimize sugar, using a natural sweetener instead, such as stevia.
- ☐ Stay hydrated.
- ☐ Take a multivitamin-mineral supplement.

Physical activity
- ☐ Walk (30 minutes, at least five days a week).
- ☐ Using a pedometer, keep track of your daily steps, and write down the number of steps at bedtime. (You'll be doing this for the next three days.)

DAY 10: Stroll Barefoot

No, I'm not suggesting you become a hippie for a day. This is actually a therapy called earthing or "barefoot therapy." It drains inflammation-causing positive electrical charges out of your body in much the same way that wires in your house are grounded to prevent the buildup of excess charge in electrical equipment. A barefoot walk fills up your body with anti-inflammatory negatively charged particles—sort of like getting a transfusion of health-giving, cell-protecting antioxidants.

When was the last time you actually walked on the earth, foot to ground? Probably a long time ago. Do it for a few minutes today. Go for a walk in your bare feet. Even walking on concrete will "ground" you, though walking on asphalt won't. (Why the difference? Concrete is a conductive substance made of water and minerals, and it retains moisture—so those negatively-charged particles pass through it, just as if you were sitting or standing on grass or open ground, we were told by Stephen Sinatra, MD, co-author of the book *Earthing*. On the other hand, asphalt is made from petrochemicals and is not conductive.)

If you can't go for a barefoot walk, sit in a chair outside with your feet planted on the ground, reading or relaxing. In winter, or if you live in an urban environment where there's little opportunity to ground, try using "grounding" devices such as foot mats and bed sheets, available at Grounded.com. For more information on this, I recommend an excellent book called *Earthing: The Most Important Health Discovery Ever!* by Clinton Ober, Stephen T. Sinatra, MD, and Martin Zucker.

Day 10: Life-Change Checklist...

Nutrition
- ☐ Eat whole, fresh, locally grown foods—especially berries and fatty fish. Snack on nuts.
- ☐ Minimize sugar, using a natural sweetener instead, such as stevia.
- ☐ Stay hydrated.
- ☐ Take a multivitamin-mineral supplement.

Physical Activity
- ☐ Walk (30 minutes, at least five days a week).
- ☐ Using a pedometer, keep track of your daily steps, and write down the number of steps at bedtime. (You did this yesterday, and you'll be doing it tomorrow, too.)
- ☐ Walk barefoot for a few minutes or sit outside with your feet on the ground.

DAY 11: Strengthen Your Muscles

Strength training. Resistance training. Weight training. Muscle training. Those are all names for the same type of exercise: using weights or resistance bands or the weight of your own body (such as a pushup) to build muscular strength. The U.S. government's Physical Activity Guidelines for Americans recommend engaging in a round of muscle training two or more days a week. And for good reason. *Recent studies show that muscle training can...*

- •**Improve bone density (preventing, slowing, or reversing osteoporosis)**
- •**Firm and trim your body**
- •**Prevent weight gain as you age**
- •**Lower blood pressure**
- •**Lower cholesterol levels**
- •**Increase self-esteem**
- •**Prevent frailty and falls in older people**

Here are some handy guidelines for muscle strengthening from Vik Khanna, a clinical exercise specialist certified by the American College of Sports Medicine...

- •**Talk to your doctor first.** Make sure you're healthy enough for muscle training.
- •**Train with a qualified expert.** Working with a fitness professional in a facility is an excellent way to start training. The Y has good trainers and is family friendly. (In other words, you're less likely to find gangs of muscle-bound guys bench-pressing hundreds of pounds!)

●**Or train on your own.** Start with a minimal amount of equipment, such as resistance bands, tubes, or light dumbbells—all of which will probably total around $50. Such equipment usually comes with an illustrated guide that shows you how to do a whole-body workout. Two excellent sites for home equipment are PerformBetter.com and Power-systems.com.

●**Work every muscle.** Muscles work in balance, so it's important to strengthen all of you. Don't just work your arms or your legs, for example. Do exercises for all of the muscles in your arms, torso, legs, and core abdomen and pelvis.

●**Train on a different day than you do your aerobic exercise, and don't train every day.** It takes 24 hours for your muscles to recover from a session of muscle training. Don't do more than every other day, and train on a different day than you do your aerobic-type exercise (walking, biking, swimming, etc).

●**Start slowly.** Add weights and resistance in very small increments, starting at around 70 percent of the heaviest weight you can lift for any individual muscle, with 10 repetitions, for two or three sets. This provides a low risk of injury and a steady path for improvement.

For example, if you can do one biceps curl with a maximum of 12 pounds, you begin the exercise with eight pounds of weight, lifting the weight 10 times in a row. Once you can lift the weight easily 12 to 15 times, increase the weight slightly, perhaps to 15 pounds, and once again do 10 repetitions. If you use resistance bands, start with extra-light bands and then move to light, medium, and heavy. Don't set a limit to your strength. You'll probably underestimate how quickly you'll gain strength. Don't be afraid to get stronger. A strong muscle is a healthy muscle. On the other hand, pain is not needed; so the saying "No pain, no gain" is insane!

Day 11: Life-Change Checklist...

Nutrition

☐ Eat whole, fresh, locally grown foods—especially berries and fatty fish. Snack on nuts.

☐ Minimize sugar, using a natural sweetener instead, such as stevia.

☐ Stay hydrated.

☐ Take a multivitamin-mineral supplement.

Physical Activity

☐ Walk (30 minutes, at least five days a week).

☐ Using a pedometer, keep track of your daily steps, and write down the number of steps at bedtime. This evening, calculate the average: the total number of steps divided by the number of days. (For example, 15,000 steps over three days equals an average of 5,000 steps, the amount logged by the average American.) This average is your baseline.

☐ Walk barefoot for a few minutes or sit outside with your feet on the ground.

☐ Start resistance training, two or more days a week.

DAY 12: Burn a Few More Calories—Make Love!

Exercise is good for your sex life. People who are physically fit see themselves as sexier and more desirable than the average Joe or Joan. They also think they're better in bed—that their sexual performance is above average. Even if those perceptions aren't correct, research shows fitter folks are having more sex. In fact, older people who exercise have about the same amount of sex as people 20 years younger. Maybe that's because guys over 50 who exercise are 30 percent less likely to develop erectile dysfunction. And a scientific paper in the *American Journal of Lifestyle Medicine* endorses exercise as a way to improve low libido in women.

But it's not only that exercise leads to more and better sex. Sex leads to exercise, because sex is exercise. Although you're in bed (maybe), you're also moving—and burning as many calories per minute as you would while playing tennis. (Talk about "courting"!) Sex is good for sweethearts and for physical hearts. In one study, men with the most frequent sexual activity had half the risk of heart attack or stroke. Sex also generates endorphins, feel-good brain chemicals that can decrease pain.

Another benefit: Along with exercise, sex triggers the production of growth hormone, also called the fountain-of-youth hormone. Growth hormone helps you look younger, melts fat, and builds muscle. But most of all, intimate sex makes us feel younger and happier, and gives us the sense that life is worth living.

I encourage you to "exercise" with your mate today!

Day 12: Life-Change Checklist...

Nutrition

☐ Eat whole, fresh, locally grown foods—especially berries and fatty fish. Snack on nuts.

☐ Minimize sugar, using a natural sweetener instead, such as stevia.

☐ Stay hydrated.

☐ Take a multivitamin-mineral supplement.

Physical Activity

☐ Walk (30 minutes, at least five days a week).

☐ Yesterday, you calculated your baseline of daily steps. Today—Day 12—you're going to start increasing your steps, until you're at 7,000 steps by Day 18. (For ways to increase your steps, see the pedometer section in Inactivity on page 47.)

☐ Walk barefoot for a few minutes or sit outside with your feet on the ground.

☐ Burn a few more calories—make love!

DAY 13: S-T-R-E-T-C-H—With Yoga

They might want to rename yoga "yogood," because it's so good for you. Scientific studies show that the poses, or asanas, of this ancient system of exercise increase flexibility, strengthen muscles, improve balance and posture, and relax the nervous system.

Those are big benefits. So it's not surprising that science also shows a long list of conditions that yoga can help, usually by easing symptoms. That list includes anxiety, asthma, cancer, depression, diabetes, fibromyalgia, headaches, heart disease, insomnia, irritable bowel syndrome, menopause, osteoporosis, sinusitis, and urinary stress incontinence. Not bad for a simple stance!

If you're interested in yoga, there are many ways to learn a simple routine, from taking a class to watching a video. (A class is best to start with, because the teacher can correct your mistakes and help prevent injury.) But here's an easy, refreshing stretch for today, courtesy of Timothy McCall, MD, author of *Yoga as Medicine: The Yogic Prescription for Health and Healing.*

1. Stand with your feet hip-width apart, or sit up in a chair.

2. Slowly inhale and lift both arms out in front of you and then over your head.

3. As you exhale, bring your arms back down.

4. Repeat the arm movements, with your breath, five more times.

It's likely you'll find this simple yoga pose is deeply refreshing and energizing, particularly if you're under a lot of stress (and who isn't).

Day 13: Life-Change Checklist...

Nutrition

☐ Eat whole, fresh, locally grown foods—especially berries and fatty fish. Snack on nuts.

☐ Minimize sugar, using a natural sweetener instead, such as stevia.

☐ Stay hydrated.

☐ Take a multivitamin-mineral supplement.

Physical Activity

☐ Walk (30 minutes, at least five days a week).

☐ Continue to increase your daily steps. *This week's goal*: Adding 2,000 to your baseline, which you calculated on Day 11.

☐ Walk barefoot for a few minutes or sit outside with your feet on the ground.

☐ Do yoga—whether it's one stretch or regular, longer sessions, at home or in class. Aim for a minimum of once a week.

DAY 14: Let Somebody Else Move Your Muscles—Get a Massage!

Financial advisors often counsel a person to "pay yourself first" before you pay your bills, as one of the best ways to save. Well, I think the "pay yourself first" principle could also save your health.

Too often, we put everybody else first. We give and give and give, and seldom receive. And we end up depleted physically, mentally, and emotionally. That's why I think you should schedule at least one day a month to "pay yourself first." This is a day that features nonstop personal pampering. A day when you receive rather than give. Maybe a day when somebody gives you a massage.

Touch is deeply nurturing and healing. Scientific studies show that massage can lower levels of stress hormones, lessening anxiety and tension. It can help relieve all kinds of pain, including back pain, headaches, and carpal tunnel syndrome. It can also improve sleep, strengthen immunity, and lower blood pressure. And we're a society that suffers from a touch deficiency—a society where you can be "connected" to 5,000 "friends" on Facebook and never get a big hug!

If giving yourself a massage doesn't fit your budget, pamper yourself in other ways. We talked with Alice Domar, PhD, author of the book *Self-Nurture*, for suggestions: Sit on a chaise lounge in the backyard with a cool drink and the latest issue of your favorite magazine. Take an afternoon nap. Make some popcorn and watch TV. Borrow a friend's puppy and romp with it in the grass. Visit an art museum. Go for a leisurely sight-seeing walk at a nearby location that you've always wanted to visit.

It's healthy to take time to pamper yourself. Need more permission? You've got it—doctor's orders!

Day 14: Life-Change Checklist...

Nutrition

- ☐ Eat whole, fresh, locally grown foods—especially berries and fatty fish. Snack on nuts.
- ☐ Minimize sugar, using a natural sweetener instead, such as stevia.
- ☐ Stay hydrated.
- ☐ Take a multivitamin-mineral supplement.

Physical Activity

- ☐ Walk (30 minutes, at least five days a week).
- ☐ Continue to increase your daily steps. *This week's goal*: Adding 2,000 steps to your daily base-line, which you calculated on Day 11.
- ☐ Walk barefoot for a few minutes or sit outside with your feet on the ground.
- ☐ Get a massage or nurture yourself in some other way.
- ☐ Burn a few more calories—make love!

Week 3

Sleep:
Ahhh—Deep, Peaceful, Restorative

DAY 15: Figure Out How Much Sleep You Need

If you've read Poor Sleep on page 33, you know that insomnia is a major problem in the United States, with as many as 100 million Americans (nearly one-third!) regularly having sleep problems such as trouble falling asleep or staying asleep or waking up too early.

And you also know that, aside from daytime fatigue, poor sleep can cause or complicate all kinds of health problems. They include anxiety and depression, diabetes, heart disease, high blood pressure, stroke, memory loss, chronic pain, and even overweight.

Maybe you're one of the many Americans with insomnia. And maybe you're also suffering from one of the ills that poor sleep can trigger or worsen. Well, this week, the 28-Day Life-

Change Cure is all about helping you get a better night's sleep. And the first step is figuring out exactly how much sleep you need. There is no "right" amount of sleep, although studies suggest that at least seven to eight hours is best for most people. (Americans get an average of about 6.5 hours.) You can tell whether you've slept enough by how you feel the next day.

- **Are you rested?**
- **Is your mind clear?**
- **Is your energy tip-top?**
- **Are your muscles limber rather than stiff?**

If you can answer yes to these questions, you slept enough. But if you answered no to one or more of them, you may need more sleep. How much more?

To find out, conduct a two-day experiment. (Friday and Saturday nights are good nights to do this, because it's more likely you'll be able to sleep longer on weekend mornings.) On the first night, try to get one more hour of sleep than usual. On the second night, try to get two more hours than usual. So, if you usually turn off the lights around midnight and get out of bed when the alarm goes off at 6:00 a.m., stay in bed seven hours: Go to bed one hour earlier or get up one hour later.

The next night, stay in bed eight hours—go to bed an hour earlier or get up an hour later.

If you feel a whole lot better with seven hours of sleep, then that's the amount you want to try to get every night. If you feel better with eight hours, aim for that amount. (And if you don't feel better with seven or eight hours, consider seeing a holistic physician to determine other possible causes for your symptoms of not feeling rested, having a foggy mind, low energy, and/or painful muscles.)

Week 3 is all about getting the amount of sleep you have determined is right for you.

Day 15: Life-Change Checklist...

Nutrition
- ☐ Eat whole, fresh, locally grown foods—especially berries and fatty fish. Snack on nuts.
- ☐ Minimize sugar, using a natural sweetener instead, such as stevia.
- ☐ Stay hydrated.
- ☐ Take a multivitamin-mineral supplement.

Physical Activity
- ☐ Walk (30 minutes, at least five days a week).
- ☐ Continue to increase your daily steps. *This week's goal*: Adding 2,000 steps to your daily baseline, which you calculated on Day 11.
- ☐ Walk barefoot for a few minutes or sit outside with your feet on the ground.
- ☐ Do resistance training.
- ☐ Burn a few more calories—make love!

Sleep
- ☐ Start a two-day experiment to find out how much sleep you really need. Tonight, try to sleep one hour longer than you usually do.

DAY 16: Make Time for Sleep

Most of us are so busy that we cut down on sleep in order to fit in all that we have to do. But cutting down on sleep is counterproductive. You want to enjoy your day and your life, and too little sleep can cause daytime fatigue and lifetime illness. How do you find the time to sleep?

My advice: Make a two-column list of what you do during the day. In one column, put the things you enjoy doing; in the other column, put the things you don't. Then see which items in the "don't enjoy" column feel good to remove—not because you've done them, but because you don't want to do them anymore and don't really have to.

For example, do you really need to spend 30 minutes or more every day watching the news or poring over newspapers to read about events you have no control over—especially if reading it makes you feel bad and there is a good probability that much of it is nonsense anyway? So read or watch the news only as long as it feels good. The world will be just fine without your fretting about it every day!

If you're a parent, do you really need to be a member of six different committees at your child's school? Give yourself permission to say no to excess committees and meetings, and attend only those that really matter and feel good to you.

So today, make a list of all the ways you typically spend time, take a close look at your list, figure out what feels good and what doesn't, and cross off the stuff you really don't want to do. If you're like me, I think you'll find that the items you crossed off—items that seem so important but that you don't really enjoy—kind of float off into the distance. After a week or so, you may find it hard to believe that you ever participated in them or cared about them. And you'll also have plenty of time for a good night's sleep!

Day 16: Life-Change Checklist...

Nutrition

- ☐ Eat whole, fresh, locally grown foods—especially berries and fatty fish. Snack on nuts.
- ☐ Minimize sugar, using a natural sweetener instead, such as stevia.
- ☐ Stay hydrated.
- ☐ Take a multivitamin-mineral supplement.

Physical Activity

- ☐ Walk (30 minutes, at least five days a week).
- ☐ Continue to increase your daily steps. *This week's goal:* Adding 2,000 steps to your daily baseline, which you calculated on Day 11.
- ☐ Walk barefoot for a few minutes or sit outside with your feet on the ground.
- ☐ Burn a few more calories—make love!

Sleep

- ☐ Make more time for sleep—by making a two-column list of what you do during the day, putting the things you enjoy in one column and the things you don't enjoy in the other. Now, cross off the stuff you really don't want to do—and stop doing it.
- ☐ You're on the second day of a two-day experiment to find out how much sleep you *really* need. Tonight, try to sleep two hours longer than you usually do.

DAY 17: Practice Good Sleep Hygiene

"Sleep hygiene" is a phrase for the habits that help you sleep. Here are a few easy habits you can start putting in place today.

- **Cut down on caffeine.** Ingesting caffeine after 4:00 p.m. can keep you awake at bedtime. That includes the caffeine in coffee, tea, cola, energy drinks, and chocolate.

- **Exercise early.** Exercising heats and stimulates the body, which isn't best for sleep. A good cutoff time is 7:00 p.m.

- **Snack at bedtime.** A high-protein snack—a slice of turkey, a handful of nuts, a hard-boiled egg, or a chunk of cheese—can soothe the brain and balance blood sugar while you sleep, helping you fall asleep and stay asleep.

- **Keep the bath hot and the bedroom cool.** A hot bath at night is sleep inducing. A cool bedroom (around 65°F) is best for deep sleep.

- **Don't work in the bedroom.** Make your bedroom a sanctuary for sleep (and sex). If you do lots of other activities there—work, exercise, pay the bills, problem solve—you'll find it less easy to relax and sleep.

- **Make a worry list—and forget about it.** If your mind is racing with worries, sit up and write them all down (keep a pad and pen on your bedside table). Once they are off your mind and onto paper, relax. You can attend to your worry list in the morning.

- **Nullify the noise.** If you live in a noisy neighborhood or your spouse snores, wear earplugs or use a white noise machine.

- **Hide the alarm clock.** Checking the time on your alarm clock isn't conducive to sleep. Turn it in another direction.

- **Consider an electricity-free zone.** For some people, electrical currents can disrupt sleep. Tonight, turn off the circuit breakers to your bedroom before bedtime and see if that helps.

Find other tips for better sleep hygiene in Insomnia and Other Sleep Disorders on page 268.

Day 17: Life-Change Checklist…

Nutrition

- ☐ Eat whole, fresh, locally grown foods—especially berries and fatty fish. Snack on nuts.
- ☐ Minimize sugar, using a natural sweetener instead, such as stevia.
- ☐ Stay hydrated.
- ☐ Take a multivitamin-mineral supplement.

Physical Activity

- ☐ Walk (30 minutes, at least five days a week).
- ☐ Continue to increase your daily steps. *This week's goal*: Adding 2,000 steps to your daily baseline, which you calculated on Day 11.
- ☐ Walk barefoot for a few minutes or sit outside with your feet on the ground.

Sleep

- ☐ What were the results of your two-day sleep experiment? If you felt a whole lot better with one more hour of sleep than you usually get, then that's the amount you want to try to get every night. If you felt better with two more hours, aim for that amount.
- ☐ Practice good sleep hygiene.

DAY 18: Correct Your Hormone Imbalances

As discussed in Hormonal Imbalances on page 90, balancing your adrenal stress hormone levels is critical to healthy energy during the day. But they also have to drop to low levels at night so you can sleep. Often, your adrenal hormone levels have trouble dropping at night (even if they are too low during the day). You can tell this is the case if your mind is wide awake and racing when your head hits the pillow. This can occur with people who are in overdrive all day (where cortisol levels are too high all day). In others, this can be even more frustrating when you're exhausted all day (from low adrenal cortisol), until your head hits the pillow. In this situation, you have too-low cortisol during the day and too high at night.

To make matters worse, when the cortisol level finally does drop, it can drop too low. This makes your blood sugar plummet, and you find yourself suddenly wide awake at 2:00 a.m. Too low? Too high? Both? It can leave you feeling like screaming. Fortunately, this is all easy to treat.

•**If you are wide awake at bedtime** (even if you feel exhausted all day), a natural mix of ashwagandha, phosphatidylserine (50 to 150 milligrams), and theanine (50 to 200 milligrams) at bedtime will lower cortisol levels at night so you can sleep. A good mix of these can be found in Sleep Tonight (by Nature's Way).

•**If you wake frequently during the night, try a bedtime snack of one to two ounces of a high-protein food.** This can be an egg, cheese, meat, or any protein (but not a high-carb/sugar treat). Protein is digested slowly over many hours, maintaining your blood sugar levels even if cortisol levels are uneven.

Day 18: Life-Change Checklist…

Nutrition

- ☐ Eat whole, fresh, locally grown foods—especially berries and fatty fish. Snack on nuts.
- ☐ Minimize sugar, using a natural sweetener instead, such as stevia.
- ☐ Stay hydrated.
- ☐ Take a multivitamin-mineral supplement.

Physical Activity

- ☐ Walk (30 minutes, at least five days a week).
- ☐ Continue to increase your daily steps. *This week's goal*: Adding 2,000 steps to your daily baseline, which you calculated on Day 11.
- ☐ Walk barefoot for a few minutes or sit outside with your feet on the ground.

☐ Today's the day for another round of resistance training.

☐ Burn a few more calories—make love!

Sleep

☐ Practice good sleep hygiene.

☐ If your insomnia pattern fits the description in Day 18—a sign of cortisol imbalance—try the sleep remedies recommended above. Also, eat a bedtime snack of one to two ounces of a high-protein food.

DAY 19: Reset Your Inner Clock

Can't fall asleep at night? Wake up in the wee morning hours and can't fall back asleep? You may have a problem with your circadian rhythms, the inner clock in your brain that sets your sleep-wake cycle to the natural cycles of light and dark. There are a couple of easy ways to reset your inner clock.

•**Get out of bed at the same time every morning, even after a poor night's sleep.** Do this starting tomorrow, and every day after that, and you'll put your inner clock on SST—Standard Sleeping Time. When it's time to sleep, you'll sleep. When it's time to wake up, you'll wake up.

If at first you find that you're sleepy during the day, you can nap. (But try not to nap after 2:00 p.m., which can interfere with nighttime sleep.) When you nap, set the alarm for 60 to 90 minutes of nap time. If you feel groggy when you wake up, splash cold water on your face.

•**Exercise regularly.** Daily aerobic exercise, such as a brisk walk, helps stabilize circadian rhythms.

•**Eat regular meals.** Eating three meals a day, every day, helps keep circadian rhythms on track. Lunch at noon and dinner no later than 8:00 p.m. are best.

•**Take melatonin, in the right amount, at the right time.** Melatonin is the hormone that regulates the circadian cycle, and it's available over the counter as a natural supplement to treat insomnia. Most people take 3 milligrams or more, which is okay but more melatonin than most people need. The best dose—the dose that your body actually makes—is one-tenth that amount: 0.3 milligram. Higher doses are not more effective.

When you are having trouble falling asleep until too late at night, you have what is called *delayed sleep phase onset.* That is when higher doses of 3 to 5 milligrams may be helpful. (I recommend Nature's Bounty Dual Spectrum 5 mg melatonin, which is widely available. I find this product works much better than most.) Melatonin works best to reset your inner clock when you take it at the same time your body starts to produce melatonin, which is five to six hours before bedtime. Another way to help melatonin do its job: After you take it, hang out in dim indoor lighting, preferably incandescent rather than fluorescent. Bright fluorescent light can stymie the hormone.

Day 19: Life-Change Checklist...

Nutrition

☐ Eat whole, fresh, locally grown foods—especially berries and fatty fish. Snack on nuts.

☐ Minimize sugar, using a natural sweetener instead, such as stevia.

☐ Stay hydrated.

☐ Take a multivitamin-mineral supplement.

Physical Activity

☐ Meet a friend for a walk (30 minutes, at least five days a week).

☐ Congratulations: You've increased your daily step count by 2,000 steps! This week, you're going to add another 2,000 steps a day—if your baseline was 5,000, you reached 7,000 on Day 18, and are now aiming to reach 9,000 by Day 25.

☐ Walk barefoot for a few minutes or sit outside with your feet on the ground.

Sleep

☐ Practice good sleep hygiene.

☐ Reset your inner clock to beat insomnia, by…getting out of bed the same time every morning (no matter how much you've slept)…exercising regularly…eating regular meals…taking melatonin.

DAY 20: Take an Herbal Formula

If insomnia is still getting the better of you, the Sandman may need a helping hand—a *natural* hand, from an herbal sleep formula. The one I routinely recommend to my patients is the Revitalizing Sleep Formula from Nature's Way. It contains six herbs and compounds that are science-proven to help you fall asleep and stay asleep. Another excellent product is a mix of essential oils called Terrific Zzzz from Terry Naturally.

Unlike prescription sleeping pills, these products are not sedating—and they're widely available. You can take these herbal mixtures every night or when needed. You can read more about the Revitalizing Sleep Formula, Terrific Zzzz, and other natural aids for sleep in Insomnia and Other Sleep Disorders on page 268.

Day 20: Life-Change Checklist…

Nutrition

☐ Eat whole, fresh, locally grown foods—especially berries and fatty fish. Snack on nuts.

☐ Minimize sugar, using a natural sweetener instead, such as stevia.

☐ Stay hydrated.

☐ Take a multivitamin-mineral supplement.

Physical Activity

☐ Walk (30 minutes, at least five days a week).

☐ Continue to increase your daily steps. *This week's goal*: Adding another 2,000. (If your daily baseline was 5,000 steps, you're aiming for 9,000 by the end of the week.)

☐ Walk barefoot for a few minutes or sit outside with your feet on the ground.

☐ Do yoga today.

☐ Burn a few more calories—make love!

Sleep

☐ Practice good sleep hygiene.

☐ Reset your inner clock to beat insomnia (see Day 19).

☐ If insomnia is still getting the better of you, consider an herbal sleep aid, taken every night or as needed.

DAY 21: Say Good Night to Sleep Disorders

There are two main types of sleep disorders other than insomnia that afflict tens of millions of Americans, keeping a lot of them awake: restless legs syndrome and obstructive sleep apnea.

●**Restless legs syndrome (RLS)/periodic limb movements of sleep (PLMS).** You probably have RLS (which keeps people awake) or PLMS (which occurs when you're asleep) if your sheets and blankets are scattered around the bed when you wake up, if your spouse complains of being kicked in bed at night, and/or if your legs are uncomfortable and restless when you're trying to fall asleep. When I see a patient with RLS and/or PLMS, I order a test for ferritin (stored iron). If it's lower than 60, I prescribe a daily iron supplement of 25 to 30 milligrams. (A lot of doctors consider ferritin "normal" if it's over 12, which is ridiculous.) Many studies show that iron deficiency is a common cause of RLS and that, over time, an iron supplement is more effective than an RLS prescription medication in solving the problem. (PLMS isn't as well studied as RLS, but I find that remedies for RLS work well for both disorders.)

I also find that taking magnesium (200 milligrams at bedtime) and vitamin E (400 IU of natural mixed tocopherols); eating a sugar-free, high-protein diet (with a protein snack at bedtime); and cutting out coffee are helpful when RLS is keeping you (and your spouse) awake.

●**Obstructive sleep apnea.** This condition is most common in people who are overweight. The soft tissue at the back of the throat sags and obstructs the airway during sleep, cutting off breathing (essentially suffocating you) and rousing you to a semi-awake state. This can happen more than a dozen times an hour, and in the morning you're exhausted but don't know why.

If you're overweight, snore, and fall asleep easily during the day, and your spouse says you stop breathing during sleep, it's almost a sure thing you have sleep apnea. Another way to tell is to videotape yourself during sleep. Just prop up your cell phone at a right angle and press record. If you snore and repeatedly stop breathing, you have sleep apnea. (Watch for RLS at the same time.) *Note*: While you could be analyzed at a sleep clinic, they cost about $1,000 to $2,000 and insurance often denies payment. Simply watching an hour of video recorded on your phone will give a clearer answer than any sleep app.

An easy remedy: If the video shows that you stop breathing mostly while lying on your back, sew a tennis ball into your pajama top at the small of your back. It keeps you from sleeping on your back, the position where apnea (and snoring) is most likely to happen.

Other remedies include losing weight, wearing an oral appliance custom-made by a dentist (the over-the-counter devices advertised on TV don't work), or using a continuous positive airway pressure (CPAP) machine, which helps you breathe during the night. (It takes three to five months to get used to the mask worn with a CPAP machine, so keep with it—even if you find yourself taking the mask off while sleeping.) You can read more Real Cure Regimen advice in Insomnia and Other Sleep Disorders on page 268.

Day 21: Life-Change Checklist...

Nutrition

☐ Eat whole, fresh, locally grown foods—especially berries and fatty fish. Snack on nuts.

☐ Minimize sugar, using a natural sweetener instead, such as stevia.

☐ Stay hydrated.

☐ Take a multivitamin-mineral supplement.

Physical Activity

☐ Walk (30 minutes, at least five days a week).

☐ Continue to increase your daily steps. *This week's goal*: Adding another 2,000. (If your daily baseline was 5,000 steps, you're aiming for 9,000 by the end of the week.)

☐ Walk barefoot for a few minutes or sit outside with your feet on the ground.

☐ Get a massage or nurture yourself in some other way.

Sleep

☐ Practice good sleep hygiene.

☐ Reset your inner clock to beat insomnia (see Day 19).

☐ Consider an herbal sleep aid as needed.

☐ Take steps to treat restless leg syndrome, periodic limb movements of sleep, or sleep apnea—the most common sleep disorders—consider the remedies suggested in Day 21 and on page 268.

Week 4

Positive Thinking and Purpose:
Love Yourself—and Love Your Life

DAY 22: Start the Day with a Positive Thought

What was the first thought that popped into your head right after you woke up this morning? Did you start worrying about all the items on your to-do list? Did you rehash an argument you had yesterday? Did you wish you were still asleep because your dreams seemed a lot sweeter than what you imagine your day will be like?

Well, if you started the day with a negative thought, you might be having the start of a really bad day. I've found that the first thought of the day makes a huge difference in how I feel the rest of the day. It seems to set the emotional tone, like a tuning fork to which the rest of the day vibrates. So when I wake up, I make sure that the first thought I think is a positive one, and I encourage you to do the same.

Here's a simple one to try out: *I feel great today.* Say it in your mind first thing.

Day 22: Life-Change Checklist...

Nutrition

- ☐ Eat whole, fresh, locally grown foods—especially berries and fatty fish. Snack on nuts.
- ☐ Minimize sugar, using a natural sweetener instead, such as stevia.
- ☐ Stay hydrated.
- ☐ Take a multivitamin-mineral supplement.

Physical Activity

- ☐ Walk (30 minutes, at least five days a week).
- ☐ Continue to increase your daily steps. *This week's goal*: Adding another 2,000. (If your daily baseline was 5,000 steps, you're aiming for 9,000 by the end of the week.)
- ☐ Walk barefoot for a few minutes or sit outside with your feet on the ground.
- ☐ Do resistance training today.
- ☐ Burn a few more calories—make love!

Sleep

- ☐ Practice good sleep hygiene.
- ☐ Reset your inner clock to beat insomnia (see Day 19).
- ☐ Consider an herbal sleep aid as needed.
- ☐ Take steps to treat restless leg syndrome or sleep apnea.

Positive Thinking

- ☐ Start the day with a positive thought.

DAY 23: Edit Your To-Do List

If you have a typical to-do list, there are more items on it than you actually have time to do—and it feels overwhelming and stressful to encounter it every day.

I've developed a way to approach my to-do list that I find relaxes me rather than stresses me out. And it's no less effective in actually getting things done than the harried, hurried way I used to deal with my to-do list many years ago. *Here's my approach...*

1. In a notebook or on your computer, create a page with three wide columns.

2. I list my problems and projects in the left-hand column.

3. In the middle column, I write what (if anything) I plan to do soon about each of those problems and projects.

4. I consider those two columns to be what I leave in the hands of God or the Universe or Spirit (or whatever name or idea is meaningful to you).

5. Every so often, I move an item from the "*Spirit*" columns to the right-hand column—"*my*" column. The items in this column are the one or two things that I want to work on right now.

6. I also keep a separate list of everyday errands and put a star next to those that must get done soon. I do the other items on my errand list if and when I feel like it.

I am constantly amazed at how the problems and projects in the "Spirit" columns move forward (on their own) as quickly as the items in "my" column. Try it yourself. I have a feeling that your to-do list will turn into a ta-da list, just like mine. Another task completed, as if by magic. Ta-da!

Day 23: Life-Change Checklist...

Nutrition
- [ ] Eat whole, fresh, locally grown foods—especially berries and fatty fish. Snack on nuts.
- [ ] Minimize sugar, using a natural sweetener instead, such as stevia.
- [ ] Stay hydrated.
- [ ] Take a multivitamin-mineral supplement.

Physical Activity
- [ ] Walk (30 minutes, at least five days a week).
- [ ] Continue to increase your daily steps. *This week's goal*: Adding another 2,000. (If your daily baseline was 5,000 steps, you're aiming for 9,000 by the end of the week.)
- [ ] Walk barefoot for a few minutes or sit outside with your feet on the ground.
- [ ] Do yoga today.

Sleep
- [ ] Practice good sleep hygiene.
- [ ] Reset your inner clock to beat insomnia (see Day 19).
- [ ] Consider an herbal sleep aid as needed.
- [ ] Take steps to treat restless leg syndrome or sleep apnea.

Positive Thinking
- [ ] Start the day with a positive thought.
- [ ] Edit your to-do list—and delegate to the Universe!

DAY 24: Feel Your Feelings

A feeling stays with you until you actually feel it. That means if you don't really feel your anger, you may find yourself simmering for decades. And if you're like most people, you'll think that your anger is caused by what's happening today, when the fact is that your suppressed anger has accumulated into a giant reservoir that spills into your psyche at the slightest provocation. Same for sadness, anxiety, and all the other unhappy emotions. When you deny a feeling, your mind magnifies it to make it bigger and clearer to you, so you can feel it and be done with it. Keep denying the feeling, and the blues turn into chronic depression; anger turns into a constant attitude of hostility, cynicism, and hatred; and worry turns into anxiety and panic.

Resisting a feeling is like trying to stop a cloud because you want it to be sunny again. Letting the cloud pass is the way back to a brighter state of mind. You're finished with the feeling when it no longer feels good. It actually feels good to fully feel anger, sorrow, or fear. That's why we call a session of much-needed, unrestrained sobbing a "good cry." And who hasn't experienced the joy of a good, self-righteous hissy fit? Or the enjoyment of a scary movie? When it no longer feels good to feel sad or angry, then the feeling has been fully experienced—you're done. Time to move on!

How do you fully feel your feelings? *Here are a couple of tips...*

•**Don't worry about the "why."** Maybe you don't know why you're feeling the way you're feeling. No problem. Trying to label or figure out a feeling actually shifts you out of the feeling and into your mind, leaving you stuck in the feeling (because you haven't felt it fully). When your mind attempts to label or explain why you are feeling a feeling, it's okay to say to your mind, "No, thank you." Then continue to feel the feeling fully, without any resistance and without needing to understand why you are feeling the way you do.

•**Relax.** You can often tell you are resisting a feeling if your body is tense or constricted—if your jaw is tight, your arms and legs are crossed, your breathing is shallow. If you notice any of this, remind yourself to do the opposite: Let your jaw slacken, uncross your arms and legs, and breathe!

Fully feeling your feelings and then letting go of them when they are done is one of the keys to happiness. (And don't forget to allow yourself to fully feel your joyful feelings, too! Many of us feel undeserving of joy, or tell ourselves that it is transient and disappointing. Allow your joy— and celebrate it!) You can read more about it in Happiness Deficiency on page 55.

Day 24: Life-Change Checklist...

Nutrition
- [ ] Eat whole, fresh, locally grown foods—especially berries and fatty fish. Snack on nuts.
- [ ] Minimize sugar, using a natural sweetener instead, such as stevia.
- [ ] Stay hydrated.
- [ ] Take a multivitamin-mineral supplement.

Physical Activity
- [ ] Walk (30 minutes, at least five days a week).
- [ ] Continue to increase your daily steps. *This week's goal*: Adding another 2,000. (If your daily baseline was 5,000 steps, you're aiming for 9,000 by the end of the week.)
- [ ] Walk barefoot for a few minutes or sit outside with your feet on the ground.
- [ ] Burn a few more calories—make love!

Sleep
- [ ] Practice good sleep hygiene.
- [ ] Reset your inner clock to beat insomnia (see Day 19).
- [ ] Consider an herbal sleep aid as needed.
- [ ] Take steps to treat restless leg syndrome or sleep apnea.

Positive Thinking
- [ ] Start the day with a positive thought.
- [ ] Edit your to-do list—and delegate to the Universe.
- [ ] Fully feel all your feelings—it's the best way to prevent chronic unhappiness.

DAY 25: Take Some Time to Relax

Excess stress can cause or complicate nearly every illness, from headaches to heart disease. That's why it's helpful to create an emotional, mental, and physical state that's just the opposite of stress—a state of relaxation. You can do that intentionally by practicing a "relaxation technique," a simple type of meditation. For those just starting with relaxation training, I recommend the classic book *The Relaxation Response*, by Herbert Benson, MD, associate professor of medicine at Harvard Medical School and director emeritus of the Benson-Henry Institute for Mind Body Medicine at Massachusetts General Hospital.

We talked with Dr. Benson, and he reiterated the simplicity and effectiveness of the book's technique, first introduced to the public in 1975. *Here's how to do it...*

1. Pick a focus word, sound, short phrase, or prayer that is firmly rooted in your belief system, such as "Amen," "Hail Mary," "Shalom," "Allah," or "Om Shanti." You can also use a neutral word, such as "One."
2. Sit quietly in a comfortable position.
3. Close your eyes.
4. Relax your muscles, progressing from your feet to your calves, thighs, abdomen, arms, shoulders, neck, and head.
5. Breathe slowly and naturally, saying your focus word, sound, phrase, or prayer silently as you exhale.
6. Assume a passive attitude. Don't worry about how well you're doing. When other thoughts come to mind, simply and gently return to your repetition.
7. Continue for 10 to 20 minutes.
8. When you stop, continue sitting quietly for a minute or so, allowing other thoughts to return. Then open your eyes and sit for another minute before rising.

Practice the technique once or twice daily, such as before breakfast and before dinner.

Day 25: Life-Change Checklist...

Nutrition
☐ Eat whole, fresh, locally grown foods—especially berries and fatty fish. Snack on nuts.
☐ Minimize sugar, using a natural sweetener instead, such as stevia.
☐ Stay hydrated.
☐ Take a multivitamin-mineral supplement.

Physical Activity
☐ Walk (30 minutes, at least five days a week).
☐ Continue to increase your daily steps. *This week's goal*: Adding another 2,000. (If your daily baseline was 5,000 steps, you're aiming for 9,000 by the end of the week.)
☐ Walk barefoot for a few minutes or sit outside with your feet on the ground.
☐ Do resistance training today.
☐ Burn a few more calories—make love!

Sleep

☐ Practice good sleep hygiene.

☐ Reset your inner clock to beat insomnia (see Day 19).

☐ Consider an herbal sleep aid as needed.

☐ Take steps to treat restless leg syndrome or sleep apnea.

Positive Thinking

☐ Start the day with a positive thought.

☐ Edit your to-do list—and delegate to the Universe.

☐ Fully feel all your feelings—it's the best way to prevent chronic unhappiness.

☐ Practice a relaxation technique every day.

DAY 26: Follow Your Bliss

The late Joseph Campbell, the world's most renowned student and expert on the vast variety of the planet's different religions, myths, and tribal cultures, was asked to summarize what he learned from all these traditions. He did so in three words: "Follow your bliss."

What did he mean, exactly? Many spiritual traditions teach that a human being is essentially a soul. And the desire of the soul is to fully experience its true divine nature—its bliss. (For those of you who are uncomfortable with the word soul, feel free to substitute the words psyche or your true self.) When you are in alignment with your psyche or soul, you feel good. When you aren't, you feel bad. It's really that simple.

If I feel good—if I'm centered and happy and joyful—I know that I am connected to my soul and its desire, and that I am as close to being authentic as I know how to be. If I feel bad, I know that I am not attuned to what my soul prefers. It's a matter of being authentic and true to yourself!

Today, follow your bliss. In other words, do what you feel good doing. And make the conscious choice to keep your attention on things that feel good. One way to do this is to practice what I call the as-if technique. Think about what would feel best to you—at work, at home, in your relationships, and in your life altogether. As you do this, keep an image in mind of the situation that feels best, and feel as if that situation were already happening. For example, you want a raise at work, keep in mind a paycheck that is 10 percent higher than your current paycheck. Or you want you and your spouse to get along better, keep in mind an image of the two of you happily relating over a candlelit dinner.

Do this for a few minutes today, and every now and then. I think you will be amazed at the results, as you look back one day and realize that the happy things you were fantasizing about have become a reality in your life. For now, knowing these changes are in progress (even if they don't happen overnight) can leave you feeling happier immediately.

Day 26: Life-Change Checklist...

Nutrition

☐ Eat whole, fresh, locally grown foods—especially berries and fatty fish. Snack on nuts.

☐ Minimize sugar, using a natural sweetener instead, such as stevia.

☐ Stay hydrated.

☐ Take a multivitamin-mineral supplement.

Physical Activity

☐ Walk (30 minutes, at least five days a week).

☐ Congratulations—you're now walking 9,000 steps a day. Next week, add another 1,000 steps per day, to get to 10,000 steps daily—a standard recommendation for optimal lifelong health and fitness.

☐ Walk barefoot for a few minutes or sit outside with your feet on the ground.

Sleep

☐ Practice good sleep hygiene.

☐ Reset your inner clock to beat insomnia (see Day 19).

☐ Consider an herbal sleep aid as needed.

☐ Take steps to treat restless leg syndrome or sleep apnea.

Positive Thinking

☐ Start the day with a positive thought.

☐ Edit your to-do list—and delegate to Spirit!

☐ Fully feel *all* your feelings—it's the best way to prevent chronic unhappiness.

☐ Practice a relaxation technique every day.

☐ Follow your bliss—do (and visualize) what makes you *happy*!

DAY 27: Release Old Traumas

When I think of old traumas, I sometimes think of the ghost Jacob Marley, the partner of Ebenezer Scrooge in *A Christmas Carol*, who hauled around chains consisting of all his bad deeds and mistakes. "I wear the chain I forged in life," said the Ghost to Scrooge. "I made it link by link, and yard by yard." Well, you don't have to be a ghost to haul around the "chain" of your past.

Many of us do it every day, hauling around a chain whose links are the emotional traumas of our experience. And like Marley's, it's a long and heavy chain. But like any chain, unbending a single link can release the entire chain—and you can feel suddenly and amazingly free. In other words, it is surprisingly easy to release yourself from the pain and burden of old traumas—even horrific traumas like physical or sexual abuse.

One of the releasing techniques that I teach patients—a simple, straightforward, and powerfully effective technique for releasing old, stored emotions—is the Emotional Freedom Technique (EFT). It was developed by Gary Craig, who simplified a technique called Thought Field Therapy, developed by Roger Callahan, PhD, author of *Five Minute Phobia Cure.*

Dr. Callahan had found that tapping certain acupressure points quickly relieved emotional distress. EFT is helpful in dissipating phobias (such as fear of flying), anxieties, traumas, anger, depression, resentment, guilt, low self-esteem, and many other uncomfortable emotions. EFT takes only a few minutes to learn and often produces permanent results. The main ingredient for success is a willingness to use it for persistent, traumatic feelings. Try it today. (See "How to Do the Emotional Freedom Technique [EFT]" in Happiness Deficiency on page 60.)

Note: For simple issues, it's fine and effective to do EFT on yourself. But for severely traumatic, complex, or deep-seated issues (such as child sexual abuse), I find it can be very helpful to work with an EFT practitioner. To locate one, visit Gary Craig's website (EFTuniverse.com). There are many books on EFT. My favorite is *Getting Thru to Your Emotions with EFT*, by Phillip and Jane Mountrose (also available as a DVD). Also, check out the EFT videos with Brad Yates on YouTube.

Although EFT will clear the emotional energy, how about the emotional traumas stored in the muscles that contribute to pain? For that, try a wonderful accompaniment to EFT: a trembling technique described in the book *Waking the Tiger*, by Peter Levine, PhD. Put simply, the body releases the traumatic energy stored in muscles by trembling. This is where the expression "shake it off" comes from. Animals do this naturally, but humans feel kind of stupid when they start trembling, and they suppress it. So, when you're by yourself and feel like you want to tremble, let it happen. You will feel lighter and clearer after each time. (You can read more about trembling on pages 59 and 61, in Happiness Deficiency.)

Day 27: Life-Change Checklist...

Nutrition

☐ Eat whole, fresh, locally grown foods—especially berries and fatty fish. Snack on nuts.

☐ Minimize sugar, using a natural sweetener instead, such as stevia.

☐ Stay hydrated.

☐ Take a multivitamin-mineral supplement.

Physical Activity

☐ Walk (30 minutes, at least five days a week).

☐ Congratulations—you're now walking 9,000 steps a day. Next week, add another 1,000 steps per day, to get to 10,000 steps daily—a standard recommendation for optimal lifelong health and fitness.

☐ Walk barefoot for a few minutes or sit outside with your feet on the ground.

☐ Do yoga today.

☐ Burn a few more calories—make love!

Sleep

☐ Practice good sleep hygiene.

☐ Reset your inner clock to beat insomnia (see Day 19).

☐ Consider an herbal sleep aid as needed.

☐ Take steps to treat restless leg syndrome or sleep apnea.

Positive Thinking

☐ Start the day with a positive thought.

☐ Edit your to-do list—and delegate to Spirit!

☐ Fully feel *all* your feelings—it's the best way to prevent chronic unhappiness.

☐ Practice a relaxation technique every day.

☐ Follow your bliss—do (and visualize) what makes you *happy*!

☐ To release old traumas, consider the Emotional Freedom Technique, described above and on page 60. Also, release traumatic energy stored in your muscles by natural trembling.

DAY 28: Forget About All Your Plans—Take the Day Off!

There is a natural flow and balance between "doing" and "being" that is largely ignored by our fast-paced society. We think doing is where it's at, and we're doing something all the time. But take a look at the patterns of nature. The activity of day is followed by the rest of night. The activity of summer is followed by the rest of winter. And that time of rest is not unimportant. It is the time of rejuvenation, of restoration, of quiet preparation for renewed creative activity. It is the time of being.

Traditional societies and religions have always acknowledged that it's important to stop, to contemplate, to pause, to rest—to be. (Even God took a break after creating the universe!)

And that's why I've made the final day of the 28-Day Life-Change Cure a day when you don't do anything. A day when you just be.

So take the day off! For pleasure and regeneration. For ease and enjoyment. For comfort and contemplation. The rest you are giving yourself is the precious gift of *being*. Think you'll find that when you return to activity—when you return to all the goals for greater health and happiness that the 28-Day Life-Change Cure and this entire book were designed to help you achieve—you'll be more creative and effective than ever.

Day 28: Life-Change Checklist...

☐ Take the day off!

Resources

Finding a Holistic Health Practitioner

Holistic physicians are much more likely than conventional physicians to be familiar with the treatments and principles discussed in this book. Below, I list the websites for several organizations of physicians who take a holistic approach to medicine. Each of these sites has a type of "Find a Practitioner" function that allows you to locate a holistic physician near you.

American Association of Naturopathic Physicians

Website: Naturopathic.org

Find an ND: Naturopathic.org (click on FindaDoctor)

American Holistic Health Association

Website: AHHA.org

Holistic Practitioners: AHHA.org/holistic-practitioners/

American College for Advancement in Medicine

Website: ACAM.org

Find a Practitioner: ACAM.org (click on Find Practitioner)

International College of Integrative Medicine

Website: ICImed.com

Find a Practitioner: ICImed.com (click on Find a Practitioner)

Academy of Integrative Health & Medicine

Website: AIHM.org/

Find a Provider: AIHM.org/directory

Supplements to Simplify Treatment

I recommend many different nutritional and herbal supplements in the Real Cure Regimens throughout this book, some of which are formulas I have developed. Most of these formulas are available in health food stores, in naturally oriented and other supermarkets, and in drugstores. They are also available on my website and other online outlets.

Jacob Teitelbaum, MD

Website: EndFatigue.com

At the website, you can also sign up for free e-mail newsletters that will keep you on the cutting edge of developments in health care.

Phone: 800-333-5287

Specific Products and Companies

Terry Naturally

Description: This is my favorite supplement company in the world. It gets its vision from Terry Lemerond, who has brought countless remarkable health-supporting supplements, including glucosamine, to the U.S. market. I consider him the "Oprah" of the supplement world!

They make countless excellent, cutting-edge products, including: Vectomega for omega-3 fish oil support; Curamin for pain; Adrenaplex for adrenal support; CuraMed, which is the only form of curcumin I will use; Sucontral D for blood sugar control; HRG 80 Red Ginseng for energy, stamina, cognitive function, and even erectile function! They have dozens of other products, every one of them superb.

Website: TerryNaturallyVitamins.com

Phone: 877-575-5155

Nature's Way (formerly Enzymatic Therapy)

Description: This is another company that produces many excellent products, including the Fatigued to Fantastic product line, which I developed. This line includes the Energy Revitalization System multinutrient powder, Adrenal Stress End, and Revitalizing Sleep Formula. These products can be found in many retail outlets (such as health food stores), at EndFatigue.com, and at other online sites. I have directed that my royalties for these products go to charity.

Website: NaturesWay.com

Phone: 800-962-8873

SHINE Ribose and SHINE Smart Energy

Description: These are two products that I designed to optimize energy and overall health. The SHINE ribose is the "gold standard" form used in my studies on ribose—but costs 50 percent less than other brands.

Smart Energy combines the ribose, ashwagandha, rhodiola, schisandra, green tea, and magnesium to turbocharge your energy, stamina, and overall vitality—beyond anything you could have imagined. I recommend taking one scoop of this along with one scoop of the Energy Revitalization System Powder each morning. Give it a month to see results—and prepare to be amazed. It will be the best 30 seconds you spend each day for overall vitality.

Available at EndFatigue.com

Sources for Services

There are many different types of services involved in some of the Real Cure Regimens, such as allergy detection and compounding pharmacies. Sources for these services are listed below.

Allergy Detection and Elimination

Nambudripad's Allergy Elimination Techniques (NAET)

Description: I recommend this uniquely effective method as part of many of the Real Cure Regimens in this book, such as in Food Allergy (page 225) and Hay Fever and Other Airborne Allergies (page 231). The website supplies information about the technique and offers help with locating practitioners worldwide.

Website: NAET.com

Compounding Pharmacies

A compounding pharmacy makes customized prescription and nonprescription medications on-site. I recommend compounding pharmacies many times in this book as the best source of a particular medication, such as bioidentical hormones or sinusitis nose sprays.

ITC Compounding & Natural Wellness Pharmacy

Description: This mail-order compounding pharmacy does a superb job of quality control and makes a wide range of bioidentical hormones, topical pain formulas, the Sinusitis Nose Spray, and much more.

Although there are many excellent compounding pharmacies, this is the one I recommend trying first.

Website: ITCpharmacy.com

Phone: 888-349-5453; 303-663-4224

Women's International Pharmacy

Description: This pharmacy—based in Madison, Wisconsin, and with a strong online presence—focuses on custom-compounded bioidentical hormones for men and women. It also offers compounded medications for pets.

Website: WomensInternational.com

Phone: 800-279-5708

Prescription Medications

I've found the best prices in the United States for prescription medications from the following companies:

Costco Pharmacy

Description: They have excellent prices on generic prescriptions.

Website: Costco.com (To see medication prices, click on Pharmacy and then on Check Drug Prices.)

GoodRx

Don't have prescription insurance? Tired of getting robbed every time you go to the pharmacy? Simply download this free app. It routinely cuts drug prices by as much as 95 percent, and lets you know the best places to go in your area for each medication.

Laboratories for Stool Cultures, Sensitivity Testing, and Bowel Infections

I recommend stool testing for parasitic and other types of infections in several chapters in this book. However, most laboratories are not equipped to do such testing reliably. The following laboratories are.

Genova Diagnostics and DiagnosTechs

Description: They do an excellent job with stool testing for ova and parasites (O&P testing) and bacterial infections, as well as many other tests. Stool testing kits are available through your doctor, who can order the testing through them. Samples are collected at home and sent to the lab. These tests are covered by many insurance policies.

Websites: GDX.net; DiagnosTechs.com

Phone: 800-522-4762; 828-253-0621 (Genova)
800-878-3787; 425-251-0596 (DiagnosTechs)

Saunas

In Cellular Toxicity (on page 109), I recommend sweating to remove toxins. Using saunas for 30 minutes, three to seven times a week, is an excellent way to systematically do that. (Shower afterward so the toxins aren't reabsorbed.) The sauna I use and recommend—a type called far infrared—is sold by:

High Tech Health

Website: HighTechHealth.com

Phone: 800-794-5355; 303-413-8500

Sinus Products

Robert Ivker, DO

Description: I consider Dr. Robert Ivker the world's top expert on healing acute and chronic sinusitis. His website includes many helpful tools and resources.

Website: SinusSurvival.com

Phone: 800-869-9159

About the Authors

Jacob Teitelbaum, MD, is a board-certified internist and nationally known expert in the fields of chronic fatigue syndrome, fibromyalgia, sleep and pain. He is also Director of the Practitioners Alliance Network (PAN), which brings health-care practitioners together for improved patient care. Dr. Teitelbaum is author of numerous books including *The Fatigue and Fibromyalgia Solution*, *Diabetes Is Optional*, the best-selling *From Fatigued to Fantastic!*, *Pain Free 1-2-3 — A Proven Program for Eliminating Chronic Pain Now*, *Three Steps to Happiness! Healing Through Joy*, the *Beat Sugar Addiction NOW!* series and the popular free iPhone and Android application "Cures A-Z." He is the lead author of four studies on effective treatment for fibromyalgia and chronic fatigue syndrome, and a study on effective treatment of autism using NAET. Dr. Teitelbaum has appeared on *Good Morning America*, CNN, Fox News Channel and the *Dr. Oz Show*. He lives in Kona, Hawaii. Endfatigue.com, Vitality101.com

Bill Gottlieb, CHC, is a health coach certified by the American Association of Drugless Practitioners. He is the author of 16 health books that have sold more than 3 million copies and have been translated into 11 languages. He is also a health journalist whose articles have appeared in many publications, including *Bottom Line Personal*, *Bottom Line Health*, *Prevention*, *Reader's Digest* and *Men's Health*. From 1976 to 1995, Bill worked at Rodale Inc., where, as editor-in-chief of Rodale Books and Prevention Magazine Health Books, he creatively conceived and edited health books that sold more than 50 million copies, including *The Doctors Book of Home Remedies* and *New Choices in Natural Healing*. He is also the author of *Speed Healing* (Bottom Line Books). He lives in northern California. BillGottliebhealth.com

Index

Index

Index